Otoacoustic Emissions:
Clinical Applications

Otoacoustic Emissions: Clinical Applications

edited by

Martin S. Robinette, Ph.D.

Department of Otorhinolaryngology
Section of Audiology
Mayo Clinic
Rochester, Minnesota

and

Theodore J. Glattke, Ph.D.

Department of Speech and Hearing Sciences
University of Arizona
Tucson, Arizona

1997
Thieme
New York · Stuttgart

Thieme
381 Park Avenue South
New York, New York 10016

OTOACOUSTIC EMISSIONS: CLINICAL APPLICATIONS
Martin S. Robinette and Theodore J. Glattke

Library of Congress Cataloging-in-Publication Data

Otoacoustic emissions: clinical applications/edited by Martin S.
   Robinette and Theodore J. Glattke.
       p.   cm.
   Includes bibliographical references and index.
   ISBN 0-86577-579-6.—ISBN 3-13-103711-3
       1. Otoacoustic emissions.   I. Robinette, Martin S.   II. Glattke,
   Theodore J.
       [DNLM: 1. Cochlea—physiology.   2. Cochlea—physiopathology.
   3. Otoacoustic Emissions, Spontaneous.   WV 250O88 1996]
   RF294.5.076086   1997
   617.8'4—dc20
DNLM/DLC
for Library of Congress   91-17977
                                                                     CIP

Dedicated to the memory
of Hallowell Davis, M.D., explorer.

Important note: Medical knowledge is ever-changing. As new research and clinical experience broaden our knowledge, changes in treatment and drug therapy may be required. The editors of the material herein have consulted sources believed to be reliable in their efforts to provide information that is complete and in accord with the standards accepted at the time of publication. However, in view of the possibility of human error by the authors, editors, or publisher of the work herein, or changes in medical knowledge, neither the editors or the publisher, nor any other party who has been involved in the preparation of this work, warrants that the information contained herein is in every respect accurate or complete, and they are not responsible for any errors or omissions or for the results obtained from use of such information. Readers are encouraged to confirm the information contained herein with other sources. For example, readers are advised to check the product information sheet included in the package of each drug they plan to administer to be certain that the information contained in this publication is accurate and that changes have not been made in the recommended dose or in the contraindications for administration. This recommendation is of particular importance in connection with new or infrequently used drugs.

Some of the product names, patents, and registered designs referred to in this book are in fact registered trademarks or proprietary names even though specific reference to this fact is not always made in the text. Therefore, the appearance of a name without designation as proprietary is not to be construed as a representation by the publisher that it is in the public domain.

Printed in the United States of America.

5   4   3   2   1

TNY ISBN 0-86577-579-6
GTV ISBN 3-13-103711-3

Contents

Preface vii

Contributors ix

Perspective

1. **Otoacoustic Emissions in Perspective** 1
   David T. Kemp

2. **New Views of Cochlear Function** 22
   Allen F. Ryan

Populations with Normal Hearing Sensitivity

3. **Spontaneous Otoacoustic Emissions** 46
   Kathryn E. Bright

4. **Transient Evoked Otoacoustic Emissions** 63
   Theodore J. Glattke and Martin S. Robinette

5. **Distortion Product Otoacoustic Emissions** 83
   Brenda L. Lonsbury-Martin, Glen K. Martin,
   and Martin L. Whitehead

6. **Ipsilateral Suppression of Transient Evoked Otoacoustic**
   Emissions 110
   George A. Tavartkiladze, Gregory I. Frolenkov,
   Alexandr V. Kruglov, and Serge V. Artamasov

Clinical Populations

7. **Influence of Middle-Ear Disease on Otoacoustic Emissions** 130
   Robert H. Margolis and Mary Beth Trine

8. **Otoacoustic Emissions and Audiometric Outcomes** 151
   Frances P. Harris and Rudolf Probst

9. **Distortion Product Emissions and Sensorineural Hearing Loss** 181
    Barry P. Kimberley, David K. Brown, and Jont B. Allen

10. **Contributions of Evoked Otoacoustic Emissions in Differential Diagnosis of Retrocochlear Disorders** 205
    Martin S. Robinette and John D. Durrant

11. **Neonatal Screening via Evoked Otoacoustic Emissions.** 233
    N. Brandt Culpepper

12. **Evoked Otoacoustic Emissions in Evaluating Children** 271
    Judith E. Widen

Instrumentation Review

13. **General Recording Considerations and Clinical Instrument Options.** 307
    T. Newell Decker

14. **Basic Instrumentation Issues in Acquiring Distortion Product Otoacoustic Emissions** 333
    Janice E. Painter

    Index 347

Preface

Otoacoustic emissions (OAEs) are acoustical signals that can be detected in the ear canal. They occur spontaneously as narrow-band tonal signals. They also occur during and after stimulation of the ear and are thought to be due to vibrations produced at various locations within the cochlea. They are detected because the vibrations travel toward the base of the cochlea, cause displacement of the ossicles, and result in motion of the tympanic membrane much like the diaphragm of a loudspeaker. The discovery of OAEs by David Kemp in 1977 heralded a revolution in thinking about how the auditory system functions and has set the stage for new appreciation of the nature of hearing impairments caused by damage to the cochlea. A tremendous amount of time was spent in the 1960s and 1970s trying to explain the discrepancy between the precision of tuning and threshold sensitivity of the ear and the predictions made from von Bekesy's reports of traveling wave dynamics that first appeared in 1928. In 1955 von Bekesy wrote "In the inner ear there is a paradoxical vibration of the cochlear partition. This is an unfortunate situation, but analysis of the movements inside the cochlea presents in part a problem of hydromechanics, a field in which plausible reasoning has commonly led to incorrect results." In spite of von Bekesy's warning, the conventional wisdom of the period became an obstacle to understanding the unique differences in inner and outer hair-cell structure, placement, innervation and functioning. Exquisite threshold sensitivity and sharp tuning were thought to be due to some type of filtering mechanism that was based on neural elements, rather than cochlear dynamics.

It seems inevitable that someone with initial training outside the field of auditory physiology would be required to develop a new perspective on the functioning of the ear. In 1948, astronomer Thomas Gold and biologist and radar expert R. J. Pumphrey published two papers that reviewed the theories and data that had been gathered in the 19th and early 20th century, and they came to a startling conclusion: "Previous theories of hearing are considered, and it is shown that only the resonance hypothesis of Helmholtz interpreted in accordance with the considerations enumerated in the first part of this paper is consistent with observation." In other words, they recognized that the traveling wave phenomenon could not account for the sensitivity and precision of the normal cochlea. In 1988, while recalling his experiences in 1948, Gold stated: "Boy! if the thing only had a positive feedback in it, all these problems would disappear, wouldn't they?" Kemp's understanding of auditory functioning from the viewpoint of a physicist and his empirical data brought the reasonable concepts advanced by Gold and Pumphrey into focus.

Contemporary theories of hearing suggest that the healthy cochlea employs an efficient mechanical process to amplify the motion patterns associated with near threshold stimulation to levels that are compatible with the sensitivity of the sensory elements in the organ of Corti. This process was called the *cochlear amplifier* by Hallowell Davis in 1983. Under normal conditions, the amplifier system produces exquisite sensitivity and frequency selectivity. Behavioral thresholds, on one hand, and direct measures of basilar membrane responses to low intensity stimuli, on the other, reveal vulnerability to insults that are known to lead to permanent hearing loss. Permanent damage to the cochlear amplifier is seen as a major factor in the production of sensorineural hearing loss. The emissions are thought to be due to the leakage of the energy produced by the cochlear amplifier back into the ear canal. Therefore, cochlear damage and hearing loss are reflected in the alteration of OAE properties.

Measurements of OAEs also provide the researcher and clinician with a glimpse of the dynamics of cochlear functioning in response to sounds of low and moderate intensity. They are extracted from background noise with familiar averaging and spectral analysis techniques, but they are unique in several respects. Under certain conditions of stimulation the energy recorded as OAEs may exceed the energy in the eliciting stimulus. Hence, the response may be very robust for stimuli of modest intensities. Precision in the place of generation of an OAE may be demonstrated by examining the interaction of OAEs and suppressor stimuli, and central nervous system influence on cochlear dynamics may be revealed with both ipsilateral and contralateral competing stimuli.

The new tools provided by emission recordings have resulted in a tremendous excitement among audiologists and others who study auditory functioning. We have at our disposal a measure of preneural function in the inner ear that can be accessed using noninvasive techniques that do not require sedation. This acoustic otoscope allows us to scan the cochlear epithelium from the base to the apex and produces acoustical images that are revealing secrets long hidden from view or obscured in electrical recordings.

This book includes contributions of several persons who have made significant contributions to the study of auditory functioning with OAE and OAE-related measurements. First and foremost, Kemp provides observations of the impact that the discovery of OAEs has had in redefining our understanding of cochlear processes and provides a glimpse, as only he can provide, of theories, evidence, and measurements that have led him to his views.

We are fortunate that the text has the benefit of Allen Ryan's interpretations of cochlear functioning to set the stage for the normal human and clinical data that follow. Katie Bright's knowledge and experiences with emission studies builds on her early experiences at the University of Arizona conducting large scale studies of normal listeners with spontaneous otoacoustic emissions (SOAEs). Bright and one of us (TJG) studied at the University of Washington in 1982 with Craig Wier to overcome some gaps in our understanding of emissions. Brenda Lonsbury-Martin and her colleagues were also gracious hosts for us in Seattle in 1982. Fran Harris worked with Lonsbury-Martin and her colleagues at Baylor University while pursuing her Ph.D. in Arizona. During that period Harris completed basic and clinical studies of distortion product emissions. Her recent collaboration with Rudi Probst in Basel has been extremely productive, and their chapter on audiometric outcomes reflects their extensive clinical experience. The contribution of Lonsbury-Martin and her colleagues provides us with an excellent overview of the properties of distortion product otoacoustic emissions (DPOAEs) in persons with normal audiometric thresholds. Barry Kimberly and his colleagues have exceptional insights into the cochlear phenomena that underlie normal and disordered distortion production emissions, and their chapter reflects their sophistication in this area.

Brandt Culpepper and Judy Widen have provided excellent reviews of issues related to neonatal screening and pediatric populations, respectively. Brandt's experiences have been enriched by her first hand knowledge of the newborn hearing screening program at Logan Regional Hospital. Widen's extensive experience at the University of Kansas is well known to persons who are familiar with the literature on pediatric audiology. Because OAEs are influenced by the fact that the stimulus must be transmitted to the cochlea via the middle ear and the response must be detected in the ear canal via reverse transmission, it is important to appreciate the interaction of middle-ear status and emission properties. Bob Margolis and his colleagues have built on their fundamental studies of immittance measurements to provide us with important details in this regard. We have been fortunate to become familiar with the work of George Tvarkaladze through his frequent visits to the United States and his kind invitations to participate in workshops in Moscow. His studies of ipsilateral emission suppression shed light on the complex interactions that occur and illustrate the dynamic nature of the suppression mechanisms. The cooperation of John Durrant in preparing a review of clinical findings in the area of differential diagnosis has strengthened the contributions of one of us (MSR) to this area. Newell Decker and Jan Painter provide us with a basis for understanding the instrumentation and analysis techniques that are employed in obtaining recordings of transiently evoked OAEs and DPOAEs.

The scientific underpinnings and practice of audiology have taken on a new dimension as the result of the addition of OAE measurements to our toolbox. These remarkable developments have been fostered to a large degree by the influence that Kemp has had on both basic and applied research involving cochlear mechanics, OAEs, and hearing loss. Like Davis, Kemp remains committed to forging applications of basic measurements into the clinical armamentarium. He has been very generous with his knowledge, patience, and time. His personal perspective on the developments of the last 18 years is an especially valuable resource for us all.

The idea for this book was spawned during 1993 by I. Kaufman Arenberg, who organized annual meetings devoted to electrocochleography and OAEs in the early 1990s and provided a forum for some of the volume contributors to share experiences. We feel fortunate to have had the opportunity to participate in those meetings and learn from our colleagues.

We find that audiology remains exciting and stimulating after a combined experience of about 70 years. We acknowledge the support of our mentors John H. Gaeth (MSR) and Arnold M. Small, Jr. (TJG), who guided us to the pathways that we have followed. We also thank Wayne O. Olsen, who helped MSR edit several chapters. Our professional journeys have been interesting and they promise to be even more so in the future.

Martin Robinette
Ted Glattke

Contributors

Jont B. Allen, Ph.D.
AT&T Bell Laboratories, Murray
  Hill, New Jersey

Serge V. Artamasov, M.D.
Research Center for Audiology
  and Hearing Rehabilitation,
  Moscow, Russia

Kathryn E. Bright, Ph.D.
Department of Communication
  Disorders, University of
  Northern Colorado, Greeley,
  Colorado

David K. Brown, Ph.D.
Department of Surgery, Faculty
  of Medicine, University of
  Calgary, Calgary, Alberta

N. Brandt Culpepper, Ph.D.
Department of Audiology,
  National Center for Hearing
  and Management; Department
  of Communicative Disorders
  and Deaf Education, Utah State
  University, Logan, Utah

T. Newell Decker, Ph.D.
Department of Special Education
  and Communication Disorders,
  University of Nebraska,
  Lincoln, Lincoln, Nebraska

John D. Durrant, Ph.D.
Department of Communication
  Sciences and Disorders and
  Otolaryngology, University of
  Pittsburgh, Pittsburgh,
  Pennsylvania

Gregory I. Frolenkov, M.D.
Research Center for Audiology
  and Hearing Rehabilitation,
  Moscow, Russia

Theodore J. Glattke, Ph.D.
Department of Speech and
  Hearing Sciences, University of
  Arizona, Tucson, Arizona

Frances P. Harris, Ph.D.
Department of
  Otorhinolaryngology,
  Kantonsspital, Basel,
  Switzerland

David T. Kemp, Ph.D.
Institute of Laryngology and
Otology, University College,
London, England

Barry P. Kimberley, M.D., Ph.D.
Minnesota Ear, Head, and Neck
Clinic, Minneapolis, Minnesota

Alexandr V. Kruglov, M.D.
Research Center for Audiology
and Hearing Rehabilitation,
Moscow, Russia

**Brenda L. Lonsbury-Martin,
Ph.D.**
Department of Otolaryngology,
University of Miami Ear
Institute, Miami, Florida

Robert H. Margolis, Ph.D.
Department of Otolaryngology,
University of Minnesota,
Minneapolis, Minnesota

Glen K. Martin, Ph.D.
Department of Otolaryngology,
University of Miami Ear
Institute, Miami, Florida

Janice E. Painter, M.S., M.B.A.
Grason-Stradler, Incorporated,
Milford, New Hampshire

Rudolf Probst, M.D.
Department of
Otorhinolaryngology,
Kantonsspital, Basel,
Switzerland

Allen F. Ryan, Ph.D.
Department of Surgery,
Department of Otolaryngology,
and Department of
Neuroscience, University of
San Diego School of Medicine,
La Jolla, California

Martin S. Robinette, Ph.D.
Department of
Otorhinolaryngology, Section of
Audiology, Mayo Clinic,
Rochester, Minnesota

**George A. Tavartkiladze, M.D.,
Ph.D.**
Research Center for Audiology
and Hearing Rehabilitation,
Moscow, Russia

Mary Beth Trine, M.S.
Southeastern Ear, Nose, and
Throat Clinic, Nashville,
Tennessee

Martin L. Whitehead, Ph.D.
Department of Otolaryngology,
University of Miami Ear
Institute, Miami, Florida

Judith E. Widen, Ph.D.
Department of Hearing and
Speech, University of Kansas
Medical Center, Kansas City,
Kansas

Otoacoustic Emissions in Perspective

DAVID T. KEMP

Introduction

From the outset, otoacoustic emissions (OAEs) have caused excitement and elicited skepticism. Their paradoxical relation to the hearing process and the sheer novelty of cell-based sound generation has stimulated research. And for those who had studied and admired the workings of the human cochlea from afar through clinical audiology or psychoacoustics, OAEs provide a direct means of communication with the sensory cells previously available only to the laboratory physiologist. For those physical scientists engaged with the physics and engineering of manmade signal detecting and processing systems, OAEs provide an opportunity to contribute to hearing research and clinical audiology in a novel way that the first auditory biophysicists would have found hard to believe.

This chapter provides a broad, perspective view of OAEs and reviews the basic framework of knowledge needed to understand OAEs. This chapter is particularly useful to those who may have seen and used OAE instrumentation, but want to understand the rationale behind the technology and to explore how OAEs fit in the developing understanding of hearing. This chapter should help to unify the multiple facets of OAEs and allow the audiologist to more clearly distinguish between fact and fiction in the many confusing, conflicting, and incomplete accounts of OAEs. Ultimately, this chapter's aim is to help the audiologist to use OAEs more effectively.

History

The progress of OAE technology from the research laboratories to the clinics has been slow. The reasons for this delay relate more to the climates in audiology, hearing research, and particularly the audiometric instrument industry in the 1980s than to any specific technical problem in OAE implementation. The current commercial OAE technology differs little from that in use for OAE research in the late 1970s and early 1980s. For example, a portable TEOAE instrument was operational and demonstrated to leading manufacturers in London in 1978 (Figure 1–1), and the first human distortion product OAE (DPOAE) recordings were reported at the Inner Ear Biology conference in Seefeld that same year (Kemp 1979a). The effectiveness of transient evoked OAEs (TEOAEs) for infant screening was practically demonstrated by Johnsen and Elberling (1982) just two years later. But these events had no immediate impact on clinical practice. And why was that? First, there were no resources for the fully working laboratory prototype OAE systems of that time to be duplicated and made available for wider evaluation. There was publication of OAEs in the scientific literature, but what was needed was publication in hardware. The industry failed to respond to this need throughout the 1980s. Second, there was an inertia in acceptance at an academic level.

To understand the hesitation of scientists to use OAEs, the progress of general auditory theory should be reviewed. The origins of the understanding of how the cochlea processes sound are in the mid-19th century. At that time the frontiers of science included the theory of music and of musical instruments. Mathematicians, such as Fourier, had succeeded in interpreting complex sounds as the summation

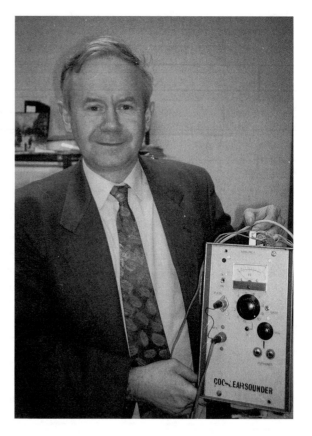

Figure 1–1. A 1995 photograph of David Kemp with the world's first routine OAE instrument, the *Cochlear Sounder* used at the ILO in London between 1977 and 1984. It performed TEOAE measurements, was battery powered, and used an analogue CCD leaky averager circuit. It displayed a real-time running average of the nonlinear OAE (updated every second). The waveform was viewed on a battery powered pocket oscilloscope screen (not shown), and data was recorded on a portable reel-to-reel tape recorder in analogue form. The taped records were later digitized prior to frequency analysis. When this unit was built the laboratory system for recording DPOAE and SOAEs comprised two racks of equipment, TEOAE recording could be achieved more simply.

of simple generic sounds or harmonics. Helmholtz had succeeded in analyzing sounds acoustically with a series of resonators and believed that the ear must use a similar process. When, with the perfection of the compound microscope, accurate drawings of the detailed structure of the cochlea were circulated it was natural for scientists, such as Helmholtz, to look for frequency-specific resonators in the ear. They thought they had found them in the fibers of the organ of corti and basilar membrane, and the place theory of hearing was born. They were not aware, however, that natural damping by the fluid in the confined spaces of the cochlea would be so severe as to destroy any tendency for musically sharp resonance in the structures of the cochlea. In working to perfect mechanical sound recording in the phonograph during the 1880s and 1890s, Edison had to confront the limitations of the physical world, and he was never able to capture the 10 octaves of vibration needed for high-fidelity sound reproduction. The scale and performance of man-made physical devices aimed at capturing and manipulating sound vibration have yet to approach the performance of the ear.

By creating an electrical analogue of sound the newly perfected telephone of the 1890s was freed of some of the limitations of mechanics because electrical currents have negligible mass and can be easily manipulated. The advent of radio technology focused attention on means of frequency separation that used electrical circuits in the early part of the century. Vacuum-tube technology not only assisted radio engineers but also allowed biological potentials to be easily studied. In the 1930's Wever and Bray identified the cochlear microphonic signal, which supported the telephone theory of hearing. However, it soon became clear that hearing is not based on a direct electric analogue of sound because, unlike copper wire, nerve fibers cannot carry such a rapidly fluctuating telephone signal. It was nevertheless an eminent telephone engineer, von Bekesy, that applied himself to the task of tracing sound vibration in its passage through the cochlea. Brilliant microscopic techniques enabled him to discover that a relatively slow (1m/s) traveling wave was created that neatly delivered incoming sound energy of different frequencies to different places along the Organ of Corti. This met one essential requirement of Helmholtz's theory, but the resolution of the frequency analysis observed in the ear was too low to account for the auditory resolution. The problem was clearly one of damping and poor frequency selectivity, exactly as encountered by radio engineers 20 years previously, and overcome, then, with the help of the vacuum tube. In the ear too much energy loss from viscous drag on the structures and fluids of the cochlea resulted in serious degrading of the cochlear traveling-wave development and a serious loss in the potential sensitivity and resolution of the cochlea system.

While most auditory physiologists from the 1940s to the early 1980s accepted the outcome of von Bekesy's experiments on the cadavers' cochleas as being relevant to normal functioning, one biophysicist Thomas Gold was not. In 1948 Gold had tried to alert auditory physiologists to the main weakness of the Bekesys work (Gold 1948, 1989). He argued that in the living ear there must be a mechanism for energy loss reduction or undamping. A sensitive and selective detector, such as the ear, could not afford to waste the energy it collects. Energy loss degrades resonant tuning, frequency resolution, and sensitivity—all vital for auditory functioning. Applying the same logic to the cochlea as radio engineers applied in the 1920s and 1930s to enhance the selectivity of radio receivers, Gold reasoned that nature would not have been so foolish as to ignore the possibility of positive feedback. Nature must have provided some biological device, such as the vacuum tube only operating with vibration, to enhance the response of the cochlea. By taking electrochemical energy from the endocochlear potential and converting it to mechanical vibration exactly in time with the incoming sound vibration, energy loss could be completely compensated for. According to Gold, von Bekesy's experiments had failed to show the true response of the cochlea because his specimens were dead and no longer exhibited active behavior. Regrettable for the field of audiology was that Gold's advice was not taken, and a somewhat disillusioned Gold turned to the more outward looking field of cosmology.

Gold had, in fact, predicted motility in the organ of Corti nearly four decades before its discovery in outer hair cells. Another startling conclusion of Gold was that maladjusted ears should be expected to emit continuous tones. Positive feedback or self reinforcement, as proposed by Gold, is a form of amplification that outside of certain limits leads to self-sustaining oscillation, unless there is tight control. Today, tonal sound generation by the ear is called *spontaneous OAEs* (SOAEs), and SOAEs are associate with overactivity rather than disease. But Gold tried and failed to record SOAEs 50 years ago because he searched for them in association with strong tonal tinnitus, a symptom only rarely associated with SOAEs. It is now believed that healthy overactivity is needed to produce SOAEs. Gold also did not consider the possibility of sound emission as a normal by-product of the hearing process because that would have contradicted the physical understanding of the forward traveling wave. He, therefore, did not predict stimulated OAEs or their association with normal functioning that is the basis for today's clinical applications of OAEs. Nevertheless, auditory theory was seriously diverted for 40 years because the insights of Gold were not given serious consideration.

The existence and nature of stimulatable acoustic emissions from the human ear was first published in 1978 (Kemp, 1978). The term *acoustic emission* is actually borrowed from materials science, where it was well known that energy locked up in the internal stresses of a metal (e.g., after welding) could be released spontaneously or in response to physical excitation. The motivation to look for stimulated OAEs in human ears was different to that of Gold's fruitless search for spontaneous tonal emissions. The search for stimulated OAEs was based on pyschoacoustical investigations of the unexplained peaks and valleys in the detailed structure of the normal audiogram first noted by Elliot (1958) and shown by Kemp's 1975 measurements in Figure 1–2. Their orderly association with aural combination tones, subjective tonal tinnitus, and other anomalies of normal hearing (Kemp & Martin, 1976; Kemp, 1979, 1980) suggested a physical explanation. The model of the phenomenon adopted at that time is still relevant. It is that wave propagation in the cochlea is virtually loss-free near threshold, and that a nonlinearity at the peak of the traveling wave turns around or scatters back some of the traveling wave energy, and returns both stimulus frequency and intermodulation signals back to the middle ear. Reverse propagation of cochlear waves was unknown at that time. As with a reverberant room, in this scenario standing waves are set up in the cochlea, which emphasizes some frequencies and suppresses others accounting for the microstructure of auditory threshold. In fact the cochlea behaves more like a

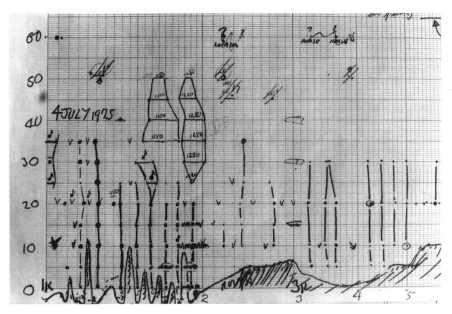

Figure 1–2. A psychoacoustic auditory phenomena map obtained in Kemp's laboratory in 1975. It shows the regular structure of auditory threshold (*ripple at the bottom* between 1K and 2K Hz) paralleled by loudness maxima (*vertical lines*), and accompanied by beats from tonal tinnitus (*horizontal zigzags* at around 1.8 K Hz), and frequency-level areas with diplacusis (outlined areas) caused by distortion products between the applied sound and the spontaneous OAE (causing the tonal tinnitus). The entire phenomena set could be modeled by assuming the listener was hearing via a 5 ft³ reverberant enclosure, assisted by a rather poor quality PA system. Only in 1977 did was there enough confidence in this hypothesis to begin to look for correlates of this distortion and reverberation in human ears, and they were found.

room with its natural acoustics enhanced by an imperfect acoustic amplification, hence the potential for feedback howl (SOAEs) and intermodulation distortion (DPOAEs). These phenomena are observable because the oval window transmits internal cochlear vibrations on to the middle ear and so to the ear canal. Standing waves, SOAEs and DPOAEs recorded by an insert microphone were the first OAE observations to be made at the London laboratory in 1977. Publication proved difficult and a more compelling demonstration of the real behavior of the cochlea was needed. This was achieved by borrowing a simple technique from architectural acoustics. A single impulse is applied to reveal the strength and duration of reverberation and, hence, the quality factor of the auditorium or the ear (Figure 1–3).

In 1978 as in 1948 it was very difficult for auditory scientists to accept this new model of cochlea behavior, but now there was experimental verification in the form of transient evoked OAEs. The cochlea was considered by most researchers to be a mechanically passive and linear system crudely sorting the vibrations received from the middle ear and delivering them to the sensory hair cells. Hair cell motility was not known. Significantly, there was no proven physical or physiological

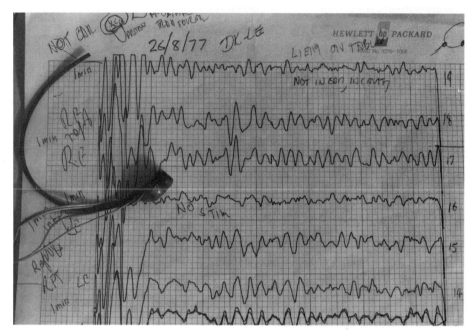

Figure 1–3. A photograph of the first recording of TEOAEs (August 26, 1977). Original data and probe shown. From the top down: *a*, room noise level; *b*, first TEOAE; *c*, TEOAE repeat; *d*, no response with no stimulus; *e*, other ear TEOAE; *f*, other ear TEOAE repeat. This experiment was performed to test a theory of the origin of DPOAEs, SFOAEs, and SOAEs, which had been studied using pure-tone stimuli and with an insert microphone for several months.

explanation for the observed high frequency selectivity of hearing. It was in this context that the first international scientific conference on the "Active and non-linear mechanical processes in the cochlea" associated with OAEs was held at the Institute of Laryngology and Otology (ILO) in London in the fall of 1979 [See Hearing Research Vol. 2 1980 for conference proceedings]. At this meeting Ake Flock reported the growing evidence for contractile behavior in outer hair cells (Flock, 1980), D. O. Kim reported the strong evidence for mechanical nonlinearity and bi-directional interaction between hair cells and cochlear mechanics (Kim, 1980), largely ignored at the time, but confirmed experimentally by Le Page and Johnstone in the Guinea pig (Le Page & Johnstone, 1980). Finally J. Zwislocki demonstrated the potential value of a better physical understanding the micro-mechanics of the organ of Corti and of the role of the tectorial membrane (Zwislocki, 1980). Back in 1979 the phenomenon of otoacoustic emissions stood enigmatically at the center of these equally important and independent "appeals" for a fresh look to be taken at cochlear mechanics.

The change had begun. Several years later audiofrequency hair cell motility was demonstrated by Brownell and a true measure of mechanical frequency selectivity was obtained (Brownell, 1983; 1984; Brownell, Bader, Bertrand & de Rebauplerve,

1985). By 1985 OAEs were accepted as a by-product of what appeared to be a biological hearing aid. Indeed, it was becoming clear that the cochlea was not the passive and sluggish responder to sound it was thought to have been after von Bekesy. Most importantly for clinical audiology, the cause and nature of moderate sensory hearing impairment was having to be completely reinterpreted. It was now to be seen as a loss in active biomechanical responsiveness in the cochlea rather than a simple loss of inner hair cell sensitivity. This was a revolutionary step forward for theories of deafness.

Confidence in the basic significance and reliability of OAEs as an exquisitely sensitive indicator of cochlear status has gradually grown, and over the last few years OAEs have finally begun to enter the main stream of hearing screening and diagnostic audiology. But the process of assimilation and development is far from over. Mystery and confusions remain, even amongst scientist and instrument manufacturers. At the heart of the problem is the fact that as an audiological tool OAEs are so different from audiometry and from the measuring of electrophysiological and myogenic responses, that borrowed understanding and terminology has led to serious misconceptions. OAEs are a completely new biological phenomenon and the multidisciplinary approach needed to understand them means that those to whom we habitually turn to for enlightenment on audiological matters, found themselves initially ill equipped to master this new technology. Until this book there have been few digestible and comprehensive texts to assist clinicians and audiologists understand and exploit OAEs to the full.

Nature of OAEs

OAEs are sounds found in the external auditory meatus that originate in physiologically vital and vulnerable activity inside the cochlea. There is abundant experimental evidence that this activity is intimately associated with the hearing process. It happens that OAEs are generated only when the organ of Corti is in near normal condition, and they can emerge (or, at least, can be detected) only when the middle-ear system is operating normally. The sounds generated by the cochlea are small but potentially audible, sometimes amounting to as much as 30 dB SPL. They can emerge spontaneously because sound already in the cochlea perpetually recirculates, but more commonly OAEs follow acoustic stimulation. No electrodes are needed to observe OAEs. They are not electrical in nature but vibratory responses. In fact, microphones are used to detect them, and they are converted to an electrical to process them more easily.

OAEs are created by motion of the eardrum driven by the cochlea through the middle ear chain. To record OAEs a healthy middle ear with good sound conduction is needed. The cochlea does not significantly radiate sound through the air of the middle ear. In fact, at frequencies below 3 kHz even the OAE vibration transmitted through the middle ear would be undetectably small were it not for the fact the ear canal is physically closed. Closing the ear canal is an essential part of the OAE technique and enables any oscillatory movement of the ear drum to more efficiently compress and rarefy the air that otherwise would flow silently in and out of the ear canal, without creating sound. The tympanic-membrane motions responsible for regular OAEs are subatomic in scale.

The need to close off the ear canal to maximize OAE level is a reminder that the specific sound level of OAEs is not an absolute physiological quantity; it is the product of the driving force within the cochlea, the conductive properties of the middle ear, and the specific volume and acoustics of the air enclosed in the ear canal. If one were to keep the cochlea the same but change the fitting of the probe or the ear-canal volume or the middle-ear characteristics, then the OAE would change in intensity, in much the same way that the recordable ABR voltage changes with electrode positioning and resistance. No great clinical significance is attached to the absolute microvolt level of the ABR, and no great significance should be attached to the precise sound levels of OAEs.

A stronger OAE does give greater confidence that there is normal hearing in an ear, and there is a significant correlation between OAE strength and hearing threshold in a mixed population of normal and impaired ears. But a person's hearing threshold is only one of many factors that influence externally recordable OAE levels. It is certainly possible to establish norms of OAE levels under specific stimulus conditions for a population, but it is not possible to translate a person's OAE level into an audiometric threshold with any useful accuracy. Ears at the extremes of OAE levels can have thresholds of 0 dB and ears with average OAEs levels can have thresholds of 20 or 30 dB SPL. There are too many undefined sources of variance and intersubject differences in OAE levels to treat OAE dB SPL as a quantitative measure. A more physiologically meaningful measure, if it could be achieved, would be to assess the energy of the returned wave impinging on the stapes. But even this measure would include the poorly understood and highly variable factor responsible for the retro-ejection of energy from the cochlear traveling wave.

One thing that is certain is that healthy cochleas do contain a mechanism capable of returning sound to the middle ear, and significantly impaired cochleas normally do not. This makes OAEs a uniquely valuable clinical tool.

Recording OAEs

In the most general terms, an OAE instrument consists of an acoustic ear-canal–probe assembly containing a loudspeaker to stimulate the ear, a microphone to record all the sounds in the ear canal, and a signal separating process that can discriminate between sounds emerging from the cochlea and other sounds, such as the stimulus and noise, to extract, analyze, and display the unique, cochlear sounds (i.e., OAEs).

The probe must physically seal the ear canal to maximize OAE collection, but also to exclude ambient noise. It must contain a sensitive microphone with low internal noise and wide bandwidth. It must also contain sound-delivery transducers— one in the case of transient-stimulus delivery and two in the case of two-tone delivery for distortion product analysis. The latter is needed because feeding two tones in with a single transducer would introduce much more distortion than the cochlea produces.

Stimulation of the ear can be achieved in an infinite number of ways, and OAEs will always be generated. The choice of stimulation determines, not only which portions of the cochlea are stimulated, but also the form of processing needed for optimum OAE extraction. Cochlear biophysics teaches that a pure tone stimulates a substantial portion of the cochlea simultaneously, not just one point, as often imagined. A pure-tone stimulus is not a totally place-specific stimulus. All of the cochlea up to the conventional *frequency place* participate to some extend in advancing the traveling wave and participate in the audition of that tone. With two-tone stimulation used for DPOAE measuring an even wider portion of the cochlea is involved, and in the case of a transient stimulus, virtually the whole of the cochlear is stimulated.

Many audiologists find it difficult to accept that frequency-specific information can be obtained from OAEs elicited by non–frequency-specific stimuli, such as transients. However, it is the cochlea that is frequency-specific in it's response, and this frequency specificity is maintained in the case of transient or tonal stimulation. Each portion of the cochlea gives its strongest response at one specific frequency; and this applies to the OAE response. The unique feature of OAEs, which tends to confuse those more familiar with neural responses, is that the response of each portion of the cochlea can be separated out from the OAE signal after it emerges from the ear, by instrumental frequency analysis. In contrast, gross neurogenic electrophysiological signals cannot be retro-analyzed for frequency specificity— hence, the peculiar need for frequency specific stimulation of an already frequency specific cochlea in diagnostic ABR work. Thanks to the cochlea and the nature of sound vibration, frequency-specific OAE recordings can be conducted with any stimulus (clicks and tones). There is an operational difference between the use of wideband (*click*) stimulation and narrowband (*tonal*) stimulation. With tonal stimulation (e.g., DPOAE recording) only part of the cochlea is being tested at any one time so that a series of measurements need to be made that cover the whole frequency range. With click-evoked OAEs data is collected from a substantial length of the cochlea simultaneously, and the response is broken down into separate frequencies afterwards.

Once the desired stimulus is selected the process of response extraction can be designed. This process is not trivial. Many other sounds exist in the ear canal besides the stimulus and OAEs. There are those sounds entering from the outside world and those generated by motion and vibration in the head, such as speech, breathing, swallowing, and blood flow. So how can one be sure that a sound recorded in the closed ear canal is a sound generated by the cochlea and not the stimulus, or some other sound? How can one be sure a sound emanating from the ear is associated with the hearing process and not some other source, such as vascular noise? These are crucial questions and are at the heart of all OAE technology, as well as the effective use of OAEs.

The problem of response-signal extraction is not unique to OAEs. The auditory brain stem response, for example, is but a small part (~ 1/30th) of the total neurogenic electrical activity found on the scalp and an even smaller part of the possible myogenic and environmental interference present. Synchronous averaging and filtering can be employed to extract OAEs from noise as with ABR. In fact, OAEs have an advantage over ABR responses here. Their level (typically 10 dB SPL) is comparable with the expected noise level in a good sound-treated room and with a quiet subject. Wilson (1980) actually succeeded in demonstrating OAEs without averaging, although with the typical patient this is not possible, 30-s to

3-min averaging is generally needed. But there is an additional problem to be overcome with OAEs. The stimulus and response are of the same nature (sound) and exist in the same place (the ear canal).

Fortunately, OAE responses can be identified and separated from the stimulus sound and the response of the middle ear system on the basis of their unique properties associated with their cochlea origin. The key properties used to extract OAEs are the inherent delay of the OAE response and the nonlinearity of the OAE-generating mechanism. The delay of OAEs is associated with the slow cochlear traveling wave velocity which is around 1 m/sec, which gives a time of 10 ms to travel 1 cm. The nonlinearity is associated with the physiologically dependent nature of the mechanisms and forces encountered by the traveling wave as it engages with the hair cells of the cochlea. Although delays and nonlinearities can also be found in electroacoustic instrumentation, these can normally be controlled to be much smaller than those found in the cochlea.

The two major classes of OAE instruments (TEOAE and DPOAE) both use these OAE properties but in different ways. With transient stimulation, time gating is very effective in separating the stimulus from the delayed OAE response from the cochlea. Most of the stimulus and middle-ear response is over in about 3 ms, and thus this time period is not included in the analysis. Depending on the frequency considered, OAEs have latencies up to 20 ms. Nevertheless, a small component of the probe and middle-ear response spills over into the recorded post-stimulus period and can pose as a short-latency OAE. It should also be noted that delayed echoes of the stimulus sound from the walls of the test room a few feet away would also show a latency greater than 3 ms. Fortunately, such reflections are exceedingly small from insert probes and are linear in behavior (unlike biological responses). To protect from any acoustic artifact in TEOAE measurements, the signal extracted by time gating is further tested for genuine cochlear origin by alternating the level of stimulation. Cancellation processing can then easily eliminate any purely proportional acoustic responses or reflections and leaves only the typically biologically saturating response of the cochlea. In effect, regular TEOAE instruments extract the distortion present in the delayed acoustic response found in the ear canal and identifies this with the cochlea. In the process of nonlinear extraction some genuine linear-OAE response is lost and thus reduces the signal to noise ratio. In summary, in TEOAE recording OAE latency is the primary identifier and OAE nonlinearity is the validator.

The other common method of OAE measurement uses the nonlinearity of OAEs as the primary separator and is called *DPOAE recording*. DPOAE processing is the reverse of TEOAE processing in that the nonlinear response component is extracted first then tested for a cochlear origin. As with TEOAEs, the level of stimulation is varied, but much more rapidly, at many hundreds of times a second. This is achieved by applying two pure tones simultaneously having a frequency ratio that results in partially overlapping of the vibration fields in the cochlea. Stimulus-level fluctuation occurs most strongly at the position in the cochlea where the two traveling waves (from f_1 and f_2) are of equal size. The ratio of stimulus frequencies and levels determines where in the cochlea the maximum beating occurs. Cochlear traveling-wave characteristics decree that for this to happen maximally at the place of reception of the higher of the two frequencies presented, the lower frequency tone must normally be stronger than the higher tone. There is no way the two tones can beat at the place for the lower frequency tone because the higher frequency tone never reaches this place. Wherever the two tones meet, the OAE generator sees a vibration of fluctuating amplitude. Being a nonlinear mechanism it fails to copy exactly the dynamics of the waveform envelope, returning an OAE signal comprised of an OAE response to each tone (the stimulus frequency emission) plus smaller OAEs at several new combination tone frequencies, including $2f_1 - f_2$, $3f_1 - 2f_2$, $2f_2 - f_1$. The new tones can be easily extracted from the on going stimulus tones by frequency analysis, but the stimulus frequency OAEs present are unfortunately lost in this method.

The creation of an intermodulation distortion product (e.g. $2f_1 - f_2$) is a mechanical process that can happen owing to nonlinearity in any instrumentation, such as a hearing instrument. The existence of the distortion product $2f_1 - f_2$ does not, therefore, on its own indicate cochlear functioning. The cochlear origin of any $2f_1 - f_2$ distortion product recorded in the ear canal needs to be confirmed, but this can be done in several ways. At the most basic level the measurement in a cavity can be repeated at the same stimulus levels to assure that there is no comparable instrumental distortion. By measuring the latency of the distortion-OAE components the involvement of the cochlear traveling wave can be confirmed. To be doubly sure a simultaneous masking tone (f_3) to confirm the frequency specific nature of the nonlinearity which is unique to the cochlea (Brown & Kemp, 1984) can be applied. In summary, with DPOAEs, cochlear nonlinearity is the primary identifier; current DPOAE instruments vary in their capacity to perform positive cochlear validation by latency. As a general rule any OAE instrument should be frequently run in a damped test cavity to assess the level of artifact production.

Once signal extraction has been completed and the extracted signal validated as an OAE, the question arises "what further analysis should be conducted and what data should be displayed to the user?" The key clinical information is the evidence for or against an OAEs being present at each frequency. Because the auditory bandwidth is around 1/3 octave, analysis of the response signal intensity at 2 or 3 points per octave should be adequate for most purposes. The next step is to interpret the observations.

The implications of a strong OAE well clear of the system noise is unambiguous. The cochlea has a functional response to incoming vibration at that frequency. By comparing the absolute level with the normal range of OAE levels, one may go further to determine if the OAE activity is significantly above or below average for the particular conditions. One cannot absolutely interpret the meaning of above-average or below-average OAEs at this time, but certainly one would want to follow-up an OAE result in the lower 5% of the normal range if there were any other indications.

If the validated OAE response is only slightly above the noise level, there is the question of what the chance is of this being a statistical artifact. This assessment is not trivial, but can be done based on the measured statistics of the noise present and the time taken for the recording. There is no fixed minimum signal-to-noise ratio that can be applied generally. Take the recommendation of the equipment suppliers and users. It is always valuable to repeat the OAE measurement and look for correlations.

If there is no detectable OAE above the noise level, the absolute level of the noise needs to be known before any conclusion can be made at all. A useful approach is to compare noise level with the normal range of OAE levels. Because noise will obscure smaller OAEs, such a comparison will reveal the probability of the noise having obscured a smaller OAE within the normal range. If so, the test was invalid and must be repeated; if not, then the test can be accepted as an absent OAE result.

In screening applications where noise and time limits the collection of ideal data, it is common to set a target for the number of frequency bands that must show an OAE for a pass to be accepted. When used as part of a clinical audiometric test battery in controlled conditions, each frequency band of interest, needs to be probed for OAEs for the time needed to obtains a statistically valid outcome. The principles remain the same.

TEOAE versus DPOAE Technology

Competitive claims that one type of OAE technology is intrinsically better than the other must be discarded. They are different and each have different advantages and disadvantages. The primary difference between the DPOAEs and TEOAEs techniques is in what the cochlea is doing while one is measuring and which parts of the whole OAE response are captured and which parts are rejected.

The DPOAE method rejects all the stimulus frequency OAEs present in the response. Current practice also tends to reject all but the $2f_1 - f_2$ distortion component of the OAE leading to a very narrow view of activity. The other components are easily accessible and may prove to have supplementary value. Figure 1–4 shows 16 separate distortion product emissions from one stimulus pair. The TEOAE method captures all components of the OAE, both linear and nonlinear, but the nonlinear validation process sacrifices the linear OAE portion leading to a loss in signal to noise ratio. This loss may be unnecessary in some applications when contamination by the stimulus is not a concern (e.g., low level TEOAE or differential measurements).

The two techniques observe the cochlear in different conditions. The cochlea is a complex organ that behaves differently to every stimulus. Unlike a passive, linear mechanical system one cannot reliably predict the performance of the cochlea under one set of conditions from its performance under another. If one wants to know how a cochlea responds to low stimulation low stimulation then must be provided. If one wants to know how the cochlea behaves under interrupted stimulation or under continuous stimulation the appropriate stimuli must be used.

With the regular TEOAE method the cochlear response is observed between stimulations in the relaxation phase, and this is obviously relevant to its behavior at low levels. TEOAEs have been shown to be able to separate normal from abnormal ears at the 20 to 30 dB HL point. Because click stimulus requires few parameters, standardization is relatively easy. Data is collected simultaneously across a wide frequency range and can be retrospectively analyzed by frequency. Data can be grouped and averaged in frequency bands as required for comparison with other data. Validation is achieved simply with the nonlinear cancellation method. Under the best conditions, TEOAEs can be observed in real time (20 ms), and even under clinical conditions a screening test can take less than 1 min. The mean time of

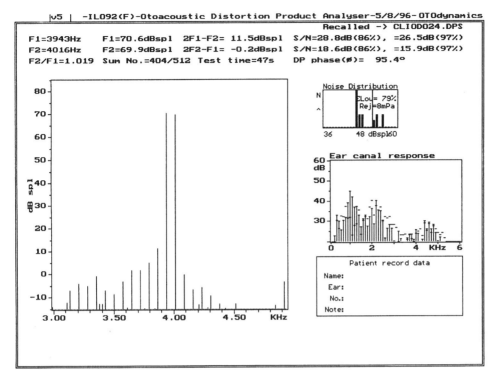

Figure 1–4. DPOAEs from a two month old healthy ear, showing multiple DPOAEs (16 are visible, 11 below, and 5 above the primary tones [F_1 = 3943 Hz, F_2 = 4016 Hz]). This is quite normal for close primary ratios. It raises the question what aspects of DPOAE give the most useful data? The figure more completely describes the cochlear nonlinear activity than the single DPOAE extracted from wider primaries.

testing, even in routine nursery newborn screening applications, is around 2 min. It has a very high specificity (+95%) on newborns with clean dry ears.

The disadvantage of the TEOAE technique is that it fails to extract responses at high frequencies partly owing to the time gating used to separate stimulus from OAE. High-frequency OAEs have the shortest latency and are lost. Also, TEOAE specificity reduces with age, possibly because of TEOAE sensitivity to clinically insignificant changes in the cochlea. This effect can be compensated, to some extent, by increasing the stimulus intensity or rate. However, the nature of a click stimulus means that the peak limits of the instrumentation are quickly reached.

The tonal stimuli used in DPOAE recording offer more scope for providing the cochlear with a greater intensity stimulus. The typical continuous stimulus levels used for clinical DPOAE measurements (60–70 dB SPL) constitute a more intense stimulus than the mean level used during standard TEOAE recording. This may account for the higher cut off point for DPOAEs (35–45 dB) and a lower sensitivity to hearing loss. Sensitivity can be restored by lowering stimulus level, but this increases the test time. A major advantage of the DPOAE technique is its ability to recover OAE responses above 6k Hz, although adult ear canal resonance may cause calibration difficulties in this region. A disadvantage of the method is that lower frequency observations are more easily influenced by low frequency noise because the DPOAE response is frequency shifted down from the test frequency (f_2) by 2/3 octave. Finally, the penalty of using the long duration pure tone stimuli needed for DPOAE recording is that the response obtained is highly specific to the particular pattern of vibration set up in the cochlea by that particular stimulus frequency ratio and intensity ratio. This is a disadvantage because interference and cancellation can occur in the cochlea. A change of a few percent in frequency, or ratio can result in a large difference in DPOAE level and result in increased variance in DPOAE levels. To smooth out interference effects, measurements should be taken closer than three per octave and at alternative ratios and then averaged. This adds an unacceptable time penalty with DPOAEs, but happens automatically with TEOAEs.

Overall, DPOAE and TEOAE techniques turn out to be rather complementary (Figure 1–5). First they reveal cochlear status in two contrasting stimulus conditions— one steady state, the other intermittent. TEOAEs are best at detecting threshold elevation below 3 k HZ; DPOAEs are best above 3 k Hz (Prieve, 1992). TEOAEs may be too sensitive to cochlear conditions in adults, and DPOAEs may be too insensitive. TEOAEs present an averaged overview of cochlear activity; DPOAEs a snap shot specific to one set of stimulus parameters. TEOAE provide a view of cochlear activity to soft stimulation; DPOAEs can be obtained at moderate and with care to higher levels of stimulation. Clearly, a combination and comparison of the two seems ideal.

Decibel Levels and Hearing Threshold

Both DPOAE and TEOAEs are excellent screening tools. One cannot accurately predict threshold levels from OAE decibel levels, but one can distinguish between good and impaired cochlear functioning. One should expect this from the nature of OAEs because the driving force responsible for OAEs is only a by-product of forces functionally associated with the progression, strengthening, and development of traveling wave vibration in the cochlea. The source of these forces is, most likely, in longitudinal contraction of the lateral walls of the outer hair cells, and they control the strength of the traveling wave, which is the primary determinant of hearing threshold. OAEs were the first experimental indication of wave amplification in the cochlea (Kemp, 1979a), but this process is now thought to be essential to overcome the natural viscous absorption of vibrational energy in the fluid motions occurring in the confined spaces within the cochlea and to achieve high frequency selectivity and sensitivity. But there are other very important factors involved in hearing threshold. The sound vibrations collected by the ear drum pass through many stages and transformations on route to the auditory cortex (Figure 1–6).

Factors assisting sensitive threshold include:

1. open external auditory meatus
2. a mobile light and stiff tympanum
3. a light and well articulated ossicular chain

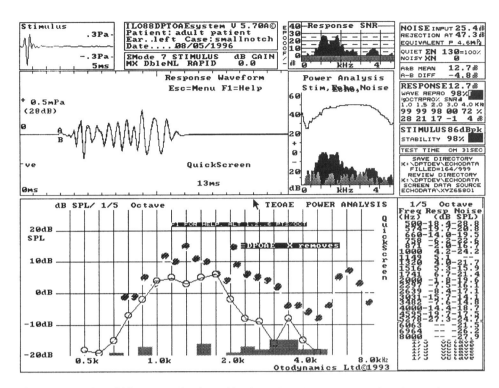

Figure 1–5. One-fifth octave display of both TEOAE (*open connected circles*) and DPOAE (*filled circles*) for the same patient ear. TEOAE and DPOAE data are very similar below 4 k Hz, when analyzed on a comparable basis. DPOAEs can, however be measured out to 8 k Hz. For the 1–4k Hz range, sometimes the DPOAE component is stronger than the nonlinear TEOAE component and sometimes the reverse is true. These data from an adult patient took 31 seconds for the TEOAE and 60 seconds for the DPOAE to reach the same frequency resolution and signal to noise level.

4. a mobile and low loss attachment of the stapes to the oval window
5. a well formed mobile and low-loss basilar membrane supporting a normal traveling wave
6. optimum electrochemical environment of the scala media
7. optimum condition of the outer hair cells
8. optimum configuration of the outer hair cells (including the medial efferent system)
9. optimum coupling of motion within the organ of Corti, especially from basilar membrane to outer hair cell to inner hair cell
10. optimum condition and function of the inner hair cells
11. optimum synaptic function at the inner hair cell—including efferent interaction
12. optimum neural transmission out of the inner ear

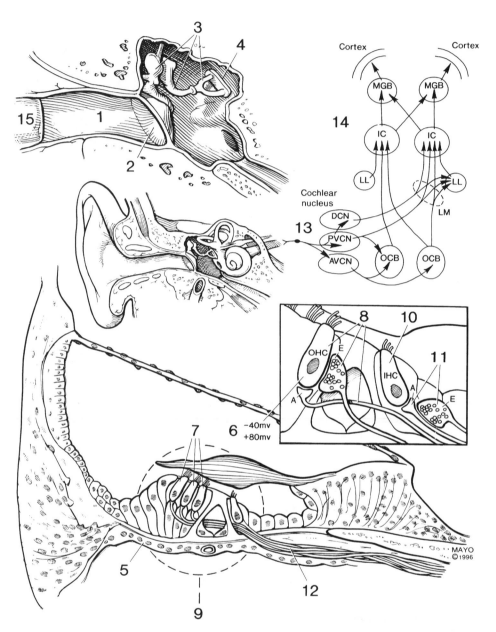

Figure 1–6. Anatomy of the human auditory system with a numerical listing of factors assisting auditory threshold sensitivity. (Factors are listed in text).

13. optimum mapping and processing of the neural signals reaching the cochlear nucleus

14. optimum function of the entire auditory pathway.

Auditory threshold depends on the sum total of activity and efficiency all these levels, but OAEs involve only some of the above factors. Because OAEs depend on sound vibration reaching the organ of Corti, they must share the factors *1, 2, 3, 4* and *5*. Because it is known that outer–hair-cell function is needed for good hearing and for OAEs factors *6, 7,* and *8* can also be included.

At this point OAE-generation diverges from the hearing process. While *9* is clearly important, the escape of vibration back in the middle ear to form OAEs is obviously not completely the same factor as the transmission of vibration to the inner hair cell to stimulate hearing. So it is changed to *9a*. Factors *10* through *14* do not affect OAE production, except that crossed olivo-cochlear bundle (COCB) activity may determine factor *8* to some extent. Additionally, for a second time factors *2* through *5* have to be included because the OAE vibration must travel to the drum by reverse passage through the cochlea and middle ear. Such a reverse process may have different acoustic parameters and it is denoted by renaming these factors *2a* through *5a*. Furthermore, the cochlea delivers a vibratory force to the ear drum, not a predefined decibel sound pressure. The sound pressure depends on the acoustics of the enclosed ear canal in which the probe microphone is situated, and this is quite different from the way the open ear canal normally affects incoming sound. This is called factor *15*.

Auditory threshold can be nominally computed by adding factors 1 through 14. However, to determine the OAE level however one must add a different set of factors

OAE level factor = 1 + 2 + 3 + 4 + 5 + 6 + 7 + 8 + 9a + 5a + 4a + 3a + 2a + 15

From this it is clear that, relative to hearing threshold, OAEs are doubly sensitive to middle ear disorders and completely insensitive to disorders affecting only inner hair-cell or afferent-neural functioning. That OAEs do, in fact, have excellent sensitivity to cochlear dysfunction indicates that cochlear dysfunction most commonly impacts on factors 6 through 8. But this is not to say that OAE level relates closely to audiometric threshold, because audiometric threshold is determined by factors not included in OAE generation.

The earliest clinical reports of OAEs focused on the similarity in form of DPOAE-frequency–grams and TEOAE spectra with audiograms in selected cased where there were well defined frequency ranges of normal and of abnormal hearing (Kemp, Bray, Alexander, & Brown, 1986). In the original publications no claim was made that audiometric threshold could actually be determined with any useful accuracy from OAEs measurements—only that OAEs could identify the frequency that at which threshold became substantially elevated. However, fueled by a clinical desire for an efficient objective auditory threshold method and by the superficial similarity between the audiogram chart and the DPOAE intensity frequency display published by many groups, expectations that OAEs did predict thresholds grew spontaneously. More refined methods involved a kind of threshold determination in which stimulus levels were reduced until the OAE was no longer detectable above the noise. There is no true physiological threshold of OAE generation because it is a preneural phenomena, but the detection threshold obtained by growth-rate measurements is a complex combination of the system noise level, averaging time and OAE input-output function. Even so, the term *DP audiogram* briefly slipped into common use before being counteracted by conscientious researchers eager to prevent clinical misunderstanding. This is not to say that the partial correlation that exists between audiometric threshold and OAE level will never be useful; but more research is required to identify and quantify the other factors involved. The possibilities can, at least, be explored.

If one were to compare a person's actual threshold and OAE level against the average population trend of OAE level with hearing loss, an OAE deficit or surplus at each frequency relative to the mean OAE level for the average ear with identical threshold could be obtained. Even ears within the normal audiometric range could depart from the mean. Such a deviation would arise from differences in the OAE and hearing pathways in this person relative to those in the average ear. An OAE-audiometric threshold (O-T) gap would have been identified. This O-T gap must originate in the combined effect of two important groups of factors. An emission group (E group) consisting of factor *9a* and *2a* through *5a* above that are uniquely associated with the OAE phenomenon and a sensory neural group (the SN group) that consists of factors *10* through *14* that do not influence OAEs. Factors *1* through *8* always apply equally to both OAEs and hearing. They comprise the conductive factors *1* through *5* (C group) and the cochlear amplifier, factors *6* through *8* (A group).

It is precisely because the OAE pathway includes the C and A groups that they are a sensitive indicator of cochlear dysfunction and are partially correlated with threshold. But it is precisely because OAEs include the E group and not the SN group that OAE levels do not strongly correlate with threshold and why an O-T gap can arise. To illustrate the implications of this take two subjects with identical audiograms, but with different OAE levels. This could arise in a number of ways. A real SN group difference between the two may be hidden by a compensatory difference in conductive efficiency (C group) or the cochlear amplifier (A group). This would be clinically interesting, but impossible to establish from the OAE recordings alone. Regular tympanometry would not assist, either, because the conductive efficiency of the middle ear and cochlea at medium to high frequency is not determinable in this way. Alternatively, the same observations could equally arise from two subjects truly having the same hearing and middle ear and sensory status, but in which the E group of factors governing the transmission of OAE vibration back to the meatus differed—something of little clinical significance. There are other combinations. The ears might be identical other than in ear canal shape (factor *15*). Until there is the means to clinically separate these factor groups, it will not be possible to fully interpret OAE decibel levels. In the future and as part of a battery of tests, however, it may be possible.

Prospects for Development in OAE Technology

If OAE decibel level can not be quantitatively interpreted, what other characteristics of OAEs are there that may reveal more about the status of a person's cochlea?

Essentially, OAEs offer objective evidence of the integrity of the entire pre-synaptic auditory system. It is an accident of biology that the most common auditory disorders affect this region. Even some retrocochlear disorders exert an negative impact on the cochlea. It is an accident of biophysics that a correlate of sound vibration in the cochlea just prior to its arrival at the sensory cells can be so easily recorded. A good analogy is with the visual inspection of the retina. The aim there is to confirm the integrity of the sensory epithelium and the quality of the inspection optics, and the intensity of the illumination assist greatly. But no one would suggest that progressively dimming the illumination until the observer could only see the retina would be a credible way to measure visual acuity for the patient. What would be more valuable would be to compare every visually observable characteristic of the patient's retina with the normal appearance. This, in a way, is the direction that developments in OAE technology are aimed.

OAEs are rich in information not yet learned or understood. The most delicate and important aspect of cochlear functioning for normal threshold appears to be that contributed by the outer hair cells, and these cells are central to OAE generation. It follows that OAEs may potentially inform clinicians of the onset and nature of cochlear conditions. Although the absolute level of OAEs is too much influenced by not essential acoustic and mechanical factors, the parameters of the nonlinear interaction and OAE latency are not.

So far OAE latency has been introduced as a validating factor only. However, norms for DPOAE latency are being established (O'Mahoney & Kemp, 1995; Moulin & Kemp, 1996a, 1996b). Although OAE latency is expected to have a strong anatomical component originating in basilar membrane properties, a vulnerable component cannot be ruled out. Certainly different species exhibit very different OAE latencies (Kemp & Brown, 1983). Clinical research should soon demonstrate if abnormal-OAE latency has diagnostic or predictive significance.

Nonlinearity is at the heart of OAE generation and hair cell physiology. The problem is to collect and assimilate enough OAE data to support an unambiguous model of cellular nonlinearities in an individual ear. Current TEOAE and DPOAE measurements only scratch the surface. During DPOAE measurements at least 80% of the available information is discarded. During $2f_1 - f_2$ production, there is also OAE emission at f_1, f_2, $3f_1 - 2f_2$, $2f_2 - f_1$, and sometimes even more. It is tempting to believe that the $2f_1 - f_2$ component is sufficient, but it is not. A way needs to be found to integrate all this data into a descriptor of the underlying OAE generator. And when this is achieved researchers have to find the time to collect data at multiple ratios and levels. The OAE instruments of the future will employ computer-driven dynamic stimuli that will actively trace key OAE parameters to characterize an ear's status.

In addition to OAEs being a probe of cochlear anatomy though OAE latency and cell physiology through nonlinearity, OAEs can also be employed as a probe of cochlear-frequency selectivity. The introduction of a third tone into a DPOAE recording allows a suppression tuning curve to be obtained. The clinical applications of this method are only just being explored as suitable instrumentation becomes available.

The level of OAEs can be an extremely sensitive indicator of change in a cochlea. Many factors may influence a person's OAE level and prevent a quantitative interpretation—each have a unique relation to auditory physiology. Changes in middle-ear or cochlear status are reliably reflected in OAE level. Contralateral activation of the medial efferent system reduces OAE levels by 10 to 20%, presumably via factor 8. Exposure to noise depresses OAEs substantially, presumably via factor 7. Loop diuretics also suppress OAEs presumably via factor 6. We could continue to identify a factor-specific agent whose effect can be calibrated using OAEs.

There is clearly scope for an immense amount of quantitative research on the peripheral auditory system using OAEs, but this work has only started.

The slow infusion of OAE technology into practical use has parallels in the introduction of tympanometry and BSER. It takes time to digest and understand new methods. In playing my part in promoting development and use of OAE technology I have become aware of the highly conservative nature of the audiometric instrument industry. At best, a lack of industrial understanding of the potential of a new technique delays its dissemination and evaluation. At worst, narrow commercialism works to limit the flexibility and capacity of instrumentation to the minimum before there has been time for the less well understood features to be accepted. The result can be that application development becomes prematurely frozen and stereotyped. Researchers lose interest in developing new clinical applications as there is no way to propagate them. OAE testing is already being stereotyped in hardware by those with least understanding of the physiology of the process and of the potential of the technique. Hopefully, commercially available OAE instrumentation will retain sufficient flexibility and power long enough to allow fruitful clinical research to proceed on some of the topics discussed in this chapter.

References

Brown, A. M., & Kemp, D. T. (1984). Suppressibility of the $2f_1 - f_2$ stimulated acoustic emissions in gerbil and man. *Hearing Research, 13*, 29–37.

Brownell, W. E. (1983). Observations on a motile response in isolated outer hair cells. In W. R. Webster & L. M. Aitken (Eds.): *Mechanisms of hearing* (pp. 5–10). Monash University Press.

Brownell, W. E. (1984). Microscopic observation of cochlear hair cell motility. *Scanning Electron Microscopy, 3*, 1401–1406.

Brownell, W. E., Bader, C. R., Bertrand, D., & de Ribaupierve, Y. (1985). Evoked mechanical responses of isolated cochlear outer hair cells. *Science, 227*, 194–196.

Elliott, E. (1958). A ripple effect in the audiogram. *Nature, 181*, 1076.

Flock, A., (1980). Contractile proteins in hair cells. *Hearing Research, 2*, 411–412.

Gold, T. (1948). Hearing II: The physical basis of the action of the cochlea. *Proceedings of the Royal Society of London. Series B: Biological Sciences, 135*, 492–498.

Gold, T. (1989). Historical background to the proposal 40 years ago of an active model for cochlear frequency analysis. In J. P. Wilson & D. T. Kemp (Eds.), *Cochlear mechanisms: Structure, function and models* (pp. 299–306). New York: Plenum.

Johnsen, N. J., & Elberling, C. (1982). Evoked acoustic emissions from the human ear: I. Equipment and response parameters. *Scandinavian Audiology, 11*, 3–12.

Kemp, D. T. (1978). Stimulated acoustic emissions from within the human auditory system. *Journal of the Acoustical Society of America, 64*, 1386–1391.

Kemp, D. T. (1979a). Evidence of mechanical nonlinearity and frequency selective wave amplification in the cochlea. *Archives of Otorhinolaryngology, 224*, 37–45.

Kemp, D. T. (1979b). The evoked cochlear mechanical response of the auditory microstructure in models of the auditory system and related signal processing techniques. *Scandinavian Audiology, 9*, 35–47.

Kemp, D. T. (1980). Towards a model for the origin of cochlear echoes. *Hearing Research, 2*, 533–548.

Kemp, D. T., & Brown, A. M. (1983). A comparison of mechanical nonlinearities in the cochleae of man and gerbil from ear canal measurements. In R. Klinke and R. Hartmann (Eds.): *Hearing: Physiological bases and psychophysics* (pp. 82–88).

Kemp, D. T., Bray, P., Alexander, L., & Brown, A. M. (1986). Acoustic emission cochleography: Practical aspects. *Scandinavian Audiology, 25* (Suppl.), 71–82.

Kemp, D. T., & Martin, J. A. (1976). Active resonant systems in audition. *Abstracts of XIIIth International Congress of Audiology* (pp. 64–65). Florence, Italy.

Kim, D. O. (1980). Cochlear mechanics: Implications of electrophysiological and acoustical observations. *Hearing Research, 2,* 297–317.

Le Page, E., and Johnstone, B. (1980). Nonlinear mechanical behavior of the basilar membrane in the basal turn of the guinea pig cochlea. *Hearing Research, 2,* 183–189.

Moulin, A., & Kemp, D. T. (1996a). Multi-component acoustic distortion product otoacoustic emission phase in humans. I: general characteristics. *Journal of the Acoustical Society of America,* in press.

Moulin, A., & Kemp, D. T. (1996b). Multi-component acoustic distortion product otoacoustic emission phase in humans. II: Implications for DPOAEs' generation. *Journal of the Acoustical Society of America,* in press.

O'Mahoney, C. F., & Kemp, D. T. (1995). Distortion product otoacoustic emission delay measurement in human ears. *Journal of the Acoustical Society of America, 97,* 3721–3735.

Prieve, B. A. (1992). Otoacoustic emissions in infants and children: Basic characteristics and clinical application. *Seminars in Hearing, 13,* 37–52.

Wilson, J. P. (1980). Recording of the Kemp echo and tinnitus from the ear canal without averaging. *Journal of Physiology, 298,* 8–9.

Zwislocki, J. J. (1980). Theory of cochlear mechanics. *Hearing Research, 2,* 171–182.

2

New Views of Cochlear Function

Allen F. Ryan

Changing Perspectives on Cochlear Physiology

The physiological responses that occur in the cochlea are the foundation of the process of hearing. The inner ear separates stimulus frequencies into different spatial regions of the auditory system, converts changes in pressure into variation in the discharge of auditory neurons, and preserves a remarkable amount of temporal information from the original acoustic signal. How these tasks are accomplished is one of the most fascinating stories in biology.

The story is also rapidly evolving. The past fifteen years has seen enormous changes in our understanding of how the cochlea functions. As originally formulated by von Bekesy (1949) the traveling wave theory dominated the study of cochlear mechanics for decades. As elegant and satisfying as the theory was, however, it was not consistent with a growing body of experimental data that suggested the presence of significant nonlinearities in cochlear responses (Goldstein, 1967; Rhode, 1971) and seemingly disproportionate effects of outer–hair-cell destruction (Harrison & Evans, 1979; Ryan & Dallos, 1975). The existence of additional processes involved in cochlear mechanics and transduction was proposed theoretically (Davis, 1983; Lynn & Sayers, 1969), but there was little direct evidence of what the processes were.

Two breakthroughs lead to a re-assessment of cochlear physiology. The first was the discovery by Kemp (1978) of otoacoustic emissions, which provided strong evidence for the existence of an active, energy-generating process in the cochlea. The second was the discovery by Brownell (1983) of outer–hair-cell motility, which provided a potential physical substrate for the active process. This chapter will review cochlear physiology in the light of these and other recent advances.

An Overview of Cochlear Anatomy

Labyrinthine Fluids and Membranes

The *cochlea* is a long, tapered cavity in the temporal bone and is filled with fluid. In mammals, including human beings, the cavity is coiled into a tight spiral. The broad end close to the middle ear is called the *base*. The narrow end of the spiral is the *apex*. This fluid space is divided lengthwise into three compartments, called *scalae*, by the basilar membrane and the Reissner's membrane (Figure 2–1). The fluid space between the Reissner's membrane and the upper bony wall of the cochlea is the *scala vestibuli*. The fluid space between the basilar membrane and the lower bony wall is the *scala tympani*. The space between the two membranes is called the *scala media* or the *cochlear duct*. Because it is bound on two sides by tissue membranes, the scala media is elastic, and it responds to pressure from either side by moving in the appropriate direction.

The *scala vestibuli* and the *scala tympani*, the two outer chambers, are filled with *perilymph*, which is a typical extracellular fluid rich in sodium and low in potassium. The scala media contains endolymph, which is a unique extracellular fluid low in sodium and high in potassium, the reverse of perilymph. The fluid-filled spaces of the inner ear are separated from the air spaces of the middle ear by

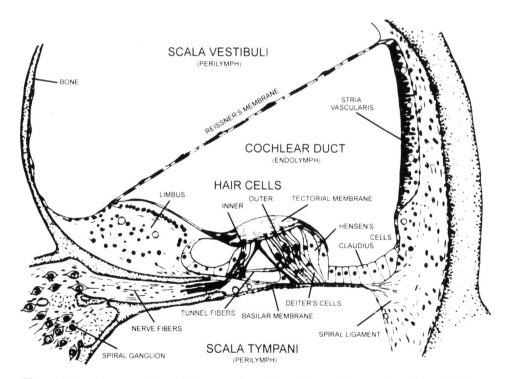

Figure 2–1.   A cross-section of the central portion of the cochlear cavity. (From H. Davis et al. [1953]. Acoustic trauma in the guinea pig. *Journal of the Acoustical Society of America*, 25, 1180. Used with permission.)

bone, except for two openings. The oval window, leading from the middle ear into the scala vestibuli, is occupied by the stapes footplate. The footplate is held in place by the flexible annular ligament, which seals the perilymph into the scala vestibuli and yet allows the stapes to move within the oval window. Therefore, any movement of the stapes is transferred through the oval window to the perilymph. The *round window* is the other opening between the cochlea and the middle ear that leads into the scala tympani on the opposite side of scala media from the oval window; it is covered by a thin, flexible membrane. When pressure is applied to the cochlear fluids through the oval window, it is transmitted through scala media to scala tympani, and the round window membrane compensates by bulging outward.

Cochlear Partition

The basilar membrane, which separates the scala media from the scala tympani, consists of connective tissue fibers embedded in an acellular matrix. Sitting on top of the basilar membrane are the structures directly responsible for sensory function in the cochlea. The structures include the sensory epithelium known as the *organ of Corti* and a gelatinous structure called *the tectorial membrane*. With the basilar membrane, the structures make up the *cochlear partition*. This composite structure is essential to cochlear function.

The cochlear partition maintains the same basic structure along the length of the cochlea. However, it changes in character as it progresses from the base of the cochlea to the apex in three ways vital to its function. First, the partition is approximately ten times wider at the base than at the apex. Second, it has more mass at the base than at the apex, owing mostly to increases in the number and size of supporting cells in the organ of Corti. Finally, the partition is stiffer at the base than at the apex, largely because of the structural properties of the basilar membrane; the change in stiffness is more than one hundredfold (von Bekesy, 1960).

Figure 2–2 shows a cross-section of the cochlear partition. The sensory cells of the organ of Corti are embedded in a matrix of supporting cells. The supporting cells, which make up the bulk of the organ, firmly anchor it and the embedded sensory cells to the basilar membrane: If the membrane moves, the sensory cells closely follow its motion. The sensory and supporting cells occur in rows that run along the length of the cochlea (Figure 2–3). The sensory cells are called *hair cells* because the top of each cell bears a cluster of *stereocilia* (sometimes described as hairs). The stereocilia occur in several rows of increasing length, and the ciliary bundles rise like a staircase above each hair cell. The stereocilia are connected to each other along the sides by fine filaments called *side links* (Pickles, Comis, & Osborne, 1994). The tip of each stereocilium is connected to the sides of the next tallest stereocilium by a longer filament known as a *tip link* (Pickles, Comis & Osborne). The tip is thought to be associated with ion channels in the hair-cell membrane.

There are two types of cochlear hair cells. A single row of flask-shaped inner hair cells are completely surrounded by supporting cells, except for the hair-bearing surface. Three rows of outer hair cells near the outer edge of the organ of Corti contact the supporting cells only at their very top and bottom. The bulk of the elongated, cylindrical body of the outer hair cell is suspended in the fluid spaces inside the organ of Corti; the spaces are filled with a fluid similar to perilymph. The

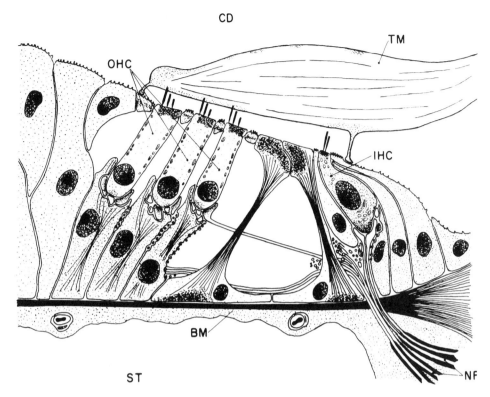

Figure 2–2. A cross-section of the cochlear partition. (From Ryan & Dallos [1996]. Used with permission.)

edges of the outer hair cells have a layer of membrane-bound compartments called *subsurface cisternea* just beneath the cell membrane (Figure 2–4). The subsurface cisternea are lined by mitochondria which suggests that they may consume energy. There are approximately 3,500 inner hair cells and 12,000 outer hair cells in the human cochlea.

Directly above the organ of Corti and separated by a narrow space is the *tectorial membrane*. The membrane is a cellular, gelatinous structure that is firmly attached at its inner edge to the cochlear wall. Otherwise, it is only loosely coupled to the organ of Corti by slender processes. The tallest stereocilia of the outer hair cells (but not of the inner hair cells) are embedded in its underside (Kimura, 1966) and facilitates the transmission of movement between the membrane and the outer hair cells. The fluid between the tectorial membrane and the hair-bearing surfaces of the hair cells is *endolymph* (Ryan, Wickham, & Bone, 1980).

Spiral Ganglion and Cochlear Innervation

The fibers of the auditory nerve enter the cochlea through the modiolus in the center of the cochlear spiral. They emerge from openings in the inner edge of the bony cochlear wall and enter the organ of Corti. Approximately 95% of these afferent fibers approach the nearest inner hair cell and form one-to-one connec-

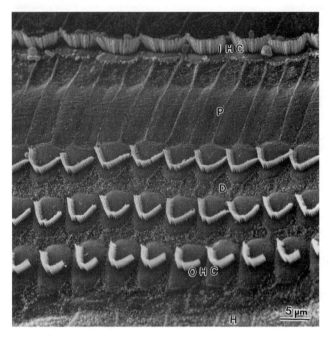

Figure 2–3. The organ of Corti as viewed from the cochlear duct, with the tectorial membrane removed, in a scanning electron micrograph. Note the sensory hairs of the single row of inner hair cells and of the three rows of outer hair cells. (From G. Bredberg, H. Ades, & H. Engstrom [1972] Scanning electron microscopy of the normal and pathologically altered organ of Corti. *Acta Oto-Laryngologica, 301* [Suppl.], 3. Used with permission.)

tions, about 20 per hair cell (Kiang, Rho, Northrop, Liberman, & Ryugo, 1982). The remaining 5% cross the organ, turn and travel down the cochlea toward the base for several hundred micrometers, and contact groups of outer hair cells. Each such fiber contacts from 20 to 50 sensory cells, and each outer hair cell may receive processes from up to 20 afferent fibers (Kiang, Rho, Northrop, Liberman, & Ryugo). Thus, the innervation patterns of the two types of hair cells are different, and most of the information transmitted to the brain originates from the inner hair cells, not the outer hair cells. The nerve fibers contact both types of hair cells at the bottom, farthest from the stereocilia. There the hair cell contains the presynaptic structures necessary to chemically transmit signals to the afferent nerve endings.

The cell bodies of auditory nerve cells lie just inside the bone of the modiolus from the organ of Corti, in the spiral ganglion. There are two types of eighth–cranial-nerve neurons in the ganglion, which correspond to the two kinds of afferent nerve fibers that independently innervate the two groups of hair cells (Kiang, Rho, Northrop, Liberman, & Ryugo). The larger and more numerous neurons innervate the inner hair cells and send large, myelinated axons to the cochlear nucleus in the brainstem. The smaller group, which innervates the outer hair cells, sends small unmyelinated axons to neurons around the periphery of the cochlear nucleus (Brown, Berglund, Kiang, & Ryungo, 1988).

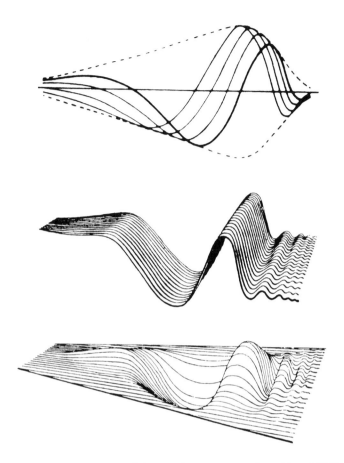

Figure 2–4.   Upper panel: Diagram of the traveling wave produced by a 200 Hz tone at four successive instants in time. The stimulus is a continuous sinusoid, i.e., a pure tone. For purposes of illustration, the cochlea has been "uncoiled" into a straight tube. The base lies on the left side of the figure. The amplitude of displacement of the partition has been greatly enlarged. The dotted lines represent the displacement envelope, within which all vibrations are confined for a given stimulus. The envelope rises slowly to a maximum and then falls rapidly thereafter. The waveforms illustrate the progression, or travel, of the wave from the base toward the apex. (From von Bekesy [1948]. Used with permission.) Lower panels: Because the edges of the basilar membrane are fixed, the traveling wave produces an alternating bulge in the center of the membrane. (From Tonndorf [1960]. Used with permission.)

A small number of the fibers in the eighth cranial nerve are efferent, i.e., they transmit impulses from the brain to the cochlea. The fibers arise from neurons whose cell bodies are located in the brain stem and mostly on the side opposite from the ear which they innervate. While there are only a few hundred efferent neurons, once the efferent fibers reach the cochlea, they branch out to form a large number of nerve endings. Two populations of efferents have been identified in the cochlea. Each population originates from different cell groups in the brain stem

(Warr & Guinan, 1979) and differs biochemically (Ryan, Schwartz, Helfert, Keithley, & Wang, 1987; Ryan, Schwartz, Keithley, & Wang, 1992). One group contacts the afferent fibers just beneath the inner hair cells (Warr & Guinan; Ryan, Schwartz, Helfert, Keithley, & Wang, 1992). The other group terminates directly on the outer hair cells (Warr & Guinan; Ryan, Schwartz, Keithley & Wang, 1992).

Stria Vascularis

The cochlea contains several tissues which participate indirectly in the transduction process by maintaining the normal ionic composition and the potentials of the cochlear fluids. These structures are located primarily on the outer wall of the cochlea. The stria vascularis, spiral prominence, and spiral ligament (Figure 2–1) consume large quantities of energy, even when the inner ear is at rest, in order to maintain homeostasis in the cochlea (Ryan, Goodwin, Woolf, & Sharp, 1992). The outer wall structures, especially, the stria vascularis are thought to be responsible for the secretion of endolymph, and for the generation of the endocochlear potential, a resting potential critical to the function of the inner ear (Offner, Dallos, & Cheatham, 1987).

Cochlear Mechanics

Traveling Wave

The cochlea is a complex hydromechanical system activated by the motion of the stapes footplate. Inward motion of the footplate produces an increase in pressure in the perilymph near the oval window. Outward motion results in lowered pressure. Because the bony cochlear capsule is inflexible, an outward or inward bulging of the round window membrane compensates for the pressure on the cochlea. However, to reach the round window, the pressure must be absorbed by and transmitted across the cochlear partition. Because the partition is flexible, it can be displaced in both directions and transfers the pressure change to the fluids in the region of the round window. The resulting energy exchange between the surrounding fluids and the moving partition initiates a characteristic wave pattern that progresses along the partition from the base to the apex. Because of its progression along the cochlea, the phenomenon is known as a *traveling wave*.

Because of the structural characteristics of the partition, the traveling wave does not maintain a uniform amplitude throughout the cochlea. From its origin at the base, it increases in amplitude while progressing toward the apex until it reaches a maximum, beyond which it declines rapidly. Moreover, the location along the cochlea at which the traveling wave reaches its largest amplitude changes with the frequency of the stimulating signal. High frequency stimuli generate the maximum wave amplitude at the base of the cochlea. For low frequencies, the maximum amplitude of displacement is toward the apex (von Bekesy, 1949).

Figure 2–4 illustrates some basic features of the traveling wave in the inner ear of human cadavers (von Bekesy, 1949). Positions of the cochlear partition are drawn for four successive instants.

The vibrations of all but the lowest audible frequencies do not travel the entire length of the cochlear partition. Instead, they die down before reaching the helicotrema. High-frequency stimuli are extinguished quite close to the base, whereas

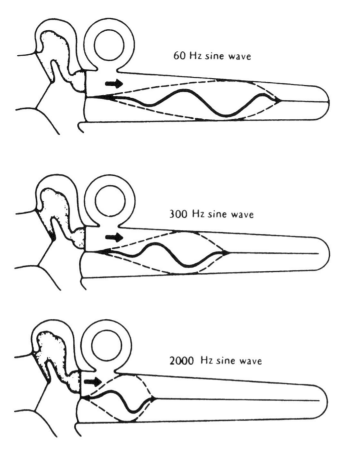

Figure 2–5. Diagram of traveling wave envelopes for three frequencies. Amplitude of displacement has been greatly exaggerated.

low-frequency stimuli are propagated further toward the apex (Figure 2–5). This difference in the behavior of the partition to different frequencies of stimulation is due to its peculiar structure. Because of the base-to-apex changes in width, mass, and, especially, stiffness, the ability of the partition to absorb energy from high-frequency changes in fluid pressure is diminished toward the apex. Thus, high-frequency energy excites only the basal region, whereas low-frequency energy is allowed to travel further along the cochlea (von Bekesy, 1949, 1960). The end result is that different frequencies of stimulation produce displacement envelope maxima at different locations along the cochlea. Different locations are thus tuned to different stimulus frequencies. The hydromechanical wave action of the cochlea maps the frequency of a given stimulus in the spatial extent and maximum amplitude of the traveling waves that the stimulus produces.

The traveling wave progresses from the base to the apex because of the differences in the physical characteristics of the basilar membrane, not because the oval window first stimulates the cochlear base. In fact, the traveling wave has an identical pattern if stimulation is provided artificially at the cochlear apex. Moreover, progression does not occur because energy is transmitted from one region of the basilar membrane to the adjacent region. An incision made entirely through the basilar membrane does not affect the nature of the traveling wave (von Bekesy, 1960).

Interaction Between the Organ of Corti and Tectorial Membrane

What happens to the cochlear hair cells when a particular region of the cochlear partition is set into motion? The effective stimulus to the cochlear hair cells is the displacement of their stereocilia from their resting position (Hudspeth & Corey, 1977; Russell, Richardson & Cody, 1986). For the outer hair cells, the displacement is thought to occur as follows: The hinge points about which the basilar and tectorial membranes rotate during the displacement of the cochlear partition are different (Figure 2–1). Also, the outer edge of the tectorial membrane is not firmly attached to the organ of Corti. The effect of this arrangement is shown schematically in Figure 2–6. Vertical displacement of the cochlear partition drags the tectorial membrane across the surface of the organ of Corti and produces a radial shearing force on the longest row of outer–hair-cell sensory hairs (Dallos, 1992) whose tips are embedded on the tectorial membrane (Kimura). Because the stereocilia are interconnected by side links (Pickles, Comis & Osborne), all the cilia on a hair cell bend with this shearing force.

The inner hair cells, which do appear not to be connected to the tectorial membrane, are probably stimulated by fluid streaming between the two membranes and through their stereociliary arrays. The fluid is set in motion by relative movement between the tectorial membrane and the organ of Corti (Dallos, 1992; Dallos, Billone, Durrant, Wang, & Raynor, 1972).

Cochlear Nonlinearities

While the traveling wave and links between the outer–hair-cell stereocilia provide an elegant mechanism for activation of the cochlear hair cells, there are reasons to conclude that they do not fully explain cochlear mechanics. One reason is the perception of combination tones, apparent tones which may be heard when two tones are presented simultaneously, even though they are not present in the acoustic signal. The perception of these tones at low stimulus intensities suggests the presence of significant nonlinearities, and can best be explained by an active process requiring energy (Ruggero, 1993). The traveling wave model proposed by von Bekesy (1949) would not produce these distortion products. None were observed in his cadaver experiments, and, therefore, combination tones were not believed to originate in the basilar membrane. More recent measurements of cochlear mechanics in living cochleas have shown distortion products to be present in the motion of the basilar membrane (Rhode; Ruggero & Rich, 1991) . Such data strongly suggested the existence of some active process which affects the motion of the cochlear partition.

Cochlear Electrical Environment

Displacement of the stereocilia produces responses in hair cells that cause transmitter release from the presynaptic area at their bases (a process known as *transduc-*

Inhibition

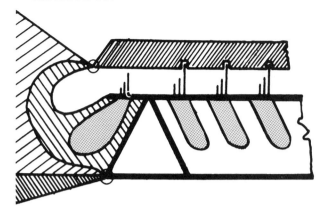

Excitation

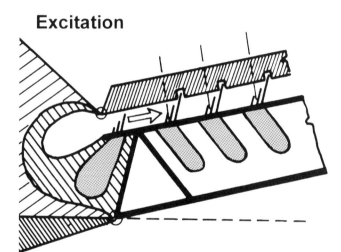

Figure 2–6. Probable pattern of shearing action between the tectorial membrane and the organ of Corti. The hairs of the inner hair cells, which are not attached to the tectorial membrane, are thought to be displaced by fluid movement. *Bottom*: Organ at rest. *Top*: During displacement toward scala vestibuli. (From Ryan & Dallos [1996]. Used with permission.)

tion.) The transmitter, in turn, generates nerve impulses in the afferent fibers of the auditory nerve. The cell membrane and intracellular responses that are the intermediate steps between stereociliary movement and transmitter release are not well understood; however, it is thought that both electrical and mechanical events are involved. To understand the available evidence regarding the nature of the hair-cell transduction process, it is first necessary to understand the electrical environment of the cochlea.

Endocochlear and Intracellular Resting Potentials

An electrode placed in the endolymph of the cochlear duct registers a constant positive potential, i.e., a voltage difference, from the rest of the body of approximately 80 mV (Offner, Dallos, & Cheatham). The resting voltage is called the *endocochlear potential*, and is thought to be maintained by a combination of active ionic pumps and selectively permeable ion channels in the cells of the stria vascularis (Marcus, Takeuchi, & Wangemann, 1992; Ryan & Watts, 1991). The pumps and channels are also responsible for the high potassium and low sodium contents of endolymph, which is a composition found in no other extracellular fluid in the body.

Microelectrodes penetrating the organ of Corti record negative resting potentials from the inside of individual cells (both supporting cells and hair cells). Outer hair cells have resting potentials of approximately −70 mV (Dallos, Santos-Sacchi, & Floc, 1982), whereas those of inner hair cells are approximately −40 mV (Russell & Sellick, 1977). This means that between the inside of the hair cell and above the upper surface of the endolymph is a potential difference (or a gradient) of 120 to 150 mV, which is an extremely high gradient for a biological system. It is likely that the potential difference initiates a continuous flow of positively charged potassium ions from the endolymph into the hair cells through ion channels on the upper surfaces of the cells. The ions move from the hair cells into the low potassium fluid that fills the spaces within the organ of Corti through potassium-selective channels in the cells' membranes.

Cochlear Evoked Potentials

COCHLEAR MICROPHONIC AND SUMMATING POTENTIAL

When the cochlea is stimulated, the resting balance of electrical potentials described is disturbed. To examine these events, electrodes are placed on either side of the scala media (one in the scala tympani and one in the scala vestibuli) and the electrical activity in the region of the cochlear partition near the electrodes is observed. Two principal responses to stimulation that can be recorded from the cochlea—the *cochlear microphonic* and the *summating potential* are shown in Figure 2–7. The cochlear microphonic and the summating potential recorded from a particular cochlear location vary with changes in stimulus frequency. Both potentials reach a maximum at a particular "best" frequency that corresponds to the displacement peak of the traveling wave envelope at that point in the cochlea (Figure 2–8). Below the best frequency the potentials decline slowly, whereas above the best frequency they exhibit a rapid decrease in amplitude.

The cochlear microphonic and the summating potential are produced primarily by the outer hair cells. If these cells are destroyed while the inner hair cells remain intact, the amplitude of the microphonic is reduced by about 40 dB (Dallos & Wang, 1974), and its character is altered in a manner consistent with the proposed stimulation of the inner hair cell by fluid movement rather than by actual partition displacement (Dallos, Billone, Durrant, Wang & Raynor).

INTRACELLULAR POTENTIALS OF HAIR CELLS

The cochlear microphonic and summating potential reflect the summed activity of a large number of sensory cells. If the responses of individual cells are recorded

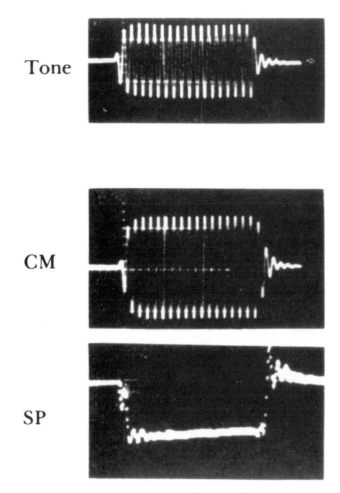

Figure 2–7.   The cochlear microphonic and summating potential response to a pure-tone stimulus. The top of the figure shows a short tone burst applied to the eardrum. The lower panels show responses recorded from the cochlea. Two features of the responses are apparent. First, the frequency of the stimulus is reproduced by the cochlea as a pattern of voltage fluctuation, like a microphone. For this reason, the electrical reproduction of the signal is known as the cochlear microphonic. Second, a sizable shift in the baseline voltage occurs. The shift is called the summating potential. The two potentials are recorded simultaneously, as a mixture. They have been electrically separated in the figure for illustration purposes. (From Ryan & Dallos [1996]. Used with permission.)

with fine microelectrodes inserted inside the cells (Dallos, 1985; Dallos, Santos-Sacchi & Flock; Russell & Sellick), both types of hair cells respond to sound with a fluctuation of the intracellular potential reminiscent of the cochlear microphonic and with a large decrease in the negative resting potential similar to the summating potential. However, the intracellular potentials recorded from individual hair cells are different from the cochlear microphonic and summating potential, because the latter reflect the combined activity of many hair cells. The evoked changes in the

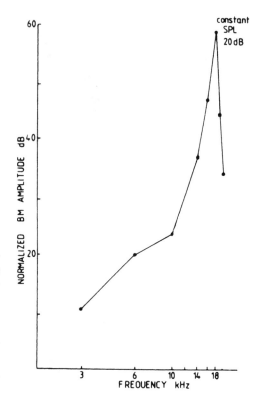

Figure 2–8. Basilar membrane displacement produced at various frequencies of stimulation at a cochlear location close to the base. (Adapted from P. Dallos, M. A. Cheatham, & J. Ferraro [1973]. Cochlear mechanics, nonlinearities and cochlear potentials. *Journal of the Acoustical Society of America, 55,* 597. Used with permission.)

intracellular potential occur for a more limited range of frequencies and peak in a narrow band of frequencies corresponding to those which produce the maximum amplitude of basilar membrane motion at that cochlear location. The individual inner and outer hair cells are sharply tuned to a specific best frequency (Dallos, Santos-Sacchi, & Flock; Russell & Sellick). A tuning curve recorded from an inner hair cell is shown in Figure 2–9. The tuning of the inner hair cells and their associated afferent nerve fibers is much sharper than that of the basilar membrane measured by von Bekesy (Figure 2–4). The outer hair cells are just as sharply tuned.

Micromechanics and Active Processes

Hair-Cell Transduction Channel

The initial process in hair-cell transduction is the deflection of the stereociliary bundle. This deflection opens mechanically gated channels on the upper surface of the hair cell. Microelectrode recordings from different locations on the surface of hair cells suggest that these channels are located near the tips of the sterocilia (Hudspeth, 1982). Opening of the channels increases the influx of potassium ions along the steep electrochemical gradient from the endolymph into the hair cell. How the mechanically gated channels are opened is not known. The most widely accepted theory is that tension on the tip links opens the channels (Pickles, Comis, & Osborne) (Figure 2–10).

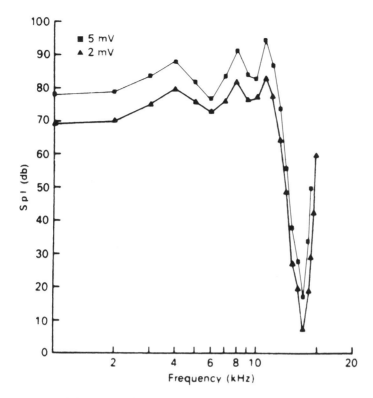

Figure 2–9. Intracellularly recorded thresholds of a cochlear inner hair cell to stimulation with pure tones at various frequencies. Note the narrowly tuned region of greatest sensitivity of the cell. (From Dallos, Evans, & Hallworth, 1991. Used with permission.)

The influx of potassium alters the intracellular potential of the hair cell and is directly recorded with intracellular electrodes or indirectly recorded as the cochlear microphonic and summating potential. It is unlikely that the extracellular potentials play any role in the transduction process. However, the intracellular potentials may cause the release of a chemical transmitter from the presynaptic zone at the lower end of the hair cell. The transmitter, in turn, stimulates the afferent ending of the auditory nerve fibers. This explanation is appealing since the mechanoreceptors on the stereocilia of the hair cell are separated from the presynaptic zone by a relatively great distance. The intracellular potentials provide a link between the two locations. This idea also corresponds to current neurophysiological theory, because it is thought that the release of transmitter chemicals in nerve cells is caused by a change in voltage in the presynaptic area.

Cochlear Amplifier and Outer–Hair-Cell Motility

COCHLEAR AMPLIFIER

The original measurements of basilar membrane motion made by von Bekesy using cadaver cochleas (Figure 2–4) are much less sharply tuned than the re-

Inhibition

Excitation

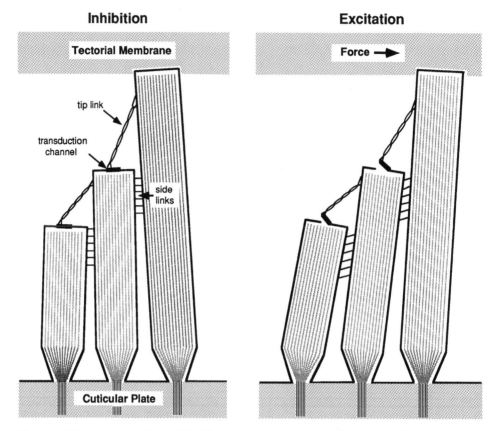

Figure 2–10. A proposed model of the mechanical receptor of the hair cell. Movement of the hair cell stereocilia in the appropriate direction puts tension on the tip links connecting adjacent stereocilia. This opens a channel, allowing ions to enter the cell and alter its electrical potential. Movement in the opposite direction closes the channel. (Adapted from J. A. Assad, & D. P. Corey [1992]. An active motor model for adaptation by vertebrate hair cells. *Journal of Neuroscience, 12,* 3291–3309. Used with permission.)

sponses of hair cells and auditory nerve fibers (Figure 2–9 & Figure 2–14). The observation and the presence of significant nonlinearities in the motion of the basilar membrane have lead to the suggestion that a *cochlear amplifier* (Davis) an active process requiring energy and located between the basilar membrane and the auditory nerve fiber, produces this additional sharpening. Recent observations of basilar membrane motion in the living cochlea (Rhode; Ruggero & Rich) revealed that the membrane is tuned just as sharply as hair cells and auditory nerve fibers (Figure 2–8). Therefore, the cochlear amplifier must be located in the basilar membrane complex itself. Because it is present only in life, it must require energy to function. Evidence from several sources indicates that the active process resides in the outer hair cells.

Approximately 95% of the afferent fibers of the auditory nerve originate on inner hair cells, whereas the extracellular cochlear microphonics and summating potentials are largely produced by the outer hair cells. The large extracellular response of

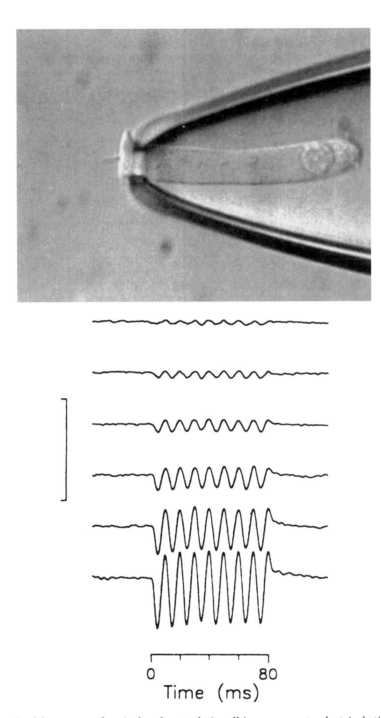

Figure 2-11. Movement of an isolated outer hair cell in response to electrical stimulation. Top panel: The hair cell is held fully inserted into a glass micro pipette. Lower panel: A sinusoidal voltage applied across the cell membrane causes length changes in the cell. The scale bar represents 400 nonometers. (Adapted from Evans et al. [1991]. Used by permission.)

the outer hair cells seems out of proportion to the 5% contribution of their afferent neurons to the auditory nerve and suggests that they have another role. In addition, selective destruction of the outer hair cells using aminoglycoside antibiotics or noise results in a loss of threshold sensitivity in the cochlea of about 40 dB (Ryan & Dallos) and a dramatic loss of tuning in eighth–cranial-nerve fibers (Harrison & Evans).

FAST OUTER–HAIR-CELL ELECTROMOTILITY

Even more powerful evidence was provided by the discovery that outer hair cells can move when they are electrically stimulated: They shorten when depolarized and lengthen when hyperpolarized (Brownell, 1983) (Figure 2–11). The electromotility is extremely fast and occurs at frequencies up to the limit of human hearing (Reuter, Gitter, Thurm, & Zenner, 1992). Studies of isolated hair cells have demonstrated that the electromotility is elicited by changes in voltage across the outer–hair-cell membrane (Santos-Sacchi, 1991) and appears to be produced by numerous molecular "motors" along the length of the cell (Dallos, Evans, & Hallworth, 1991). The preservation of electromotility, even when intracellular proteins are digested with proteolytic enzymes, indicates that the molecules are embedded in the cell membrane of the outer hair cell (Kalinic, Holley, Iwasa, Lim, & Cachar, 1992).

Observations on isolated hair cells have also shed light on the origin of nonlinearities in the responses of the cochlea. Nonlinearities have been observed in the

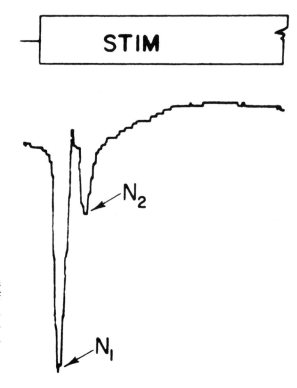

Figure 2–12. Compound action potential response at the onset of a pure-tone stimulus of 8000 Hz. (From P. Dallos [1973]. *The auditory periphery: Biophysics and physiology.* New York: Academic Press. Used with permission.)

electromotility of individual outer hair cells (Evans, 1990; Evans, Hallworth & Dallos, 1991; Santos-Sacchi, 1993). These nonlinearities appear to originate in the electromotile response itself and nonlinearities inherent in the transducer channel, which provides the voltage changes that drive motility (Santos-Sacchi, 1993).

SLOW MOTILITY AND OUTER–HAIR-CELL EFFERENT INNERVATION

Stimulation of the hair cells can also cause a second form of electromotility, gradual changes in length that occur over the course of seconds (Ohnishi, Hara, Inoue, et al., 1992). Similar "slow" motility can be elicited by pharmacological agents including acetylcholine, the neurotransmitter released by the efferent nerve endings terminating on the outer hair cells (Zenner, Reuter, Plinkert, Zimmerman & Gitter (1989), suggesting that activation of the efferents at the bases of the outer hair cells produces this response. Slow motility may not be produced by the same molecular mechanisms that produce fast motility. Several mechanisms have been proposed, including the interaction of actin and myosin (Zenner, 1988), osmotic changes within the cell (Dieler, Shehata-Dieler & Brownell, 1991) or changes in the subsurface cisternea (Dieler, Shehata-Dieler & Brownell, 1991).

THE ROLE OF OHC MOTILITY IN THE ORGAN OF CORTI

The discovery of active outer–hair-cell responses has revolutionized our understanding of cochlear mechanics and the transduction process. In the outer hair cells the receptor potentials, in addition to or even instead of causing transmitter release as in the inner hair cells, are thought to be responsible for driving the voltage-dependent motility motors (Iwasa & Kachar, 1989); Santos-Sacchi & Dilger (1988). How the mechanical responses of individual outer hair cells interact with the motion of the cochlear partition is not yet clear. However, the outer hair cells are interconnected by the cytoarchitecture of the organ of Corti (Figure 2–2), and thus if many cells move in synchrony their mechanical responses can sum. Since the tallest stereocilia are embedded in the tectorial membrane, they can influence the motion of that structure as well. Measurements of the force generated by individual outer hair cells indicate that the activation of large numbers of cells in concert should be able to change the mechanical responses of the cochlear partition (Iwasa & Chadwick, 1992). One result of this is thought to be amplification of basilar membrane motion in a narrow frequency range. That is, the outer hair cells are thought to be the cochlear amplifier. This interpretation is consistent with the loss of threshold sensitivity and tuning that is observed in the cochlea after outer–hair-cell loss (Dallos & Wang, 1974; Harrison & Evans, 1979; Ryan & Dallos, 1975).

The implication is that outer hair cells by themselves can induce basilar membrane motion, which has important implications for the origin and significance of otoacoustic emissions. In fact, using an isolated cochlear preparation, it has recently been shown that electrical stimulation of large numbers of outer hair cells can induce detectable motion in the basilar membrane (Mammo & Ashmore, 1993).

INTERACTIONS BETWEEN INNER AND OUTER HAIR CELLS

If the outer hair cells are the cochlear amplifier, the question remains as to how these cells interact with the inner hair cells to amplify their responses given that they are separate, both spatially and in their innervation, from the inner hair cells.

Two primary modes of interaction have been proposed: electrical and mechanical. Because the outer hair cells produce large extracellular potentials, several researchers have suggested that the potentials influence the inner hair cell (Harris, 1979; Ryan & Dallos, 1975) before intracellular recordings were obtained from hair cells. However, once intracellular recordings were made and the membrane properties of the hair cells had been directly measured (Dallos, Santos-Sacchi, & Flock, 1982; Russel & Sellick, 1977), it became clear that membrane resistance of the cells was too great for the extracellular potentials to have the necessary influence upon the inner hair cells (Dallos, 1983).

This line of reasoning suggests that the outer hair cells mechanically influence inner–hair-cell responses. Outer–hair-cell motility, by increasing the motion of the cochlear partition and perhaps by changing the motion of the tectorial membrane, must enhance the signal to the inner hair cells. The mechanism of amplification is not known; however, the influence must be frequency-specific, because the amplification appears to be produced almost exclusively in a narrow frequency region and results in the sharply-tuned "tip" of hair cell and the eighth–cranial-nerve fiber–tuning curves. There is evidence that outer–hair-cell responses to mechanical stimulation are tuned (Brundin, Flock, & Canlon, 1989), but this occurs only when mechanical stimulation is applied to the hair-cell body, not to the stereocilia (Evans & Dallos, 1993). Moreover, electrical stimulation, which is presumably the natural mode by which motility is elicited, does not appear to produce tuned mechanical responses (Brownell, 1983).

Neuronal Responses

Hair-Cell Synapses

The final stage of transduction is the release of a chemical transmitter from the hair-cell base, which stimulates the afferent endings of the fibers of the auditory nerve. Small vesicles that presumably contain transmitter have been identified in the hair cells. The transmitter substance released by hair cells to activate eighth–cranial-nerve fibers is not yet known with certainty. There is considerable evidence that glutamate, which operates as an excitatory neurotransmitter in other sensory systems, is the hair-cell transmitter. For example, glutamate receptors have been shown to be produced at high levels in the neurons of the spiral ganglion that contact the inner hair cells (Ryan, Brumm & Kraft 1991; Kuriyama, Albin, & Altschuler, 1993).

The efferent synapses at the bases of the outer hair cells have been shown to contain the neurotransmitter acetylcholine. Other transmitters have also been detected in these efferents, which may function as modulators of acetylcholine. The transmitter used by the synapses on the afferent neurons beneath the inner hair cells is also thought to be acetylcholine in association with other neuroactive substances.

Single Fiber Responses of Cochlear Afferent and Efferent Neurons

The end products of the transduction process are transmitted to the brain stem as discharge patterns in the fibers of the auditory nerve. The activity in the 30,000 auditory afferent fibers is normally examined in one of two ways.

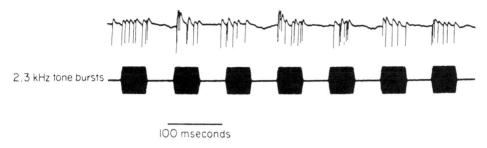

2.3 kHz tone bursts

100 mseconds

Figure 2–13. Discharges of a single eighth–cranial-nerve fiber in response to repetitive tone bursts. (From Dallos [1983]. Used with permission.)

First, if a relatively large electrode is placed near the cochlear (the round window is a common recording site) and a brief stimulus, such as a click or the leading edge of a tone burst is applied repeatedly to the ear, an electrical response known as *the compound action potential* is observed (Figure 2–13). It is produced by the synchronous discharge of hundreds of neurons. The compound action potential corresponds roughly to wave I of the auditory-brainstem evoked response, is the basis for electrocochleography, and can serve as a useful index of auditory nerve and cochlear function. Through the use of masking, it can also provide information regarding how small groups of single fibers carry information to the brain stem (Harris, 1979).

Second, if a fine microelectrode is inserted into the nerve, the responses of single fibers can be recorded. Auditory nerve fibers are often found to be spontaneously active, discharging even in the absence of sound stimulation to the ear. Because the amplitude of nerve impulses cannot change, the fiber can convey information only by varying the rate, the timing, or both of its impulses. An example of a single-fiber response to tone stimulation is shown in Figure 2–13.

Each fiber responds to a limited range of stimulus frequencies that includes the best frequency, which is the frequency to which the fiber is most sensitive. The frequency selectivity can be demonstrated graphically by charting the intensity necessary to produce a response from a single fiber at various frequencies. Several tuning curves are illustrated in Figure 2–14. Their similarity to the frequency selectivity of hair cells can be seen by comparison with Figure 2–9.

As expected, the best frequency of a fiber is determined by its point of origin along the cochlea: high-frequency fibers are at the base, and low-frequency fibers are at the apex. The spatial separation of achieved in the inner ear is preserved in the auditory nerve and passed on to the auditory centers in the brain. High-frequency fibers are found on the outside of the nerve. Progressively lower-frequency fibers occur toward the center (Kiang, Watanabe, Thomas, & Clark, 1965). Therefore, information about the frequency content of an acoustic signal is transmitted to the brain by the particular nerve fibers that are activated.

Frequency information can also be encoded by auditory nerve fibers in a different manner. At relatively low frequencies, a fiber can discharge in synchrony with the stimulus. For example, it might produce an impulse for every cycle of a sinusoidal stimulus, or perhaps an impulse every few cycles, but always in phase

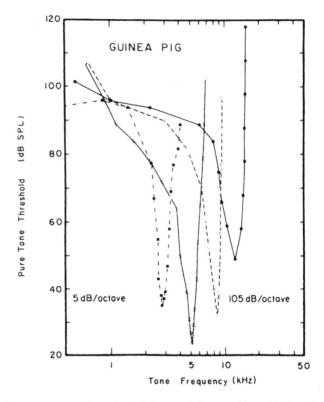

Figure 2–14. Tuning curves of single eighth–cranial-nerve fibers. Each point represents the lowest intensity that would produce a response from the fiber at that frequency. Note the similarity to the inner hair cell potential function of Figure 11. (From E. F. Evans [1970]. Narrow tuning of cochlear nerve fibre responses in the guinea pig. *Journal of Physiology*, *206*, 14. Used with permission.)

(in the same region of the waveform). Because auditory nerve fibers rarely discharge at rates of more than 200 discharges per second, frequency information could be carried in this manner by a single fiber only at frequencies up to 200 Hz. By sampling the rates of several fibers that discharge on different cycles, the brain is able to process the information at higher frequencies. However, it is generally agreed that the stimulus-locked discharge does not occur at frequencies greater than 3000 or 4000 Hz (Kiang, Watanabe, Thomas, & Clark, 1965). Synchronized discharges are elicited by the cycle-by-cycle potentials, known as the *ac potentials*, of the inner hair cells. In contrast, the dc-receptor potential is responsible for eliciting responses that are not synchronized to the cycles of stimulus, in the manner seen at high frequencies.

The intensity of auditory stimuli is also encoded by the responses of eighth–cranial-nerve fibers by increases in the discharge rate of individual fibers and by increases in the number of discharging fibers (Kiang, Watanabe, Thomas, & Clark, 1965).

Although it is clear that there are two categories of afferent nerve fibers in the auditory nerve, it has as yet proven impossible to record the responses of the spiral ganglion neurons associated with the outer hair cells (Brown, Berglund, Kiang, & Ryungo (1988). This may reflect the difficulty of recording from fine nerve fibers. However, it is also possible that these neurons do not respond to sound. The outer hair cells may function exclusively as modifiers of cochlear micromechanics, rather than as receptor cells, and their afferent innervation may be vestigial. Alternatively, their afferent innervation may carry information about the mechanical state of the cochlear duct, rather than responses to sound.

The physiological responses of the efferents which innervate the outer hair cells have been studied (Brown, 1989; Liberman & Brown, 1986). They may respond to stimulation of the cochlea which they innervate, the opposite ear, or both. They have higher thresholds than the afferents, but are similarly tuned. They innervate regions of the cochlea that transduce their best frequencies. Few efferents show spontaneous discharge. The responses of the efferents that innervate the afferent fibers beneath the inner hair cells have not been studied, because the fibers are small and unmyelinated.

Summary and Conclusions

Great strides have recently been made in the understanding several aspects of function in the cochlea. The location and possible mode of action of the mechano-receptors of the hair cells have been established. An active cochlear amplifier has been tentatively identified in the outer hair cell, and a likely candidate for the hair-cell neurotransmitter has been identified.

However, there are many questions about cochlear physiology that remain unanswered: What is the molecular nature of the cellular motor which produces outer–hair-cell motility? How is the frequency selectivity of the cochlear amplifier achieved? How does the active process of the outer hair cell fit into the motion of the cochlear partition. How do outer hair cells interact mechanically with inner hair cells? What functions are served by the efferent and afferent innervation of the outer hair cell?

Many auditory scientists (Brownell, 1990) believe that the outer hair cells are the source of otoacoustic emissions. Additional evidence has come from the observation of spontaneous vibrations in the outer hair-cell region of isolated cochlear preparations (Keilsen, Khanna, Ulfendahl, & Teich, 1992) and the demonstration of changes in otoacoustic emissions caused by stimulation of the efferent neurons leading the outer hair cells (Mott, Norton, Neely, & Warr, 1989). Therefore, otoacoustic emissions provide a window on the amplifier which provides the exquisite sensitivity and frequency resolution of the outer cochlea.

References

Brown, M. C. (1989). Morphology and response properties of single olivocochlear fibers in the guinea pig. *Hearing Research, 40,* 93–110.

Brown, M. C., Berglund, A. M., Kiang, N. Y.-S. & Ryungo, D. K. (1988). Central trajectories of type II spiral ganglion neurons. *Journal of Comparative Neurology, 278,* 581–590.

Brownell, W. E. (1983). Observations on a motile response in isolated outer hair cells. In W. Webster and L. Aitkin (eds.), *Mechanisms of hearing* (pp. 5–10). Clayton, Australia: Monash University Press.

Brownell, W. E. (1990). Outer hair cell electromotility and otoacoustic emissions. *Ear and Hearing, 11,* 82–92.

Brundin, L,. Flock, A., & Canlon, B. (1989). Sound-induced motility of isolated cochlear hair cells is frequency-specific. *Nature, 342,* 814–816.

Dallos, P. (1992). The active cochlea. *Journal of Neuroscience, 12,* 4575–4585.

Dallos, P. (1983). Some electrical circuit properties of the organ of Corti: I. Analysis without reactive elements. *Hearing Research, 12,* 89–119.

Dallos, P. (1985). Response characteristics of mammalian cochlear hair cells. *Journal of Neuroscience, 5,* 1591–1608.

Dallos, P., Billone, M. C., Durrant, J.D., Wang, C-Y., & Raynor, S. (1972). Cochlear inner and outer hair cells: Functional differences. *Science, 177,* 356–358.

Dallos, P., Evans, B. N. & Hallworth, R. (1991). Nature of the motor element in electrokinetic shape changes of cochlear outer hair cells. *Nature, 350,* 155–157.

Dallos, P., Santos-Sacchi, J., & Flock, A. (1982). Intracellular recordings from cochlear outer hair cells. *Science, 218,* 582–584.

Dallos, P., & Wang, C-Y. (1974). Bioelectric correlates of kanamycin intoxication. *Audiology, 13,* 277–289.

Davis, H. (1983). An active process in cochlear mechanics. *Hearing Research, 9,* 79–90.

Dieler, R., Shehata-Dieler, W. E., & Brownell, W. E. (1991). Concomitant salicyalte-induced alterations of outer hair cell subsurface cisternea and electromotility. *Journal of Neurocytology, 20,* 637–653.

Engstrom, H. (1960). Cortilymph: The third lymph of the inner ear. *Acta Morphologica Neerlando-Scandinavia, 3,* 192–204.

Evans, B. N. (1990). Fatal contractions: Ultrastructural and electromechanical changes in outer hair cells following transmembranous electrical stimulation. *Hearing Research, 45,* 265–282.

Evans, B. N., & Dallos, P. (1993). Stereocilia displacement induced somatic motility of cochlear outer hair cells. *Proceedings of the National Academy of Sciences, 90,* 8347–8351.

Evans, B. N., Hallworth, R., & Dallos, P. (1991). Outer hair cell electromotility: The sensitivity and vulnerability of the DC component. *Hearing Research, 52,* 288–304.

Geisler, C. D. (1974). Model of crossed olivocochlear effects. *Journal of the Acoustical Society of America, 56,* 1910–1912.

Goldstein, J. L. (1967). Auditory nonlinearity. *Journal of the Acoustical Society of America, 41,* 676–689.

Harris, D. (1979). Action potential suppression, tuning curves and thresholds: Comparison with single fiber data. *Hearing Research, 1,* 133–141.

Harrison R. V., & Evans, E. F. (1979). Cochlear fibre responses in guinea pigs with well defined cochlear lesions. *Scandinavian Audiology,* (Suppl.) 83–92.

Hudspeth, A. J. (1982). Extracellular current flow and the site of transduction by vertebrate hair cells. *Journal of Neuroscience, 2,* 1–10.

Hudspeth, A. J., & Corey, D. P. (1977). Sensitivity, polarity, and conductance change in the response of vertebrate hair cells to controlled mechanical stimuli. *Proceedings of the National Academy of Sciences, 74,* 2407–2411.

Iwasa, K. H., & Chadwick, R. S. (1992). Elasticity and force generation of cochlear outer hair cells. *Journal of the Acoustical Society of America, 92,* 3169–3173.

Iwasa, K. H., & Kachar, B. (1989). Fast in vitro movement of outer hair cells in an external electrical field: Effect of digitonin, a membrane permeabilizing agent. *Hearing Research, 40,* 246–254.

Kalinic, F., Holley, M., Iwasa, K. H., Lim, D. J., & Kachar, B. (1992). Force generation mechanism in the plasma membrane of auditory sensory cells. *Proceedings of the National Academy of Sciences, 89,* 8671–8675.

Keilsen, S. E., Khanna, S. M., Ulfendahl, M., & Teich, M. C. (1992). Spontaneous cellular vibrations in the guinea pig cochlea. *Acta Oto-Laryngologica, 113,* 591–597.

Kemp, D. T. (1978). Stimulated acoustic emissions from within the human auditory system. *Journal of the Acoustical Society of America, 64,* 1386–1391.

Kiang NY-S., Rho, J. M., Northrop, C. C., Liberman, M. C., & Ryugo, D. K. (1982) Hair cell innervation by spiral ganglion cells in adult cats. *Science, 217,* 175–177.

Kiang NY-S., Watanabe, T., Thomas, E. C., & Clark, L. F. (1965). *Discharge patterns of single fibers in the cat's auditory nerve.* Cambridge, MA: M.I.T. Press.

Kimura, R. S. (1966). Hairs of the cochlear sensory cells and their attachment to the tectorial membrane. *Acta Oto-Laryngologica, 61,* 55–72.

Kuriyama, H., Albin, R. L., & Altschuler, R. A. (1993). Expression of NMDA-receptor mRNA in the rat cochlea. *Hearing Research, 69,* 215–220.

Liberman, M. C., & Brown, M. C. (1986). Physiology and anatomy of single olivocochlear neurons in the cat. *Hearing Research, 24,* 17–36.

Lynn P. A., & Sayers, B. M. (1970). Cochlear innervation, signal processing and their relation to auditory time-intensity effects. *Journal of the Acoustical Society of America, 47,* 525–532.

Mammano, F., & Ashmore, J. F. (1993). Reverse transduction measured in the isolated cochlea by laser Michaelson interferometry. *Nature, 365,* 838–841.

Marcus, D. C., Takeuchi, S., & Wangemann, P. (1992). Ca^{2+}-activated nonselective cation channel in apical membrane of vestibular dark cells. *American Journal of Physiology, 262,* 1423–1429.

Mott, J. B., Norton, S. J., Neely, S. T., & Warr, W.B. (1989). Changes in spontaneous otoacosutic emissions produced by acoustic stimulation of the contralateral ear. *Hearing Research, 38,* 229–242.

Offner, D.L., Dallos, P., & Cheatham, M. A. (1987). Positive endocochlear potential: Mechanism of production by marginal cells of the stria vascularis. *Hearing Research, 29,* 117–124.

Ohnishi, S., Hara, M., Inoue, M., Yamashita, T., Kumazawa, T., Minato, A., & Inagaki, C. (1992). Delayed shortening and shrinkage of cochlear outer hair cells. *American Journal of Physiology, 263,* 1088–1095.

Pickles, J. O., Comis, S. D., & Osborne, M. P. (1984). Cross-links between stereocilia in the guinea pig organ of Corti and their possible relation to mechanical transduction. *Hearing Research, 15,* 103–112.

Reuter, G., Gitter, A. H., Thurm, U., & Zenner, H. P. (1992). High frequency radial movements of the reticular lamina induced by outer hair cell motility. *Hearing Research, 60,* 236–246.

Rhode, W. W. (1971). Observations of the vibrations of the basilar membrane in squirrel monkeys using the Mossbauer technique. *Journal of the Acoustical Society of America, 49,* 1218–1231.

Ruggero, M. A. (1993). Distortion in those good vibrations. *Current Biology, 3,* 755–758.

Ruggero, M. A., & Rich, N.C. (1991). Application of a commercially manufactured Doppler shift laser velocimeter to the measurement of basilar membrane vibration. *Hearing Research, 51,* 215–230.

Russell, I. J., Richardson, G. P., & Cody, A. R. (1986). Mechanosensitivity of mammalian auditory hair cells in vitro. *Nature, 321,* 517–519.

Russell, I. J., & Sellick, P. M. (1977). Intracellular studies of hair cells in the mammalian cochlea. *Journal of Physiology, 284,* 261–290.

Ryan, A. F., Brumm, D., & Kraft, M. (1991). Occurence and distribution of non-NMDA glutamate receptor mRNAs in the cochlea. *Neuro Report, 2,* 543–646.

Ryan, A. F., & Dallos, P. (1975). Absence of cochlear outer hair cells: Effect on behavioural auditory thresholds. *Nature, 253,* 44–46.

Ryan, A. F., and Dallos, P. (1996). The physiology of the cochlea. In J. Northern (Ed.), *Hearing disorders* (3rd ed., pp. 15–31). Boston: Allyn and Bacon.

Ryan, A. F., Goodwin P., Woolf N. K., & Sharp, F. (1982).Auditory stimulation alters the pattern of 2-deoxyglucose uptake in the inner ear. *Brain Research, 234,* 213–225.

Ryan, A. F., Schwartz, I. R., Helfert, R. H, Keithley, E., & Wang, Z. X. (1987). Selective retrograde labeling of lateral olivocochlear neurons in brainstem based on preferential uptake of 3H-D-aspartic acid in the cochlea. *Journal of Comparative Neurology, 255,* 606–616.

Ryan, A. F., Schwartz, I. R., Keithley, E. M., & Wang, Z.X. (1992).Selective retrograde transport of nipecotic acid identifies the cells of origin of endings which preferentially accumulate GABA. *Journal of Comparative Neurology, 326,* 337–346.

Ryan, A. F., & Watts, A. G. (1991). Expression of genes coding for α and β isoforms of Na/K-ATPase in the cochlea of the rat. *Cellular and Molecular Neuroscience, 2,* 179–187.

Ryan, A. F., Wickham, M. G., & Bone, R. C. (1980). Studies of ion distribution in the inner ear: Scanning electron microscopy and x-ray microanalysis of freeze-dried cochlear specimens. *Hearing Research, 2,* 1–20.

Santos-Sacchi, J. (1991). Reversible inhibition of voltage-dependent outer hair cell motility and capacitance. *Journal of Neuroscience, 11,* 3096–3110.

Santos-Sacchi, J. (1993). Harmonics of outer hair cell motility. *Biophysics Journal, 65,* 2217–2227.

Santos-Sacchi, J., & Dilger, J. P. (1988). Whole cell currents and mechanical responses of isolated outer hair cells. *Hearing Research, 35,* 143–150.

Smith, C. A. (1975). The inner ear: Its embryological development and microstructure. In D. B. Tower (Ed.), *The nervous system: Vol. 3. Human communication and its disorders.* (pp. 1–18). New York: Raven Press.

Tonndorf, J. (1960). Shearing motion in scala media of cochlear models. *Journal of the Acoustical Society of America, 32,* 238–244.

von Bekesy, G. (1949). The vibration of the cochlear partition in anatomical preparation and in models of the inner ear. *Journal of the Acoustical Society of America, 21,* 233–245.

von Bekesy, G. (1960). *Experiments in hearing* (E. G. Wever, trans. & ed.). New York: McGraw-Hill.

Warr, W. B., & Guinan, J. J. (1979). Efferent innervation of the organ of Corti: Two separate systems. *Brain Research, 173,* 152–155.

Zenner, H. P. (1988). Motility of outer hair cells as an active, actin-mediated process. *Acta Oto-Laryngologica, 105,* 39–44.

Zenner, H. P., Gitter, A. H., Rudert, M., & Ernst, A. (1992). Stiffness, compliance, elasticity and force generation of outer hair cells. *Acta Oto-Laryngologica, 112,* 248–253.

Zenner, H. P., Reuter, G., Plinkert, P. K., Zimmerman, U., & Gitter, A. H. (1989). Outer hair cells possess acetylcholine receptors and produce motile responses in the organ of Corti. In J. P. Wilson & D. T. Kemp (Eds.), *Cochlear mechanisms* (pp. 93–98). London: Plenum.

3

Spontaneous Otoacoustic Emissions

KATHRYN E. BRIGHT

Introduction

Spontaneous otoacoustic emissions (SOAEs) are low-level, tonal signals measured in the external ear canal in the absence of any known stimulus. They are usually inaudible to the persons from whose ears they are detected, and their presence suggests that cochlear hearing sensitivity is normal near the frequency of an SOAE.

SOAEs are recorded by coupling a sensitive, miniature microphone to the external ear canal. The noise in the ear canal is preamplified and high-pass filtered to eliminate physiological noise below 300 to 500 Hz. The signal is then delivered to a spectrum analyzer or FFT software for spectral analysis (either on- or off-line). Multiple samples are collected and averaged in an effort to decrease the random noise in the ear canal, although some high-amplitude SOAEs may be identified without averaging. Most investigators require a reproducible spectral peak at least 3 dB above the noise floor to identify an SOAE. As illustrated in Figure 3–1, a spontaneous emission is a definite, tone-like maximum in the spectrum. Whether or not an SOAE can be measured depends on the detection apparatus and data collection and analysis techniques. A number of complicated hardware and software combinations have been developed for detecting SOAEs (Penner, Glotzback, & Huang, 1993; Talmadge, Long, Murphy, & Tubis, 1993).

As early as 1948, Thomas Gold predicted an active, ongoing feedback mechanism in the cochlea. He even speculated that the feedback mechanism could become unstable and produce a spontaneous ringing; however, it was not until Kemp documented the presence of SOAEs in 1979 that the importance of Gold's hypothesis was realized. Today, there is strong evidence that the generation of SOAEs depends on normal cochlear function. Both spontaneous and evoked otoacoustic emissions are believed to be byproducts of the *cochlear amplifier*, which is the process in the cochlea responsible for the sharp frequency selectivity, high sensitivity, and wide dynamic range that the cochlea is known to possess (Kemp, 1986). The exact mechanism responsible for the generation of SOAEs is unknown, although it is likely that an SOAE originates from nonlinear outer–hair-cell activity

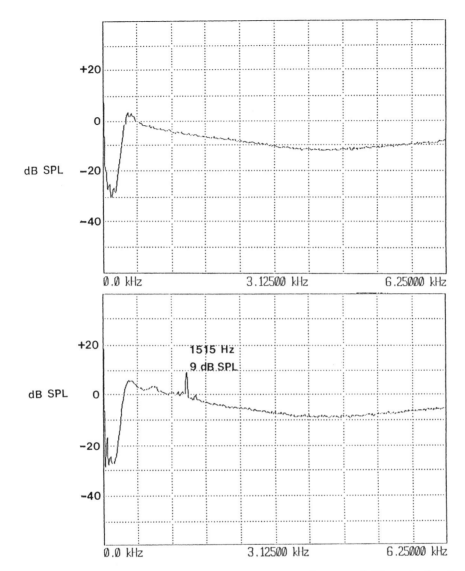

Figure 3–1. *Top*: Spectral average of noise in the external ear canal. The noise has been filtered below 400 Hz. *Bottom*: Spectral average of external canal noise that includes a spontaneous otoacoustic emission at 1515 Hz.

at the place in the cochlea tuned to its frequency (Keilson, Khanna, Ulfendahl, & Teich, 1993).

Kemp (1986) and Manley (1993) have suggested that SOAEs derive from minor structural irregularities within the cochlea that are not significant enough to affect audiometric thresholds. For example, aberrations in outer–hair-cell arrangement, such as an occasional fourth row, might cause a natural reflection of energy. Lonsbury-Martin, Martin, Probst, and Coats (1988) provided evidence to support the theory. They histologically evaluated the cochleas from a rhesus monkey who exhibited bilateral SOAEs and noted the presence of a fourth row of outer hair cells, as well as disruption in the outer–hair-cell stereocilia at the apical ends of the cochleas. The data, as well as the facts that (a) SOAEs in humans are seen only in frequency regions where the hearing is normal and (b) that SOAEs are vulnerable to the same insults that damage outer hair cells, suggest that there may be "natural imperfections" in the organ of Corti that are the physical basis for the oscillations known as SOAEs. The imperfections are not associated with damage in the cochlea, but might cause a perturbation that initiates a reverse traveling wave (Kemp, 1986).

Characteristics

SOAEs are continuous and narrowband with bandwidths near 1 Hz (Wit & van Dijk, 1990). They are present at relatively stable amplitudes and frequencies so that amplification of the signal and averaging of the spectrum of the noise in the external auditory meatus are all that is required to establish the presence of a spontaneous emission. They are vulnerable to cochlear insults known to affect outer cells—namely hypoxia (Evans, Wilson, & Borerwe, 1981), ototoxic drugs (Long & Tubis, 1988a; McFadden & Plattsmier, 1984), and noise (Norton, Mott, & Champlin, 1989).

In human ears, SOAEs have not been recorded in the presence of hearing loss greater than 25 to 30 dB HL (Bonfils, 1989; Bright & Glattke, 1986; Moulin, Collet, Delli, & Morgon, 1991; Probst, Lonsbury-Martin, Martin, & Coats, 1987), although they may be detected in some ears with mild sensorineural hearing loss. When this is the case, the ear must have a mean hearing loss greater than 25 dB HL (Moulin, Collet, Delli, & Morgon), and the SOAE is associated with a frequency region where there is preservation of hearing sensitivity (> 15 dB HL) (Bright & Glattke; Probst, Lonsbury-Martin, Martin & Coats). In addition, Moulin, Collet, Delli, and Morgon reported that they never found SOAEs in 63 subjects when the threshold at 1000 Hz was greater than 10 dB HL.

Prevalence and number of SOAEs

Estimates of the prevalence of SOAEs depend on the instrumentation and data collection procedure used to obtain them. This is illustrated by the fact that since the early 1980s prevalence figures have risen steadily with improvements in technology. Specifically, the sensitivity of the microphone, the level of the noise floor and attempts to reduce it, and the criteria for identifying a spectral peak as an SOAE are critical elements of the measurement process (Penner, Glotzback, & Huang). Early studies showed a prevalence of about 35 to 40%, and recent data has suggested that, with careful control of extraneous noise, the prevalence is as high as 72% of persons with normal hearing (Penner, Glotzback, & Huang; Talmadge, Long, Murphy, & Tubis, 1993). In addition, prevalence figures differ depending on whether the number of ears of a sample are counted or whether it is the number of persons with SOAEs that are counted. The term *prevalence* refers to the number (or the ratio) of persons with a specific characteristic in a given population at a certain time. Therefore, counting the number of ears is not an appropriate measure of prevalence.

It is not uncommon for multiple SOAEs to be present in the same ear, and they may be detected in one or both ears of the same subject (Bright & Glattke). Recent data suggest that, on average, approximately four SOAEs are detected for each emitting ear (Lonsbury-Martin, Harris, Stagner, Hawkins, & Martin, 1990; Talmadge, Long, Murphy, & Tubis; Whitehead, Baker, & Wilson, 1989). When they are observed in both ears, they are not necessarily the same frequency, although the presence of an SOAE in one ear makes it more likely that an SOAE will be found in the opposite ear (Bilger, Matthies, Hammel, & Demorest, 1990).

Two interesting and unexplainable observations have been reported. First, approximately twice as many women as men exhibit SOAEs (Bilger, Matthies, Hammel, & Demorest; Martin, Probst, & Lonsbury-Martin, 1990; Probst, Coats, Martin, & Lonsbury-Martin, 1986; Strickland, Burns, & Tubis, 1985). Second, SOAEs are more often observed in right ears than in left ears (Bilger, Matthies, Hammel, & Demorest; Penner, Glotzback, & Huang; Strickland, Burns, & Tubis). In addition, women exhibit more bilateral SOAEs and are more likely to exhibit multiple SOAEs. Some researchers have suggested that the smaller ear canal volumes of female ears might be responsible for the gender difference; but it is not likely given the fact that infants and children show the same gender differences (Probst, Coats, Martin, & Lonsbury-Martin). Bilger, Matthies, Hammel, and Demorest presented a compelling argument for a genetic (possibly X-linked) component to explain the differences in prevalence between the genders.

If there is a genetic tendency for SOAEs, it is likely that differences in SOAE prevalence would be noted between racial groups. Whitehead, Kamal, Lonsbury-Martin, and Martin (1993) reported significant differences between three racial groups (with 20 subjects in each). Although they reported no significant differences in prevalence of SOAEs between the groups (possibly because of the small number of subjects), Blacks exhibited the most SOAEs, Whites exhibited the fewest number of SOAEs, and Asians exhibited an intermediate number. In addition, there were differences in the characteristics of the SOAEs between the groups; specifically, the Asian group had higher-frequency SOAEs, on average, than the other groups, and five SOAEs from Asian women had broad bandwidths, between 20 and 55 Hz.

SOAEs occur with the same prevalence in neonates, children, and young adults (Burns, Arehart, & Campbell, 1992; Bonfils, Francois, Avan, Londero, Trotoux, & Narcy, 1992; Kok, van Zanten, & Brocaar, 1993; Strickland, Burns, & Tubis). Burns, Arehart, and Campbell found no difference in prevalence between 1-month-old infants and adults, and Bonfils, Francois, Avan, Londero, Trotoux, and Narcy reported a similar prevalence in preterm infants. In addition, the same gender- and ear-related patterns have been noted for infants and children as for adults— namely females and right ears exhibit more SOAEs. Although Strickland, Burns, and Tubis reported a prevalence of only 38% of infants and 40% of children aged 5 to 12, their data are similar to the data obtained from adults at that time and probably reflect the less sensitive measurement conditions available. Because the prevalence pattern is similar in infants, prepubescent children, and adults, it is likely that differences in prevalence associated with gender and age are not caused by hormonal differences or by pathological conditions, such as noise-induced hearing loss.

For subjects over 60 years of age, the prevalence of SOAEs appears to decrease, even when hearing loss remains within normal limits (Bonfils; Stover & Norton,

1993). In contrast, the prevalence of other types of OAEs do not appear to change significantly with advancing age when hearing sensitivity is controlled (Stover & Norton, 1993). In addition, the total number of SOAEs observed in aged ears decreases, although other SOAE features such as frequency and amplitude characteristics are not altered (Moulin, Collet, Delli & Morgon).

Frequency and Amplitude Characteristics

The majority of SOAEs from adult ears fall within the frequency region from 1000 to 2000 Hz, which probably reflects the contribution of middle ear–resonance characteristics. The majority of SOAEs from infant and newborn ears are somewhat higher in frequency (3000–4000 Hz) than those from adults (Burns, Arehart, & Campbell; Kok, van Zanten, & Brocaar; Strickland, Burns, & Tubis). SOAEs for both adults and infants can, however, be measured at frequencies higher than 7000 Hz (Burns, Arehart, & Campbell; Lind & Randa, 1990; Penner, Glotzback, & Huang; Rebillard, Abou, & Lenoir, 1987; Ruggero, Rich, & Freyman, 1983; Talmadge, Long, Murphy, & Tubis). SOAEs below 500 Hz are not typically measured because of the filters that are used to eliminate low-frequency physiological noise during recording.

SOAE frequencies remain relatively stable over short periods. Lind and Randa repeated SOAE measurements 20 seconds after the first measurement and noted a shift in frequency of less than 1 Hz. In test sessions of one hour or less, frequency shifts on the order of 10 Hz or less (<1%) are consistently reported (Frick & Matthies, 1988; Penner, Glotzback, & Huang; Ruggero, Rich, & Freyman; Zurek, 1981). Such stability has been interpreted as evidence that SOAEs are generated at specific sites on the basilar membrane (Martin, Probst, & Lonsbury-Martin, 1990).

Perhaps, more interesting is the observation that SOAE frequencies shift with circadian and monthly periodicity (Bell, 1992; Haggerty, Lusted, & Morton, 1993; Penner, Brauth, & Jastreboff, 1994). Both Bell and Haggerty, Lusted, and Morton reported that several of their subjects exhibited monthly fluctuations in SOAE frequencies consistent with menstrual cycles; their subjects also exhibited daily fluctuations that affected most, if not all, of the SOAEs from a single subject systematically, even when the SOAEs were from opposite ears. That is, when one SOAE shifted in frequency, other SOAEs from the same subject shifted in the same direction and by roughly the same amount. Each subject seemed to have a characteristic frequency fluctuation pattern for both daily and monthly fluctuations.

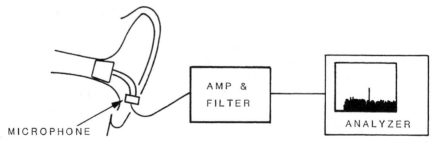

Figure 3–2. Schematic of basic instrumentation for measuring spontaneous emissions.

Some subjects exhibited frequency shifts as high as 27 to 36 Hz over an 8-week period (Haggerty, Lusted, & Morton). Whether the daily and monthly frequency fluctuations are the result of changes in cerebral spinal fluid pressure (Bell) or some other metabolic or hormonal change remains to be seen.

In a longitudinal study of adult subjects with SOAEs, Kohler and Fritz (1992) illustrated the transient nature of some SOAEs over relatively long periods of time (3 years, 6 months to 7 years, 2 months). Specifically, they observed that high-frequency SOAEs tended to disappear over time and new low-frequency SOAEs developed. In addition, all of the shifts in frequency were downward. These observations are consistent with the fact that higher-frequency SOAEs are seen in infants and children than in adults.

With regard to amplitude, the majority of SOAEs recorded from human ears are measured at levels between −12 and 20 dB SPL, with mean amplitudes for adults near −3 to 0 dB SPL (Burns, Arehart, & Campbell; Penner, Glotzback, & Huang; and for infants near 10 dB SPL (Burns, Arehart, & Campbell; Kok, van Zanten, & Brocaar). Burns, Arehart, and Campbell reported a systematic decrease in SOAE amplitude for infants who were tested between 1 month and 24 months of age. By 24 months, the average SOAE amplitude had decreased to 0 dB SPL from 8.5 dB SPL at 1 month.

SOAE amplitudes can fluctuate by as much as 10 to 15 dB over short periods (Penner, Glotzback, & Huang; Rabinowitz & Widin, 1984; Ruggero, Rich, & Freyman; Zurek) although most SOAEs are fairly stable in amplitude (<3 dB fluctuation) (Frick & Matthies; Lind & Randa; Rabinowitz & Widin). Unstable SOAEs are typically noted in ears that have more than five SOAEs (Burns, Arehart, & Campbell). It is unclear why some SOAEs are more amplitude-stable than others are, even in the same ear. Fluctuation of the noise floor, slight changes in probe placement, humidity changes in the ear canal, middle ear changes, and true fluctuations in the SOAE are factors that may be responsible for amplitude variations.

External Influences

SOAEs are affected in a complex way by a number of external conditions. Observation of how SOAEs vary in the presence of pure tones, ear canal pressure changes, and contralateral acoustic stimuli provide us with a better understanding of SOAEs and their role in cochlear physiology.

INTERACTIONS WITH PURE TONES

Many of the following observations are anecdotal and illustrate the complexity of the cochlea. First, a low-level pure tone with frequency near an SOAE frequency can cause beats or roughness to be perceived by a person previously unaware of the SOAE. Second, an external tone may cause the frequency of the SOAE to shift either up or down when it is sufficiently close the SOAE frequency (Rabinowitz & Widin; Zurek) Third, SOAEs may be suppressed by pure tones near the frequency of the SOAE (Frick & Matthies; Harris & Glattke, 1992; Rabinowitz & Widin; Ruggero, Rich, & Freyman; Zizz & Glattke, 1988). Tuning curves that show the amount of suppression for various combinations of suppressor level and frequency are similar to the V-shaped physiological and psychophysical tuning curves known to reflect frequency specificity in the cochlea (Harris & Glattke; Zizz & Glattke). Fourth, it is possible to synchronize the phase of an SOAE to that of a pure tone near the frequency of the SOAE (Wilson, 1980; Wilson & Sutton, 1981), and synchronization tuning curves can be plotted which are similar in shape and amount of tuning to the suppression tuning curves. All the observations suggest that SOAEs are cochlear phenomena that, when present, may be used to evaluate the fine tuning ability of the cochlea.

More complex interactions have been observed between SOAEs and external pure tones. For example, the interaction of two external tones may cause a previously-suppressed SOAE to be released from suppression (Rabinowitz & Widin). While introducing one external tone may suppress an SOAE, introducing a second pure tone that will suppress the first tone allows the SOAE to be released from suppression. Similarly, Burns, Strickland, Tubis, and Jones demonstrated that when multiple SOAEs are present in an ear, suppression of one of the SOAEs by an external tone may cause a second SOAE to increase in amplitude and shift its frequency.

MIDDLE EAR PRESSURE

Because SOAEs must be transmitted to the ear canal via the middle ear, it is necessary to know the effects of the middle-ear status on SOAEs. Kemp (1981) reported that changes in middle ear compliance induced by applying either posi- tive or negative pressure to the ear canal caused a shift in the frequency of the SOAE of up to 50 Hz. Wilson and Sutton (1981) noted similar results with changes in external canal pressure. They reported that the frequency shifts could occur in either direction, although the frequency usually increased. The amplitudes of the emissions increased or decreased with changes in pressure. Schloth and Zwicker (1983) demonstrated that changes in ear canal pressure for one subject caused a previously inaudible emission to become audible.

Similar results were reported recently for subjects who were seated in a pressure chamber, thereby eliminating some of the technical difficulties of changing ear canal pressure while measuring otoacoustic emissions (OAEs) (Hauser, Probst, & Harris, 1993). As expected, SOAEs in the frequency range between 1000 and 2000 Hz were most affected, and most of the SOAEs showed an increase in frequency and a decrease in amplitude with either positive or negative changes in pressure. For some SOAEs, however, an increase in amplitude was noted, and in two subjects new emissions appeared when the pressure was changed.

CONTRALATERAL STIMULATION

As with other types of OAEs, stimulation of the opposite ear with tonal or broad- band signals causes observable changes in SOAEs (Harrison & Burns, 1993; Mott, Norton, Neely, & Warr, 1989; Moulin, Collet, & Morgon, 1992; Rabinowitz & Widin). The most noticeable change in evoked emissions during contralateral stimulation is a change in amplitude, while for SOAEs frequency shifts are most noticeable, with the frequency of an SOAE shifting upward by 2 to 20 Hz. In addition, small changes in amplitudes of SOAEs may be observed depending on the level of the contralateral stimulation. Because outer hair cells receive most of the efferent innervation in the cochlea coming from olivocochlear fibers (primarily from the medial superior olive), several investigators have suggested that changes in OAEs from contralateral stimulation might provide information about the status of the efferent system. It is not clear, however, the extent to which middle-ear muscle contraction affects these observations; changes in middle ear stiffness induced by positive and negative pressure also create subtle shifts in frequency and amplitude of an SOAE.

To assess the contribution of middle ear muscle contractions, Burns, Harrison, Bulen, and Keefes (1993) evaluated one subject who had multiple bilateral SOAEs and was able to voluntarily contract her middle ear muscles. The voluntary, nonacoustic activation of middle ear muscles caused changes in her SOAEs that are similar to those seen with contralateral acoustic stimulation. The results suggest that any changes in SOAEs attributed to the efferent pathway may be confounded by changes in middle ear muscle activity even with low-level stimuli.

IPSILATERAL FATIGUING STIMULI

Temporary threshold shift (TTS) is a well-documented consequence of exposure to intense acoustic stimuli. For tonal stimuli, TTS is greatest at frequencies one-half to one octave above the frequency of the exposure stimulus. Several studies provide results that suggest that SOAEs approximately one-half to one octave above exposure tones are significantly altered as well (Cianfrone, Mattia, Cervellini, & Musacchio, 1993; Kemp, 1981, 1982, 1986). In addition, the time course of SOAE change is similar to that seen with TTS. For 4 minutes following exposure, Norton, Mott, and Champlin tracked SOAE changes at 2-second intervals and then tracked changes at 30- to 60-second intervals beyond 4 minutes. For many of their subjects they noted significant reduction in SOAE amplitude immediately following exposure and a biphasic recovery with a second decrease in amplitude at 2 minutes after exposure. The phenomenon is strikingly similar to the "bounce" in TTS recovery patterns, which is a reversal in recovery that occurs at 2 minutes after exposure.

Several conclusions can be drawn from studies of SOAEs following exposure to fatiguing stimuli: (a) TTS and changes in SOAEs following exposure to intense stimuli both arise from alterations in OHC activity, (b) SOAEs must be the result of normal physiological activity in the cochlea, and (c) SOAEs may be a unique, objective measurement of TTS not previously available to investigators.

Multiple SOAEs

Multiple SOAEs from a single ear are common. Several investigators have reported that female subjects are more likely to have multiple SOAEs than male subjects (Bilger, Matthies, Hammel, & Demorest; Strickland, Burns, & Tubis; Zurek). In ears with more than one SOAE, the minimum frequency difference is about 100 Hz and is rarely less than 50 Hz (Dallmayr, 1985; Schloth, 1983; Talmadge, Long, Murphy, & Tubis). Talmadge, Long, Murphy, and Tubis suggested that the minimum separation between SOAEs corresponds to about one-twelfth octave (or a distance of about 0.4 mm on the basilar membrane).

In some ears, SOAES may be harmonics of other SOAEs (Talmadge, Long, Murphy, & Tubis) In addition, lower frequency SOAEs may be cubic-distortion products caused by the interaction of two other SOAEs (Burns, Strickland, Tubis, & Jones, 1984; Talmadge, Long, Murphy & Tubis). That is, two SOAEs serve as the "primary" tones (f_1 and f_2) and produce a third SOAE at $2f_1 - f_2$. The frequency of a distortion product SOAE will fluctuate with frequency changes in one of the primary SOAEs, and suppression of a primary causes suppression of the distortion product SOAE as well. Similarly, Frick and Matthies were able to generate distortion products in two ears by introducing an external tone that served as one primary with an existing SOAE serving as the other primary.

Burns, Strickland, Tubis, and Jones described interactions, that they called "linked-noncontiguous" SOAEs. A subject with multiple SOAEs may exhibit one subset of the total number of SOAEs on one occasion and a second subset on another occasion. The same SOAEs comprise each of the two subsets consistently.

Relation between SOAES and Tinnitus

Subjective Tinnitus

When SOAEs were first measured it was hoped they would prove to be a physiological correlate to the sensation of tinnitus (Wilson & Sutton, 1981). Subsequent studies have shown a significant lack of correlation between the presence of SOAEs and tinnitus (Penner, 1990; Penner & Burns, 1987; Probst, Lonsbury-Martin, Martin, & Coats; Rebillard, Abou, & Lenoir; Tyler & Conrad-Armes, 1982; Zurek, 1981). Although there have been a few anecdotal reports of SOAEs associated with tinnitus (Penner, 1988, 1989, 1992; Penner & Coles, 1992), Penner (1990) estimated that only about 4% of tinnitus sufferers exhibit related SOAEs. The finding is consistent with the fact SOAEs generally are not recorded above 4000 Hz while the majority of persons with tinnitus match it at frequencies above 4000 Hz. Evidence for lack of correlation between tinnitus and SOAEs comes from suppression and masking studies in which the suppression of SOAEs has not been shown to alter the perception of tinnitus and masking of tinnitus does not obliterate SOAEs (Penner, 1992; Penner & Burns).

Penner reported three female subjects who had annoying tinnitus that was associated with SOAEs (Penner, 1988, 1989, 1992; Penner & Coles). In all three cases, introduction of tones to suppress the SOAEs also caused the tinnitus to become inaudible. Two of the three subjects described the tinnitus as varying in frequency and had SOAEs that fluctuated in level. Penner has suggested that most SOAEs are inaudible because the auditory system adapts to the constant signal, whereas in a few persons, the SOAE may become audible and annoying if it is fluctuant in nature.

Objective Tinnitus

There are a few documented cases in which a tonal objective tinnitus has been reported (Coles, Snashell, & Stephens, 1975; Glanville, Coles, & Sullivan, 1971; Huizing & Spoor, 1973; Mathis, Probst, Demin, & Hauser, 1991; Yamamoto, Tagaki, Hirono, & Yagi, 1987). An interesting observation by Glanville, Coles, and Sullivan was that three members of the same family, the father and two children, were found to have objective tinnitus, presumably traced to a dominant autosomal gene. For all three family members, the primary component of the objective tinnitus was high-frequency ($\geq$ 3500 Hz) and was associated with an abnormality in the audiogram (high-frequency hearing loss of 40–60 dB HL). In a follow-up study of two of the family members 13 years after the original report, the frequencies of the sounds emanating from the four ears were relatively unchanged and SOAE measurements were completed (Wilson & Sutton, 1983). Each of the ears exhibited multiple spontaneous otoacoustic emissions in the frequency range from 1.4 to 17 kHz. The most prominent emissions fell in the frequency range between 5000 Hz and 8500 Hz and were measured at levels of approximately 40 dB SPL.

Similarly, Mathis, Probst, DeMin, and Hauser described the case of a child who was first noted to have a tone emanating from his left ear at 6 months of age. Subsequent testing at 3 years of age revealed a high-level SOAE of 55 dB SPL at 5643 Hz and the presence of a bilateral high-frequency, sensorineural hearing loss.

These high-level SOAEs have been described as a rare form of spontaneous emission that do not display the same properties as SOAEs measured from normally hearing ears. They differ from typical SOAEs in the following ways: (a) They are associated with abnormal audiograms, (b) they occur at frequencies where hearing loss is observed, (c) they are of frequencies and amplitude levels significantly higher than those observed for other SOAEs, and (d) in animal subjects they are associated with cochlear lesions. The striking differences suggest that the mechanism responsible for high-level emissions is not the same as that thought to account for low-level SOAEs.

SOAES in Animals

Comparative studies of both mammalian and non-mammalian species provide an understanding of how structural differences or common features among animals might contribute to the production of SOAEs. Unfortunately, relatively few animals have been found with SOAEs. Among mammals, monkeys are most similar to human beings with regard to prevalence and SOAE characteristics (Lonsbury-Martin & Martin, 1988; Martin, Lonsbury-Martin, Probst, & Coats, 1985). Although significantly less prevalent in monkeys (5–9%) than in human beings (> 70%), SOAEs from various species of monkeys exhibit frequency and amplitude properties almost identical to those found in humans.

In other mammals, systematic searches for SOAEs have been unsuccessful (Probst, Lonsbury-Martin, & Martin, 1991). SOAEs have been reported anecdotally for dogs (Decker & Fritsch, 1982; Ruggero, Kramek, & Rich, 1984) guinea pigs (Evans, Wilson, & Borerwe; Ohyama, Wada, Kobayashi, & Takasada, 1991), chinchillas, (Clark, Kim, Zurek, & Bohne, 1984; Zurek & Clark, 1981), a bat (Kossl & Vater, 1985), and a pony (Mayhew, Preston, Hannant, Washburn, Johnson, & Phillips, 1995). Many of these SOAEs were identified because they were audible when a listener was close to the animal's pinna. Virtually all of the SOAEs reported from non-primate mammals had robust amplitudes (> 20 dB SPL), and exhibited characteristics similar to those described for objective tinnitus or high-level SOAEs. In the animals from whom histopathological or behavioral results were available, the SOAEs were associated with cochlear lesions or hearing loss.

The SOAEs observed from the chinchilla ears were detected only after repeated exposure to excessive noise. Of 28 chinchilla ears exposed to noise, one chinchilla had two SOAEs in one ear and a second chinchilla had a single SOAE. The SOAEs were high-level and measured at levels of 17 to 40 dB SPL and had frequencies between 4650 Hz and 6470 Hz. One of the SOAEs was associated with behavioral threshold shifts that extended across all test frequencies but one. For the two SOAEs present at time of sacrifice, clear histopathological changes in the cochlea were noted, specifically discrete loss of outer hair cells. However, similar changes were also present in ears without SOAEs (Clark, Kim, Zurek, & Bohne).

It is interesting to compare histopathological results from the two chinchillas with high-level SOAEs (Clark, Kim, Zurek, & Bohne) with the results reported for a monkey who exhibited low-level bilateral SOAEs (Lonsbury-Martin, Martin, Probst, & Coats). In the chinchillas, the SOAEs developed after noise exposure, and resulted in areas of clear damage in the organ of Corti. In the monkey, the SOAEs had characteristics similar to those observed in normal human ears and were thought to be associated with normal structural irregularities in the organ of Corti, such as a fourth row of outer hair cells. Because some human cochleas exhibit the same types of abnormalities, it may be that these regions of irregularity are implicated in SOAE production. Thus, some researchers have speculated that (a) the two types of SOAEs are really manifestations of the same generator and (b) in some ears a low-level oscillation occurs as the result of a natural imperfection, but in other ears higher-level oscillations are generated by a more severe imperfection due to damage.

Finally, some non-mammalian ears produce SOAEs with a fairly high prevalence. In frogs 71% of ears had measurable SOAEs (van Dijk, Wit, & Segenhout, 1989), and in bobtail lizards 83% of ears exhibited SOAEs (Koppl & Manley, 1993). For both animals, as temperature increases (Koppl & Manley; Manley & Koppl, 1994), frequencies of SOAEs increase; and in frogs the SOAEs are seasonal and disappear in the winter.

Clinical Implications

Because SOAEs are not measurable in all normal ears and because they appear at discrete and unpredictable frequencies, they are not the emission of choice for clinically assessing cochlear functioning. The presence of an SOAE, however, suggests that hearing is within normal limits in the frequency region of the cochlea tuned to the SOAE frequency (Bright & Glattke; Probst, Lonsbury-Martin, Martin, & Coats) and that the average threshold for that ear is greater than 25 dB HL (Moulin, Collet, Delli, & Morgon). The presence of an SOAE may also affect behavioral test results and measurements of other types of OAEs.

Effects on Behavioral Tests

THRESHOLD

A microstructure audiogram reflects fluctuation in thresholds with small changes in stimulus frequency (>50 Hz). Adjacent threshold maxima and minima may differ by as much as 12 to 14 dB, and for many subjects a distinct pattern of irregular maxima and minima of thresholds exists that is reliable over time (Long, 1984). For persons with normal hearing, behavioral thresholds at SOAE frequencies are more sensitive than thresholds at adjacent frequencies. That is, SOAEs often occur near

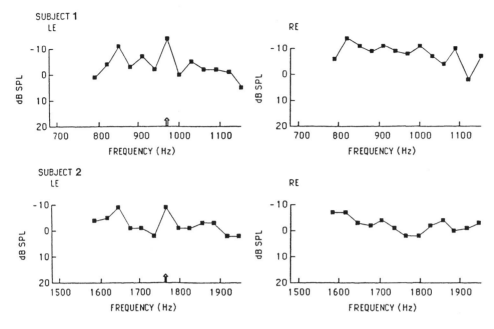

Figure 3–3. Microstructure audiogram results from two subjects. Data points occur at 30-Hz intervals. The arrows represent frequencies at which a spontaneous emission was obtained for each subject. No SOAEs were measured for the same frequency region from the subjects' right ears.

frequencies where there is a minimum in audiogram microstructure (Figure 3–3) (Bright, 1985; Long & Tubis, 1988). Not all threshold minima, however, are associated with SOAEs and not all SOAEs produce threshold minima. The implication is that subtle changes in behavioral thresholds may be the result of changes in SOAEs. Furthermore, stimulating an ear that has multiple SOAEs with an external tone may suppress some SOAEs and enhance others (Rabinowitz & Widin). When conducting experiments that include precise threshold measurements, identification of SOAE frequencies may be helpful for interpretation of results.

In addition, McFadden and Mishra (1993) reported an overall enhancement of hearing sensitivity across test frequencies for ears with SOAEs. The amount of enhancement, although slightly better in right ears, averaged 3 dB.

FREQUENCY SELECTIVITY

In addition to enhanced sensitivity, frequency selectivity is improved near SOAE frequencies (Bright; Michey & Collet, 1994). The improvement has been documented by psychophysical tuning curves obtained from ears with and without SOAEs. As shown in Figure 3–4, a tuning curve obtained near an SOAE frequency is sharper than one in the same ear at a higher frequency or one from the opposite ear with no SOAE. As with threshold measurements, experimenters should identify the presence of SOAEs before interpreting results when seeking subtle changes in tuning of the cochlea.

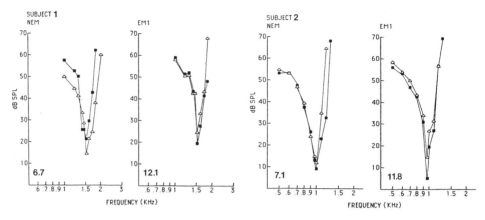

Figure 3–4. Psychophysical tuning curves (PTCs) from two subjects, each with a spontaneous otoacoustic emission in one ear and no SOAE in the opposite ear. *NEM*, non–emission ear; *EM1*, center frequency at SOAE frequency. Squares and triangles represent data obtained during two data-collection sessions. Mean *Q* values 10 dB above the PTC tip are noted on each graph.

Interaction with Other OAEs

SOAEs influence both transiently evoked otoacoustic emissions (TEOAEs) and distortion-product–evoked otoacoustic emissions (DPOAEs) (Cianfrone, Mattia, & Altissimi, 1990; Gobsch & Tietze, 1993; Kemp, 1979; Norton & Neely, 1987; Probst, Coats, Martin, & Lonsbury-Martin; Wier, Pasanen, & McFadden, 1988). Specifically, an SOAE may become synchronized to the evoking stimulus and cause a TEOAE response to persist beyond the 20- to 40-msec window that is typical (Kemp, 1979; Probst, Coats, Martin, & Lonsbury-Martin). In addition, clear spectral peaks at SOAE frequencies are apparent in TEOAE spectra (Norton & Neely, 1987) and DPOAE responses are enhanced near the frequency of an SOAE (Cianfrone, Mattia, & Altissimi; Moulin, Collet, Veuillet, & Morgon, 1993; Wier, Pasanen, & McFadden). Moulin, Collet, Veuillet, and Morgon demonstrated in a study of 135 subjects that the gender effect for both TEOAEs and DPOAEs was significantly reduced when ears with SOAEs were eliminated from the data pool. Additionally, the amplitudes of both TEOAEs and DPOAEs were significantly higher in ears with SOAEs even when the frequency bands immediately surrounding the SOAE frequency were eliminated from the analyses. The finding is consistent with McFadden and Mishra's report concerning a general enhancement of behavioral thresholds in ears with SOAEs.

Summary and Conclusions

SOAEs allow a fascinating glimpse of cochlear activity. While not inherently useful as a clinical tool, they provide supplemental information that is often helpful in interpretation of other test results. They appear to indicate that the cochlea functions normally, and their presence may even signal enhanced functioning. The ease with which SOAEs can be measured belies the complexity of the system that is responsible for their production. Further study of SOAEs and their interactions with physiological and psychoacoustic events will undoubtedly enhance our knowledge of the auditory system as well as provide an appreciation of the exquisite complexity of the system.

References

Bell, A. (1992). Circadian and menstrual rhythms in frequency variations of spontaneous otoacoustic emissions from human ears. *Hearing Research, 58,* 91–100.

Bilger, R. C., Matthies, M. L., Hammel, D. R., & Demorest, M. E. (1990). Genetic implications of gender differences in the prevalence of spontaneous otoacoustic emissions. *Journal of Speech and Hearing Research, 33,* 418–432.

Bonfils, P. (1989). Spontaneous otoacoustic emissions: Clinical interest. *Laryngoscope, 99,* 752–756.

Bonfils, P., Francois, M., Avan, P., Londero, A., Trotoux, J., & Narcy, P. (1992). Spontaneous and evoked otoacoustic emissions in preterm neonates. *Laryngoscope, 102,* 182–186.

Bright, K. E. (1985). Microstructure audiograms and psychophysical tuning curves from ears with spontaneous otoacoustic emissions. Unpublished doctoral dissertation, University of Arizona, Tucson, AZ.

Bright, K. E., & Glattke, T. J. (1986) Spontaneous otoacoustic emissions in normal ears. In M. J. Collins, T. J. Glattke, & L. A. Harker (eds.): *Sensorineural hearing loss* (pp. 201–208). Iowa City, IA: University of Iowa Press.

Burns, E. M., Arehart, K. H., & Campbell, S. L. (1992). Prevalence of spontaneous otoacoustic emissions in neonates. *Journal of the Acoustical Society of America, 91,* 1571–1575.

Burns, E. M., Harrison, W. A., Bulen, J. C., & Keefes, D. H. M. (1993). Voluntary contraction of middle ear muscles: Effects on input impedance, energy reflectance and spontaneous otoacoustic emissions. *Hearing Research, 67,* 117–127.

Burns, E. M., Strickland, E. A., Tubis, A., & Jones, K. (1984). Interaction among spontaneous otoacoustic emissions. I. Distortion products and linked emissions. *Hearing Research, 16,* 271–278.

Cianfrone, G., Mattia, B. & Altissimi, G. (1990). Distortion product otoacoustic emissions and spontaneous otoacoustic emission suppression in humans. In F. Grandori, G. Cianfrone, D. T. Kemp (eds.): *Cochlear mechanisms and otoacoustic emissions* (pp. 127–138). Basel, Switzerland: Kruger.

Cianfrone, G., Mattia, M., Cervellini, M., & Musacchio, A.A. (1993). Some effects of tonal fatiguing on spontaneous and distortion-product otoacoustic emissions. *British Journal of Audiology, 27,* 123–130.

Clark, W. W., Kim, D. O., Zurek, P. M., & Bohne, B. A. (1984). Spontaneous otoacoustic emissions in chinchilla ear canals. Correlation with histopathology and suppression by external tones. *Hearing Research, 16,* 299–314.

Coles, R. R. A., Snashell, S. E., & Stephens, S. D. G. (1975). Some varieties of objective tinnitus. *British Journal of Audiology, 9,* 1–6.

Dallmayr, C. (1985). Spontane oto-akustische emissionen: Statistik und reaktion auf akustische stortone. *Acustica, 59,* 67–75.

Decker, T. N., & Fritsch, J. H. (1982). Objective tinnitus in the dog. *Journal of the American Veterinary Medical Association, 180,* 74.

Evans, E. F., Wilson, J. P., & Borerwe T. A. (1981). Animal models of tinnitus. In D. Evered & G. Lawrenson (eds.): *Tinnitus: Ciba foundation symposium* (pp 108–138). Pitman Books: London.

Frick, L. R., & Matthies, M. L. (1988). Effects of external stimuli on spontaneous otoacoustic emissions. *Ear and Hearing, 9,* 190–197.

Glanville, J. D., Coles, R. R. A., & Sullivan, B. M .(1971). A family with high-tonal objective tinnitus. *Journal of Laryngology and Otology, 85,* 1–10.

Gobsch, H., & Tietze, G. (1993). Interrelation of spontaneous and evoked otoacoustic emissions. *Hearing Research, 69,* 176–181.

Gold, T. (1948). Hearing II.: The physical basis of the action of the cochlea. *Proceedings of the Royal Society (London), 135,* 492–498.

Haggerty, H. S., Lusted, H. S., & Morton, S. C. (1993). Statistical quantification of 24-hour and monthly variabilities of spontaneous otoacoustic emission frequency in humans. *Hearing Research, 70,* 31–49.

Harris, F. P., & Glattke, T. J. (1992). The use of suppression to determine the characteristics of otoacoustic emissions. *Seminars in Hearing, 13,* 67–79.

Harrison, W. A., & Burns, E. M. (1993). Effects of contralateral acoustic stimulation on spontaneous otoacoustic emissions. *Journal of the Acoustical Society of America, 94,* 2649–2658.

Hauser, R., Probst, R., & Harris, F. P. (1993). Effects of atmospheric pressure variation on spontaneous, transiently evoked, and distortion product otoacoustic emissions in normal human ears. *Hearing Research, 69,* 133–145.

Huizing, E. H., & Spoor, A. (1973). An unusual type of tinnitus. *Archives of Otolaryngology, 98,* 134–136.

Keilson, S. E., Khanna, S. M., Ulfendahl, M., & Teich, M. C. 1993). Spontaneous cellular vibrations in the guinea-pig cochlea. *Acta Oto-Laryngologica, 113,* 591–597.

Kemp, D. T. (1979). Evidence of mechanical nonlinearity and frequency selective wave amplification in the cochlea. *Archives of Otorhinolaryngology, 224,* 37–45.

Kemp, D. T. (1981). Physiologically active cochlear micromechanics: One source of tinnitus. In D. Evered & G. Lawrenson (eds.): *Tinnitus: Ciba foundation symposium* (pp. 54–81). Pitman Books: London.

Kemp, D. T. (1982). Cochlear echoes: Implications for noise-induced hearing loss. In R. P. Hamernik, D. Henderson, & R. Salvi (eds.): *New perspectives on noise-induced hearing loss* (pp. 189–207). Raven: New York.

Kemp, D. T. (1986). Otoacoustic emissions, travelling waves and cochlear mechanisms. *Hearing Research, 22,* 95–104.

Köhler, W., & Fritze, W. (1992). A long-term observation of spontaneous otoacoustic emissions (SOAEs). *Scandinavian Audiology, 21,* 55–58.

Kok, M. R., van Zanten, G. A., & Brocaar, M. P. (1993). Aspects of spontaneous otoacoustic emissions in healthy newborns. *Hearing Research, 69,* 115–123.

Köppl, C., & Manley, G. A. (1993). Spontaneous otoacoustic emissions in the bobtail lizard: I. General characteristics. *Hearing Research, 71,* 157–169.

Kossl, M., & Vater, M. (1985). Evoked acoustic emissions and cochlear microphonics in the mustache bat, *Pteronotus parnellii. Hearing Research, 19,* 157–170.

Lind, O., & Randa, J. S. (1990). Spontaneous otoacoustic emissions: Incidence and short-time variability in normal ears. *Journal of Otolaryngology, 19,* 252–259.

Long, G. R. (1984). The microstructure of quiet and masked thresholds. *Hearing Research, 15,* 73–87.

Long, G. R., & Tubis, A. (1988). Investigations into the nature of the association between threshold microstructure and otoacoustic emissions. *Hearing Research, 36,* 125–138.

Long, G. R., & Tubis, A. (1988a). Modification of spontaneous and evoked otoacoustic emissions and associated psychoacoustic microstructure by aspirin consumption. *Journal of the Acoustical Society of America, 84,* 1343–1353.

Lonsbury-Martin, B. L., Harris, F. P., Stagner, B. B., Hawkins, M. D., & Martin, G. K. (1990). Distortion product emissions in humans: II. Relations to acoustic immittance and stimulus frequency and spontaneous otoacoustic emissions in normally hearing subjects. *Annals of Otology, Rhinology and Laryngology, 99* (Suppl. 147), 15–29.

Lonsbury-Martin, B. L., & Martin, G. K. (1988). Incidence of spontaneous otoacoustic emission in macaque monkeys: A replication. *Hearing Research, 34,* 313–318.

Lonsbury-Martin, B. L., Martin, G. K., Probst, R., & Coats, A. C. (1988) Spontaneous otoacoustic emissions in a nonhuman primate: II. Cochlear anatomy. *Hearing Research, 33,* 69–94.

Manley, G. A. (1993). Frequency spacing of acoustic emissions. A possible explanation. In W. R. Webster & L. M. Aitkin (eds.): *Mechanisms of hearing* (pp. 36–39). Clayton, Australia: Monash University Press.

Manley, G. A., & Köppl, C. (1994). Spontaneous otoacoustic emissions in the bobtail lizard. III. Temperature effects. *Hearing Research, 72,* 171–180.

Martin, G. K., Lonsbury-Martin, B. L., Probst, R., & Coats, A.C. (1985). Spontaneous otoacoustic emissions in the nonhuman primate: A survey. *Hearing Research, 20,* 91–95.

Martin, G., Probst, R., & Lonsbury-Martin, B. L. (1990). Otoacoustic emissions in human ears: Normative findings. *Ear and Hearing, 11,* 106–120.

Mathis, A., Probst, R., DeMin, N., & Hauser, R. (1991). A child with an unusually high level spontaneous otoacoustic emission. *Archives of Otolaryngology, Head and Neck Surgery, 117,* 674–676.

Mayhew, I. G., Preston, S. E., Hannant, D., Washburn, J. R., Johnson, C. B., & Phillips, T. J. (1995). Spontaneous otoacoustic emission in a pony. *Veterinary Record, 136,* 149.

McFadden, D., & Mishra, R. (1993). On the relation between hearing sensitivity and otoacoustic emissions. *Hearing Research, 71,* 208–213.

McFadden, D., & Plattsmier, H. S. (1984). Aspirin abolishes spontaneous otoacoustic emissions. *Hearing Research, 16,* 251–260.

Michey, C., & Collet, L. (1994). Interrelations between psychoacoustical tuning urves and spontaneous and evoked otoacoustic emissions. *Scandinavian Audiolology, 23,* 171–178.

Mott, J. B., Norton, S. J., Neely, S. T., & Warr, W. B. (1989). Changes in spontaneous otoacoustic emissions produced by acoustic stimulation of the contralateral ear. *Hearing Research, 38,* 229–242.

Moulin, A., Collet, L., Delli, D., & Morgon, A. (1991). Spontaneous otoacoustic emisions and sensori-neural hearing loss. *Acta Oto-Laryngologica, 111,* 835–841.

Moulin, A., Collet, L., & Morgon, A. (1992). Influence of spontaneous otoacoustic emissions (SOAE) on acoustic distortion product input/output functions: Does the medial efferent system act differently in the vicinity of an SOAE? *Acta Oto-Laryngologica, 112,* 210–214.

Moulin, A., Collet, L., Veuillet, E., & Morgon, A. (1993). Interrelations between transiently evoked otoacoustic emissions, spontaneous otoacoustic emissions and acoustic distortion products in normally hearing subjects. *Hearing Research, 65,* 216–233.

Norton, S. J., Mott, J. B., Champlin, C. A. (1989). Behavior of spontaneous otoacoustic emissions following intense ipsilateral acoustic stimulation. *Hearing Research, 38,* 243–258.

Norton, S. J., & Neely, S. T. (1987). Tone-burst-evoked otoacoustic emissions from normal-hearing subjects. *Journal of the Acoustical Society of America, 81,* 1860–1872.

Ohyama, K., Wada, H., Kobayashi, T., & Takasada, T. (1991). Spontaneous otoacoustic emissions in the guinea pig. *Hearing Research, 56,* 111–121.

Penner, M. J. (1988). Audible and annoying spontaneous otoacoustic emissions. *Archives of Otolaryngology, Head and Neck Surgery, 114,* 150–153.

Penner, M. J. (1989). Empirical tests demonstrating two co-existing sources of tinnitus: A case study. *Journal of Speech and Hearing Research, 32,* 458–462.

Penner, M. J. (1990). An estimate of the prevalence of tinnitus caused by spontaneous otoacoustic emissions. *Archives of Otolaryngology, Head and Neck Surgery, 116,* 418–423.

Penner, M. J. (1992). Linking spontaneous otoacoustic emissions and tinnitus. *British Journal of Audiology, 26,* 115–123.

Penner, M. J., Brauth, S. E., & Jastreboff, P. J. (1994). Covariation of binaural, concurrently-measured spontaneous otoacoustic emissions. *Hearing Research, 73,* 190–194.

Penner, M. J., & Burns, E. M. (1987). The dissociation of SOAEs and tinnitus. *Journal of Speech and Hearing Research, 30,* 396–403.

Penner, M. J., & Coles, R. R. A. (1992). Indications for aspirin as a palliative for tinnitus caused by SOAEs: A case study. *British Journal of Audiology, 26,* 91–96.

Plinkert, P. K., Gitter, A. H., & Zenner, H. P. (1990). Tinnitus associated spontaneous otoacoustic emissions. *Acta Oto-Laryngologica, 110,* 342–347.

Penner, M. J., Glotzbach, L., & Huang, T. (1993). Spontaneous otoacoustic emissions: Measurement and data. *Hearing Research, 68,* 229–237.

Probst, R., Coats, A. C., Martin, G. K., & Lonsbury-Martin, B. L. (1986). Spontaneous, click- and toneburst-evoked otoacoustic emissions from normal ears. *Hearing Research, 21,* 261–275.

Probst, R., Lonsbury-Martin, B. L., & Martin, G. K. (1991). A review of otoacoustic emissions. *Journal of the Acoustical Society of America, 89,* 2027–2067.

Probst, R., Lonsbury-Martin, B. L., Martin, G., & Coats, A. C. (1987). Otoacoustic emissions in ears with hearing loss. *American Journal of Otolaryngology, 8,* 73–81.

Rabinowitz, W. M., & Widin, G. P. (1984). Interaction of spontaneous otoacoustic emissions and external sounds. *Journal of the Acoustical Society of America, 76,* 1713–1720.

Rebillard, G., Abou, S., & Lenoir, M. (1987). Les oto-émissions acoustiques II. Les oto-émissions spontanees: Resultats chez des sujets normaux ou présentant des acouphénes. *Annals of Otolaryngololology, 104,* 363–368.

Ruggero, M. A., Kramek, B., & Rich, N. C. (1984). Spontaneous otoacoustic emissions in a dog. *Hearing Research, 13,* 293–296.

Ruggero, M. A., Rich, N. C., & Freyman, R. (1983). Spontaneous and impulsively evoked otoacoustic emissions: Indicators of cochlear pathology? *Hearing Research, 10,* 283–300.

Schloth, E. (1983). Relation between spectral composition of spontaneous otoacoustic emissions and fine-structure of threshold in quiet. *Acustica, 53,* 250–256.

Schloth, E., & Zwicker, E. (1983). Mechanical and acoustical influences on spontaneous otoacoustic emissions. *Hearing Research, 11,* 285–293.

Stover, L., & Norton, S. J. (1993). The effects of aging on otoacoustic emissions. *Journal of the Acoustical Society of America, 94,* 2670–2681.

Strickland, A. E., Burns, E. M., & Tubis A. (1985). Incidence of spontaneous otoacoustic emissions in children and infants. *Journal of the Acoustical Society of America, 78,* 931–935.

Talmadge, C. L., Long, G. R., Murphy, W. J., & Tubis, A. (1993). New off-line method for detecting spontaneous otoacoustic emissions in human subjects. *Hearing Reseach, 71,* 170–182.

Tyler, R. S., & Conrad-Armes, D. (1982). Spontaneous acoustic cochlear emissions and sensorineural tinnitus. *British Journal of Audiology, 16,* 193–194.

van Dijk, P., Wit, H. P., & Segenhout, J. M. (1989). Spontaneous otoacoustic emissions in the European edible frog (*Rana esculenta*): Spectral details and temperature dependence. *Hearing Research, 42,* 273–282.

Whitehead, M. L., Baker, R. J., & Wilson, J. P. (1989). The bilateral symmetry and sex asymmetry of spontaneous otoacoustic emission (SOAE) incidence in human ears. *British Journal of Audiology, 23,* 149.

Whitehead, M. L., Kamal, N., Lonsbury-Martin, B. L., & Martin, G. K. (1993). Spontaneous otoacoustic emissions in different racial groups. *Scandinavian Audiology, 22,* 3–10.

Wier, C. C., Pasanen, E. G., & McFadden, D. (1988). Partial dissociation of spontaneous otoacoustic emissions and distortion products during aspirin use in humans. *Journal of the Acoustical Society of America, 84,* 230–237.

Wilson, J. P. (1980). Evidence for a cochlear origin for acoustic re-emissions, threshold fine-structure and tonal tinnitus. *Hearing Research, 2,* 233–252.

Wilson, J. P., & Sutton, G. J. (1981). Acoustic correlates of tonal tinnitus. In D. Evered & G. Lawrenson (eds.): *Tinnitus: Ciba foundation symposium* (pp. 82–107), London: Pitman Books.

Wilson, J. P., & Sutton, G. J. (1983). A family with high-tonal objective tinnitus: An update. In R. Klinke & R. Hartmann, (eds.): *Hearing: Physiological bases and psychophysics* (pp. 97–103). Berlin, Springer-Verlag.

Wit, H. P., & van Dijk, P. (1990). Spectral line width of spontaneous otoacoustic emissions. In F. Grandori, G. Cianfrone, D. T. Kemp (eds.): *Cochlear mechanisms and otoacoustic emissions* (pp. 110–116). Basel, Switzerland: Kruger.

Yamamoto, E., Tagaki, A., Hirono, Y., & Yagi, N. (1987). A case of 'spontaneous otoacoustic emission'. *Archives of Otolaryngology, Head and Neck Surgery, 113,* 1316–1318.

Zizz, C. A., & Glattke, T. J. (1988). Reliability of spontaneous otoacoustic emission suppression tuning curve measures. *Journal of Speech and Hearing Research, 31,* 616–619.

Zurek, P. (1981). Spontaneous narrowband acoustic signals emitted by human ears. *Journal of the Acoustical Society of America, 69,* 514–523.

Zurek, P. M., & Clark, W. W. (1981). Narrow-band acoustic signals emitted by chinchilla ears after noise exposure. *Journal of the Acoustical Society of America, 70,* 446–450.

Zwicker, E., & Schloth, E. (1984). Interrelation of different oto-acoustic emissions. *Journal of the Acoustical Society of America, 75,* 1148–1154.

4

Transient Evoked
Otoacoustic Emissions

Theodore J. Glattke
Martin S. Robinette

Introduction

Transient evoked otoacoustic emissions (TEOAEs) are complex acoustic events that can be recorded in nearly all persons who have normal hearing. Kemp's (1978) initial report of TEOAEs described several of their properties. As he noted, when a click stimulus is used to elicit the response, the emission waveform is idiosyncratic and is likely to be dominated by different frequency components at different moments in time. Kemp (1978) noted that energy in the frequency region near 1500 Hz dominated the response to acoustic click stimuli and that the response amplitude was related to the stimulus magnitude in a complex way. However, TEOAE responses from individuals with normal thresholds have signatures that are unique. Responses obtained from stimuli that are near perceptual threshold may reflect energy levels that approach the energy in the applied stimulus (Wilson, 1980). As the stimulus intensity increases, the response amplitude increases at a slower rate, growing by about 20 to 30 dB for a stimulus increment of 60 to 70 dB (Kemp, 1978). The pattern of growth of the response is compatible with the leakage of energy into the ear canal from the operation of the "cochlear amplifier" (Davis, 1983), which provides substantial gain for low intensity stimuli and reaches saturation for stimuli in the mid-intensity range (Johnstone, Patuzzi, & Yates, 1986). As Wilson noted, "an AGC system is operating or some frequency filtering follows the saturation process as the waveforms do not show clipping (Wilson, 1980a, p. 235)."

Many of the early investigations of TEOAEs focused on demonstrations that emissions were caused by mechanical activity that originated in the cochlea, rather than electrical or mechanical artifacts or oscillation of the middle ear. Hence, Kemp (1978) compared responses obtained from passive couplers and ears with hearing loss to those obtained from ears with normal thresholds. The recording apparatus was mechanically and electrically isolated following many of the steps described by Wever and Bray (1930) who identified the presence of microphonic potentials detected by electrodes placed near the cochlea nearly 50 years prior to the discovery of emissions by Kemp. Kemp (1978) reported that the responses could be altered in animals after administration of loop diuretics and noise exposure. Kemp's initial report also described the suppression of emissions that were elicited by tone bursts. The interaction between the suppressor tone, presented continuously and ipsilateral to the stimulus, and the resulting TEOAEs revealed a high degree of frequency selectivity. The general finding indicating the presence of a sharply tuned mechanical system associated with the production of emissions has been replicated by several subsequent investigations (Harris & Glattke, 1992). For example, Wit and Ritsma (1979) confirmed Kemp's observations regarding suppression of responses elicited by tone bursts and displayed a suppression tuning curve for stimuli at 1700 Hz. The tuning curve patterns associated with the suppression phenomenon are similar to those based on electrophysiologic recordings from single cells in the auditory periphery and psychophysical procedures (Kemp, 1979a).

By the end of the 1970s, the literature regarding emission characteristics included a modest number of manuscripts (Kemp, 1978, 1979a, 1979b; Wit & Ritsma, 1979) that described a wide range of emission properties and paved the way for a virtual explosion of applied research based on the phenomenon. For example, Johnsen and Elberling (1982, 1983) presented data gathered from small groups of young adults and neonates; Elberling, Parbo, Johnsen, and Bagi (1985) addressed clinical applications; and Kemp, Bray, Alexander, and Brown (1986) used the phrase "acoustic emission cochleography" to describe proposed clinical-test protocols that were evaluated on about 130 ears. Although important exceptions have occurred (Bonfils & Uziel, 1989; Prieve et al., 1993; Wilson, 1980), most of the published studies of TEOAEs have employed computer-based averaging procedures that are similar to those used in clinical electrophysiological studies and many of the clinical investigations of TEOAEs have used the ILO 88 equipment produced by Otodynamics (Kemp, Ryan, & Bray, 1990).

ILO 88 Analysis and Display

An example of a TEOAE obtained with ILO 88 equipment from a subject with normal hearing is illustrated in Figure 4–1. The data display contains information about the stimulus, recording situation and properties of the response. The key elements of the display are outlined in Table 4–1.

Characteristics of TEOAEs Elicited with Default Stimuli

Clinical appraisal of electrophysiological responses, such as the auditory–brainstem response (ABR) and electrocochleographic recordings obtained from the eighth cranial nerve, rely on estimates of response threshold, latency and amplitude to estimate the integrity of the auditory system. Kemp (1978) noted the highly nonlinear nature of the response, and he and his coworkers noted that the minimum intensity at which a TEOAE can be detected rarely corresponds with perceptual threshold (Kemp, Ryan, & Bray, 1990). Kemp (1978) noted that the apparent

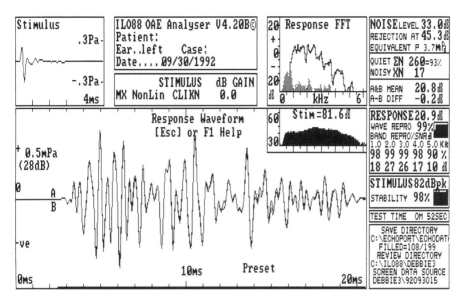

Figure 4–1. Normal TEOAE response Figure.

"threshold" of the response is critically dependent upon the noise in the recording situation as well as the status of the ear under test. For example, although a newborn may have robust emissions, physiological noise produced by the neonate may preclude detection of the emissions at "threshold" levels. Similarly, an ear with strong emission responses may reveal little attenuation of the response with significant reductions of the stimulus intensity, as little as 0.1 dB per 1 dB change (Kemp, Ryan, & Bray, 1990). Thus, it is impossible to estimate threshold of hearing from the apparent threshold of the emission response or extrapolate from detected responses to presumed threshold based on amplitude measurements. Kemp (1978), Prieve et al. (1993), Grandori and Ravazzani (1993), Stover and Norton (1993), and Prieve and Falter (1995) have examined the complex interaction between click-stimulus intensity and response characteristics, including threshold. As Kemp, Ryan, and Bray noted, researchers are far from having a standard against which response threshold, latency, and growth characteristics can be evaluated in a clinical setting. In this sense, the TEOAEs share difficulties encountered in the interpretation of cochlear microphonic potentials that, like the emissions, are intimately related to the status of the hair cells in the cochlea (Glattke, 1983).

The most common clinical application of TEOAEs involves click stimuli presented at moderate intensities (80 dB peak equivalent SPL or about 45 dB above perceptual threshold). The default stimulus employed by the ILO 88 equipment was selected to screen for hearing loss: If no response can be obtained, then it is likely the patient has a hearing loss. Generally, the spectrum of a TEOAE elicited from a healthy ear reflects the spectrum of the stimulus. TEOAEs obtained in response to click stimuli are expected to have broad response spectra. The amplitudes of TEOAEs vary directly with the amplitudes of the stimuli, but the relations

Table 4–1.   Key Elements of the ILO 88 Display

Stimulus	This includes an illustration of the stimulus waveform that was sampled prior to the onset of data collection. The duration of the electric pulse applied to the transducer was 80 µs. The time axis spans 5 ms and the decay of the transducer reponse can be seen to extend over a 2–3 ms period. The amplitude scale is indicated in Pascals (Pa). The registration of 0.3 Pa is equivalent to 83.5 dB SPL. The stimulus waveform illustrated in the panel is biphasic and decays rapidly after completion of the initial pulse. The peak amplitude in Figure 4–1 is slightly less than 0.3 Pa.
Patient/Software	The center panels identify the version of the software used to display the data (V4.20B in Figure 4–1, and information about the patient, ear tested and stimulus mode. The designation MX NONLIN CLICKN indicates that the ILO 88 default nonlinear stimulus mode was used to obtain the data. In this mode of operation, the responses are gathered from a stimulus sequence illustrated in Figure 4–2. Responses are gathered for sets of four stimuli. Three are presented in one phase at the indicated amplitude and the fourth is presented in the opposite phase at a level that is 3 times greater than each of the three previous stimuli. The sum of the responses to the four stimuli consists of waveforms that follow the stimulus precisely (*linear components*) and components that do not change in a simple fashion with stimulus intensity or phase (*nonlinear components*). Because the power in the fourth stimulus is equal to the sum of the powers of the first three and because the phase of 4th stimulus is inverted, the sum of the linear components will be 0, and only the nonlinear portions of the transducer and ear response will remain. This mode of stimulus presentation results in an average response that reduces stimulus artifacts and linear portions of the ear's response to the transients. Although little empirical data exist, Kemp, Bray, Alexander, and Brown (1986) estimated that, using this stimulus method, the linear stimulus artifacts and response components could be reduced by 40 dB while the desired nonlinear portion of the emission would be reduced by only 6 dB. In the default setting, the ILO 88 software obtains a response for one group of transient stimuli and stores that result in a memory buffer identified as *A*. The response for the next group of stimuli is stored in a buffer identified as *B*. The sampling process continues until response from 260 sets of stimuli have been stored in each of the two memory areas. Therefore, the A and B waveforms each represent the mean of responses to 260 × 4 transients or 1040 stimuli, and the total number of stimuli employed in the default condition is 2080.

The *dB Gain* value noted in the stimulus description panel indicates the gain employed to reach the nominal stimulus level. The default stimulus level is approximately 80 dB peak equivalent SPL, but other values can be selected. |
| Response Waveform | The display illustrates the time-averaged waveforms sampled for a 20.48 ms period following the onset of the transient stimulus. Tracings are plotted for the A and B memory locations and each tracing consists of 512 data points. Each data point corresponds to a period of 40 µs. The first 2.5 ms, or 63 data points, have been eliminated to reduce the contribution of a stimulus artifact to the average response waveform. The vertical scale in the response waveform panel is set at 0.5 mPa at the positions of the + and − symbols. This represents a gain of 600 (55 dB) over the representation of the stimulus waveform, i.e., if the wave- |

Table 4–1.   (*Continued*)

Waveform Response (*cont.*)	form in the stimulus window oscillates over a period that extends beyond 2.5 ms, the ringing activity will appear as a large series of oscillations in the response waveform because of the amplification employed for the response window.
Response FFT	This display provides illustrations of the fast Fourier transforms (FFT) that are based on the A and B waveforms. The resolution of the FFT analysis is approximately 49 Hz per line. The open histogram reflects the spectrum of the response that is common to the A and B tracings. This is considered to be the true emission response. The cross-hatched display represents the spectrum of the difference between the A and B waveforms, or the noise that remains in the average waveform. The horizontal scale extends from 0 to 6000 Hz. The vertical scale extends from below −20 dB to approximately +20 dB SPL. In the example, the major concentration of energy in the common or correlated portions of the A and B waveforms is in the frequency region between 1000 and 2500 Hz, where the response level reaches approximately 5 dB SPL. Response amplitude is attenuated in the high-frequency region.
Stim	This display provides a tabular representation of the peak equivalent SPL of the stimulus at the onset of the sampling. The spectrum of the stimulus is illustrated by the solid histogram. The horizontal scale of the stimulus spectrum is identical to the horizontal scale for the response FFT. The vertical scale extends from 30 dB SPL to above 60 dB. For a typical transient stimulus with a peak level of 80 dB SPL, the spectrum level (or level per cycle) will be 40–45 dB SPL.
Noise	The tabular value of the noise is the average SPL detected by the microphone during the samples that were not rejected by the software.
Rejection at ____ dB	The software permits the examiner to select a rejection threshold to reduce unwanted noise. The default rejection threshold is 47 dB SPL and the range available to the examiner extends from 24–55 dB SPL. The rejection level can be adjusted continuously throughout the sampling period and the tabular value is the threshold selected by the examiner at the end of the sampling. The rejection threshold value also is shown in mPa.
Quiet > N	This entry is the number of responses accepted for the A and the B waveforms. As illustrated in Figure 4–2, a response consists of the sum of the acoustic events recorded for a set of four transient stimuli. The percentage of all samples accepted for the average waveform is also listed in tabular form.
Noisy XN	This entry is a tally of the number of response sets that were rejected during the sampling procedure. In Figure 4–1, responses to 17 stimulus sets were rejected and so the acceptance rate was 93%.
A & B Mean	This is the sound pressure level of the average of the A and B waveforms.
A–B Diff	This is the average difference between the A and B waveforms and is the level of energy represented by the cross-hatched area of the *Response FFT* window. It is computed by taking the difference between the A and B waveforms on a point-by-point basis minus 3 dB.
Response	This value is the overall level of the correlated portions of the A and B response waveforms and is obtained from the FFT displayed in the *Response FFT* window. In Figure 4–1, the *A & B Mean* and the *Response* values are essentially identical because the *A–B Diff* is less than 1% of the power in the average waveforms.

(*continued*)

Table 4–1.   (*Continued*)

Wave Repro	This entry is actually the value of the cross correlation between the A and B waveforms expressed as a percentage. The correlation is recomputed after every 20 stimulus sets and the value of the correlation is represented in the small histogram to the right of the percentage. The result in Figure 4–1 is 99%, reflecting a near-perfect correlation, which is compatible with the very small *A–B Diff* value.
Band Repro % SNR dB	The reproducibility and signal to noise ratio values are listed below column headings of 1.0–5.0 kHz. To obtain the results, the A and B waveforms are filtered into bandwidths of approximately 1000 Hz centered at the indicated frequencies. The correlations are recomputed and the difference between the powers computed for the FFTs represented by the open and cross-hatched histograms in the *Response FFT* window are represented as the signal to noise ratio at each frequency.
Stimulus ___ dB pk	The stimulus intensity is measured after every 16 stimulus sets. The tabular value listed at this location is the result of the final computation. The final result may be different than the value obtained at the outset of the sampling procedure. The initial value is tabulated in the portion of the display containing the stimulus spectrum.
Stability ___ %	This entry and the accompanying histogram reflects changes that occur in the stimulus intensity. The single-percentage entry expresses that greatest difference detected between the first and any subsequent stimulus throughout the sampling period as a percentage, rather than dB value (1 dB ≈ 10%). The small histogram to the right of the entry chronicles the history of the stimulus intensity measurements.
Test time	This entry records the duration of the test.

between stimulus and response are complicated by the fact that TEOAEs result from highly nonlinear phenomena. From the outset, reports of properties of TEOAEs elicited from normal ears have emphasized the idiosyncratic nature of the responses. Unfortunately, few studies have provided tabular summaries of the data provided by the ILO 88 software or grouped data in terms of age, gender, and right-left differences. The following data were obtained using ILO 88 default stimulus conditions: (a) 80 μs transients; (b) nominal stimulus level of 80 to 83 dB peak equivalent SPL; and (c) nonlinear mode, unless noted otherwise. (See Figure 4–2.)

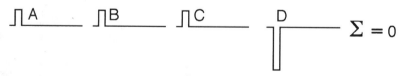

Figure 4–2.   Illustration of "nonlinear" stimulus mode. The stimuli are presented in groups of four. The first three in each group are presented in one phase. The fourth is produced in the opposite phase and at an amplitude that is three times greater than each of the preceding transients. The sum of the stimuli in each group and any portion of the transducer or ear response that follows the stimuli exactly will be zero. Any differences due to nonlinear behavior of the transducer or ear will be preserved.

Responses Obtained From Children

An example of a TEOAE response obtained from a newborn is provided in Figure 4–3. The noise produced during recordings obtained from cooperative newborns usually is concentrated in the low frequency region and results from activity related to respiration and swallowing or sucking. In Figure 4–3, the pattern of "noise" or the uncorrelated portion of the *Response FFT* display is consistent with noise generated by the baby. A poor coupling between the microphone or excessive noise in the test facility would be reflected in a spectrum that de-emphasizes the contribution of low-frequency, physiological components. As Harris and Probst (1991) noted, the whole-reproducibility score is influenced strongly by the low frequency components present in the A and B waveforms. This results from the fact that the cross correlation is between the A and B waveforms is based on all the data points representing the A and B waveforms between 2.5 and 20.48 ms. Because it

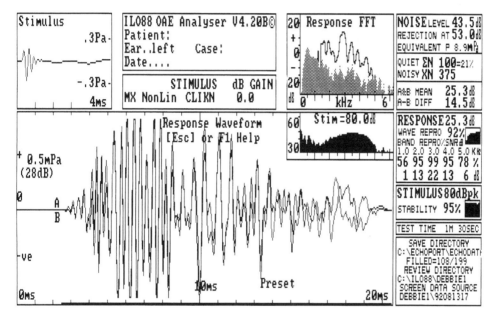

Figure 4–3. TEOAE response obtained from a newborn. The stimulus waveform reveals a slight ringing action and the stimulus spectrum reflects loss of energy in the low frequency region. The response waveforms were robust, and the noise levels were substantial. Note that the rejection threshold was set to a level of 53 dB (or 6 dB above the default setting) and set very near to the maximum permitted by the software. Consistent with the high level of noise during the recording period, only about 21% of the samples were accepted, and the sampling was terminated after 100 quiet samples were obtained.

The uncorrelated portions of the average waveforms also contribute to a robust average (14.5 dB) which falls well below the power in the correlated portion of the after waveforms. Hence the tabular value of the Response remains high. Reproducibility was high but not at the same value in Figure 4–1. Poor reproducibility in the low frequency region was a major factor in reducing the overall reproducibility score.

has a relatively long period, a low-frequency component with a duration of one or two cycles will involve proportionally more data points than a similar contribution from a response in the high frequency region. As Whitehead, Jimenez, Stagner, McCoy, Lonsbury-Martin, and Martin (1995) and Hills and Glattke (1996) have found, restricting the time window over which the ILO 88 cross-correlation is computed may enhance the apparent signal to noise ratio and associated reproducibility scores.

The amplitude of responses recorded from neonates has been reported to exceed the amplitude of those obtained from adults by 10 dB or more and the 95th percentile for TEOAE response amplitude has been estimated to be 26 dB SPL (Kemp, Ryan, & Bray; Kemp & Ryan, 1993). Kok, van Zanten, and Brocaar (1992) reported that the magnitude of the TEOAE grows idiosyncratically with age during the first few days of life of normal newborns. Van Zanten, Kok, Brocaar, and Sauer (1995) also studied emission characteristics in 144 low-birthweight children and reported that TEOAE amplitudes appeared to grow by approximately 10 dB between the postconceptional ages of 31 and 42 weeks. They observed that TEOAE amplitude reached maximum values for infants at a postconceptional age of 47 weeks. Kok, van Zanten, Brocaar, and Jongejan (1994) examined a similar group of children and noted that the responses of low-birthweight infants approached the levels found in healthy newborns when they were tested between 37 and 66 weeks after conception. Kok, Van Zanten, Brocaar, and Wallenburg (1993) reported data gathered from a large group of healthy newborns. A portion of their effort was devoted to determining the prevalence of TEOAEs as a function of hours aged. Using an objective criterion based on a whole reproducibility score greater than 50%, they report success rate in obtaining TEOAEs of approximately 75% of the ears tested when the infants were less than 36 hours old. The success rate rose to about 95% for infants greater than 108 hours old. (The success rate reported apparently reflects the result of a single attempt to obtain a response. Recent experiences in neonatal screening programs suggest that a pass rate greater than 90% can be expected for infants less than 24-hours old if multiple attempts are made to screen children within the first–24-hour period.)

Kok et al. (1993) also provided a comparison of response amplitudes obtained from the newborns with those obtained from a small group of adults with normal hearing. The median response amplitude for the neonates was approximately 16 dB SPL for those who were 24 hours old. Median response amplitude rose to approximately 20 dB and 22 dB SPL for tests conducted at the ages of 48 and 72 hours, respectively. The corresponding median value for adults included in their investigation was approximately 12 dB. The findings from a number of other studies are similar (Collet, Gartner, Veuillet, & Moulin, 1993: Johnsen, Bagi, Parbo, & Elberling, 1988; Norton & Widen, 1990; Smurzynski, 1994; Smurzynski, Jung, Lafreniere, Kim, Kamath, Rowe, Holman, Leanard, 1993; Smurzynski, Jung, Leonard, & Kim, 1993; Thornton, Kimm, Kennedy, & Cafarelli-Dees, 1994; Uziel & Piron, 1991; Zorowka, Schmitt, Eckel, & Lippert, 1993). The robust TEOAE-response amplitude in normal newborns has been a primary factor in the success of neonatal screening programs. No significant differences in response amplitude have been reported between right and left ears or between male and female ears in the neonatal.

An interesting trend in the property of the amplitude of the TEOAE default stimulus was noted by Kok, van Zanten, Brocaar and Wallenburg. The stimulus value registered for normal neonates who failed to reveal an emission was significantly greater than for those who did produce an emission response. They speculated that the middle-ear–fluid may have resulted in an increased impedance and in greater reflectance of energy from the tympanic membrane in the neonates who failed to produce an emission response.

Neonatal TEOAEs have been reported to reveal a boost in the energy in the high frequency region when compared with the responses obtained from adults with normal hearing (Kemp, Ryan, & Bray; Norton & Widen; Smurzynski, 1994; Lafreniere, Jung, Smurzynski, Leonard, Kim, & Sasek, 1991). As Norton and Widen noted, the increase may be due to obvious differences in size and shape of the middle- and outer-ear systems and their effects on the resonance characteristics of the ear, rather than changes in cochlear mechanics. For example, the resonance of the middle ear in neonates would be at a higher frequency than the resonance of the middle ear in older children or adults. This difference could produce for improved forward and reverse transmission of energy in the region above 1500 Hz and could support the improvement in the high-frequency portion of the emission.

A few studies have explored the relation between spontaneous otoacoustic emissions (SOAEs) and TEOAEs in neonates. Morlet et al. (1995) noted that SOAEs were recorded in 84% of 93 preterm and full-term infants. The average TEOAE amplitude was greater in the ears with SOAEs (23.42 dB SPL) than in those without an SOAE (19.38 dB SPL).

TEOAE responses for default stimulus conditions in more than 350 children with normal pure-tone thresholds better than or equal to 20 dB HL for frequencies of 250 through 4000 Hz have been described by Glattke, Pafitis, Cummiskey, and Herer (1995). An example of a TEOAE response obtained from a cooperative child 6 years of age is provided in Figure 4–4.

In the Glattke et al. (1995) study, responses were considered to be present if the reproducibility score 50% or greater. They found that responses were present in 87% of ears with normal thresholds using the whole reproducibility score, and were present in 95% of the same ears using the reproducibility score at 2000 Hz. Glattke et al (1995) reported that the average values of the *A + B* and *Response* outcomes were 11.9 and 10.9 dB SPL, respectively, for children with normal pure tone thresholds. Whole-reproducibility averaged 77.3%, but the average reproducibility value for the 1000 Hz bandwidth centered at 2000 Hz was 87%. This is consistent with Kemp's 1978 report regarding the frequency region of the most robust portion of the response, and the outcome of other parametric studies, such as that reported by Prieve et al. (1993). In contrast to reports regarding the properties of responses in newborns, Glattke et al. (1995) reported a slight difference in results when responses were compared for right and left ears. In general, responses from right ears were slightly more robust (~1 dB) than those obtained from the left ear. The average noise level in the recordings summarized by Glattke et al (1995) was 36.4 dB SPL.

Responses Obtained From Adults

Robinette (1992) reported the outcome of a systematic examination of responses obtained from 265 adults who ranged in age from 20 to 80 years and whose

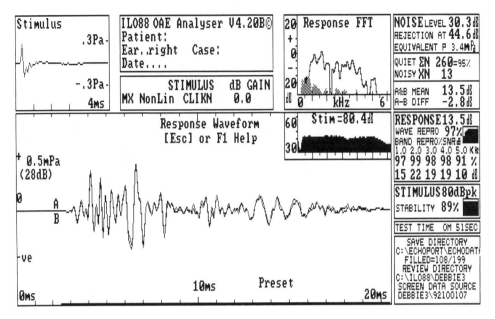

Figure 4–4. TEOAE response obtained from a cooperative 6-year-old child. The stimulus was recorded at approximately 80 dB at the outset and termination of the sampling procedure. The noise level was recorded at approximately 30 dB, and the rejection level was set at 44.6 dB (below the default setting). Approximately 95% of the samples were accepted for averaging purposes. The average power in the A and B waveforms is 13.5, and the intensity of the uncorrelated portions of the A and B waveforms is at −2.8 dB, more than 16 dB below the overall average power. As a result, intensity of the response was unaltered. Reproducibility was excellent, stimulus stability was 89%, and changes in stimulus intensity were minimal (approximately 1 dB) during the sampling. The figure reveals a clear dispersion of the individual frequency components of the response. Robust high-frequency components emerged within the first 6 ms after the stimulus. They were followed by mid- and low-frequency components, although rapid fluctuations indicating the presence of sustained activity in the high frequency region can be observed throughout the average waveforms.

audiometric thresholds were better than or equal to 25 dB HL between 500 and 6000 Hz. Robinette reported that "observable TEOAEs" were found for all normal ears. The oldest patient in the group of subjects with normal thresholds produced TEOAEs with an *A + B amplitude* of approximately 12 dB SPL, which is equivalent to the average value found for children by Glattke et al. (1995). However, the average values of *A + B amplitudes* reported by Robinette (1992) decreased from 9.7 dB SPL for the 20-to-29-year-old group to 7.2 dB SPL for the subjects with normal who were 60 to 80 years of age. Robinette (1992) noted that TEOAEs were more robust in women than in men and more robust in the right ear than in the left. The average noise level reported by Robinette was approximately 32.3 dB SPL for adults, approximately 4 dB below the average noise found for children by Glattke et al. (1995). An example of a response obtained from a 28-year-old female subject is provided in Figure 4–5.

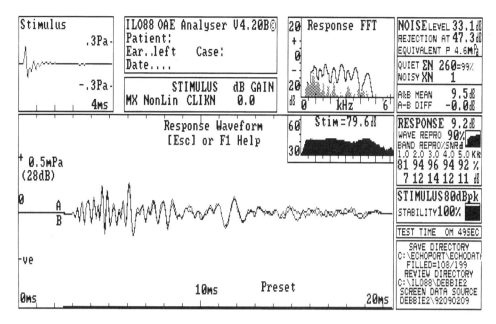

Figure 4–5. TEOAE response obtained from a 28-year-old woman. The clear-frequency dispersion illustrated in Figure 4–4 is apparent in this example. High-frequency response components emerge and decay between 2.5 and 6 ms after stimulus onset. Robust mid-frequency components are apparent in the interval between 7 and 9 ms, and lower frequency energy appeared at about 10.5 ms. The stimulus level was stable at approximately 80 dB. Noise level was 33.1 dB and the average SPL of the A and B waveforms was 9.5 dB. The mid-frequency reproducibility scores are greater than the whole reproducibility and the reproducibility score at 1000 Hz.

The literature contains conflicting statements regarding the properties of TEOAEs in adults grouped according to age at the time of test. For example, Bonfils, Bertrand, and Uziel (1988), Collet, Gartner, Moulin, and Morgon (1990), and Robinette—all noted either that the probability of recording a TEOAE or the amplitude of the TEOAE is reduced when results from older adults are compared with those obtained from younger adults. Stover and Norton concluded that, even though hearing thresholds may be within the range of what is considered to be audiometrically normal, TEOAE characteristics change with slight changes in threshold for all age groups. Older subjects are more likely to have audiometric thresholds at the upper limit of the normal range and, as a result, are also likely to have less robust TEOAE-responses than young adults' responses. Stover and Norton's investigation employed stimulus generation and response analysis techniques that were based on specialized laboratory equipment, not the ILO 88 system. They measured TEOAE amplitude and thresholds for click stimuli that ranged between approximately 10 and 70 dB SPL; they interpreted their data to suggest that both age and hearing sensitivity contribute to the changes seen in emissions obtained from older subjects, and changes in hearing sensitivity offered considerable confounding influence on attempts to study age effects.

Glattke, Robinette, Pafitis, Cummiskey, and Herer (1994) merged data files from three clinical sites to develop an impression of the properties of TEOAEs in normal-hearing subjects aged from 2 to 83 years. The TEOAE records obtained using default-stimulus conditions were examined for 505 subjects with pure-tone thresholds of 20 dB or better for 250 through 4000 Hz. Measures of the *A + B average*, the *A − B Difference*, and the *Response* (Figure 4–1) all declined with increasing age. When a very strict criterion was used to identify normal thresholds (≤ 10 dB HL) the TEOAE response amplitude differences were minimized. The correspondence between very slight changes in audiometric threshold and reduction in TEOAE amplitude are illustrated in Figure 4–6. As can be determined, the response was markedly attenuated in older subjects with thresholds that would be considered to be normal (< 25 dB HL) but with slight elevations in thresholds above 10 dB HL. Spectral analysis of the TEOAE response indicated that the signal to noise ratio

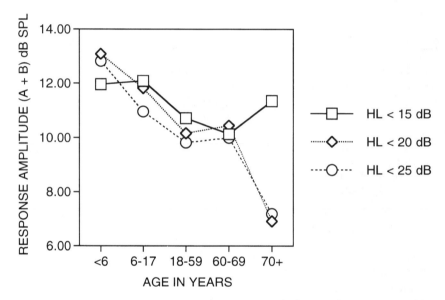

Figure 4–6.   Average TEOAE response amplitude (*A + B*) for 505 subjects grouped by age. Hearing level for the frequencies 250 through 4000 Hz is the parameter. There is a slight decrement of the (*A + B*) measurement with age if no audiometric threshold exceeds 20 dB HL and age is less than 70 years. However, the *A + B amplitude* is markedly attenuated for persons who are 70 years or older and whose HL is normal but exceeds 10 dB at one or more frequencies. As can be determined, the response was markedly attenuated in older subjects with thresholds that would be considered to be normal (<25 dB HL) but with slight elevations in threshold above 10 dB HL. Spectral analysis of the TEOAE response indicated that the signal to noise ratio remained robust (>7 dB) for 1000–Hz bandwidths centered at 1000, 2000, 3000 and 4000 Hz for all age groups. Measures of response amplitude were slightly more robust for the right ears than for left ears and for female subjects than for male subjects, following Robinette's (1992) observation. The differences emerged in the second decade of life in the data set analyzed by Glattke et al. (1994). (Adapted from Glattke et al., 1994. Used with permission)

remained robust (> 7 dB) for 1000-Hz bandwidths centered at 1000, 2000, 3000, and 4000 Hz for all age groups. Measures of response amplitude were slightly more robust for the right ears than for left ears and for female than for male subjects, following Robinette's earlier observation (1992). These differences emerged in the second decade of life in the data set that was analyzed by Glattke et al. (1994). The separation of the response amplitude measure by gender is illustrated in Figure 4–7.

Prieve and Falter (1995) examined TEOAE responses obtained using ILO 88 equipment and software in a group of 20 young (19–29 years) and older (40–61 years) adults with hearing thresholds better than or equal to 15 dB from 250 through 8000 Hz. They also determined whether the subjects' ears exhibited "synchronized" spontaneous otoacoustic emissions (SSOAEs). SSOAEs are recorded using ILO 88 software by presenting a series of click stimuli at 70 dB peak equivalent SPL and recording over a period of 80 ms following each stimulus. Repeated samples are submitted to averaging procedures and the resulting waveform is segmented into 4 intervals extending from 0 to 20, 20 to 40, 40 to 60 and 60 to 80 ms. If the A and B waveforms for the 60 to 80 ms interval contain highly correlated components, the long-latency responses are considered evidence of spontaneous activity synchronized to the transient stimuli. Prieve and Falter analyzed TEOAE responses for several stimulus intensities and concluded that, after correcting for the presence of SSOAEs that could not be recorded from older male subjects, there were no significant differences between the two groups' TEOAE threshold or amplitude. Kulawiec and Orlando (1995) studied the relations among gender, SOAEs, and TEOAE amplitude in 81 children and young adults. More SOAEs were found in right ears than in left ears, and the differences between right and left and female and male TEOAEs noted in previous studies were found again in the Kulawiec and Orlando investigation.

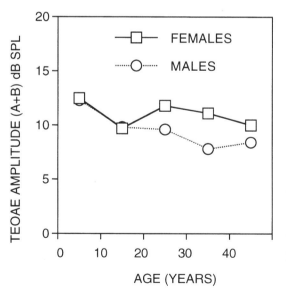

Figure 4–7. Average TEOAE response amplitude (A + B) for a 505 subjects grouped by age and gender. The data points on the extreme right represent subjects older than 45 years of age. Note that the measures interweave for children below the age of 10 and they persist for all age groups above preteen years and that the separation between male and female subjects occurs in the teen age years. (Adapted from Glattke et al., 1994. Used with permission)

Taken together, the data of Robinette, Stover and Norton, Glattke et al. (1994), and Prieve and Falter support the impression that TEOAEs obtained under default conditions from persons whose pure-tone thresholds are better than 25 dB HL are likely to be attenuated with increasing age. Beginning in the teenage years, male subjects exhibit smaller responses than are found for female subjects, and the responses obtained from right ears are slightly larger than those found for left ears. As in infants, the presence of spontaneous emissions influences the outcome of TEOAE measurements. If an SOAE is present, a TEOAE is present and is likely to be more robust than in another ear that does not reveal an SOAE. If very strict criteria are used to define normal hearing, then the response amplitude differences associated with age can be minimized. This has important implications for using TEOAEs to monitor the status of the auditory periphery in adults, inasmuch as it suggests that a slight change in an old adult's hearing may herald a substantial loss in TEOAE amplitude, but a similar threshold shift in a young person may not change the TEOAE amplitude. Finally, it appears that the prevalence of SOAEs is greater in women and that SOAES occur more often in right ears beginning in the teen years; therefore responses are likely to be more robust in women and in right ears, regardless of the age of the subject.

TEOAE Responses to Tone Bursts

Click stimuli provide an efficient means of evaluating the response of the ear to a broad spectrum, and they maximize the probability of detecting a response after a brief sampling period. Under default-stimulus conditions, the energy in any specific frequency region is approximately 45 dB below the peak stimulus intensity. The normative data that are emerging indicate that the most effective stimulus and the most robust response components are found in the mid-frequency region. There are a number of reasons to use studies of otoacoustic emissions to explore cochlear responses to stimuli that are more restricted in frequency dispersion. For example, it may be desirable to study ears at risk for high-frequency hearing loss due to noise exposure or ototoxic medications with stimuli that are concentrated in the high-frequency region. Attempts to define the configuration of hearing loss across audiometric frequencies may be enhanced if standard methods are developed to extract responses to low-frequency stimuli.

Kemp's (1978) initial study of TEOAEs included the examination of responses to tone bursts. Spectral analyses of the responses to tones were not provided, but it is clear from the average response waveforms that responses to low intensity tonal stimuli at 800, 1100, and 1800 Hz contained significant energy at the stimulus frequencies. Elberling, Parbo, Johnsen, and Bagi, as well as Probst, Coats, Martin, and Lonsbury-Martin (1986), employed spectral analyses to examine TEOAEs from ears with normal thresholds in response to tone bursts. The responses were characterized by idiosyncratic behavior, but spectral peaks were dominated by stimulus frequencies. Norton and Neely (1987) noted that the spectra of TEOAEs elicited by tone bursts were similar to those of the stimuli and that the latencies of the TEOAEs were compatible with contemporary theories of traveling wave behavior in the cochlea.

An example of a TEOAE in response to a tone burst at 3000 Hz is provided in

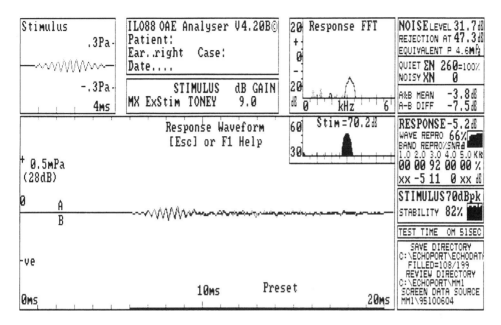

Figure 4–8. TEOAE response obtained from a young adult for tone burst stimuli. The stimulus consisted of a burst with a 2 ms rise and decay, no plateau, and a peak equivalent SPL of 70 dB. The stimulus duration was approximately 4 ms. The first 6 ms of the average response waveform has been blanked out to reduce the stimulus artifact. The average of the A & B waveforms is −3.8 dB SPL and the uncorrelated portion of the average waveforms, at −7.5 dB, reduces the *Response* value to −5.2 dB SPL. It is clear from the ILO 88 analysis that both stimulus and response spectra were restricted to narrow frequency regions.

Figure 4–8. Similar stimuli have been used in parametric studies by Xu, Probst, Harris and Roede (1994) to examine the responses of listeners with normal thresholds to single and multiple-component stimuli. Stover and Norton reported input/ output functions for TEOAEs generated in response to tone bursts and noted that the responses tend to saturate when stimulus levels reach approximately 50 dB peak equivalent SPL.

Effects of Contralateral Stimulation on TEOAEs

Properties of TEOAEs are known to be altered in the presence of contralateral stimulation. The principal result of the presentation of contralateral stimuli during the capture of a TEOAE is an attenuation of the TEOAE response. This phenomenon is illustrated by the examples in Figure 4–9.

Early descriptions of the effects of contralateral stimulation on distortion product otoacoustic emissions (DPOAEs) were provided by Brown (1988) and on SOAEs, by Kujawa and Glattke (1989) and Mott, Norton, Neely, and Warr (1989). Collet, Kemp, Veuillet, Duclaux, Moulin, and Morgon (1990) described a number of features of the alteration of TEOAEs in human subjects. Berlin et al. (1993) exam-

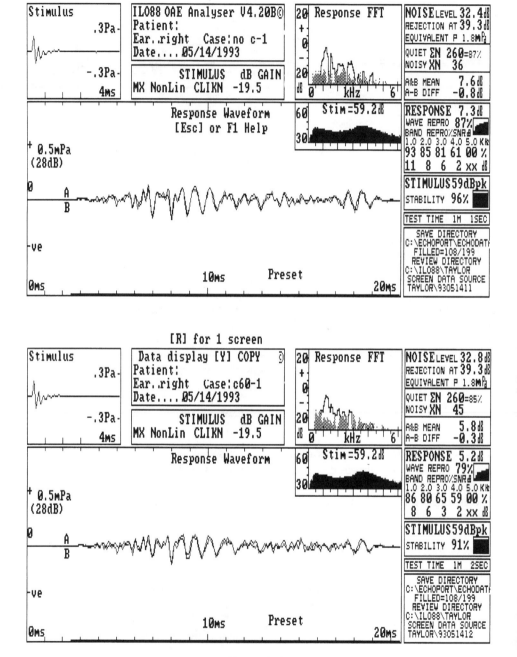

Figure 4–9.

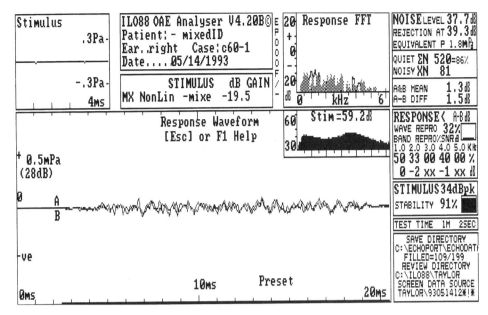

Figure 4–9. TEOAE responses obtained from a young adult. *A:* TEOAE obtained under standard stimulus conditions, except that the stimulus was attenuated to approximately 60 dB peak equivalent SPL. *B:* The stimulus was repeated while broad-band noise was presented to the contralateral ear at a level of 60 dB SPL (approximately 30 dB SL). The differences between the upper- and lower-TEOAE responses are found in a slight reduction in the *A & B Mean* value from 7.6 to 5.8 dB and a corresponding reduction in the computed *Response* from 7.3 to 5.2 dB. *C:* A response waveform that was computed as the difference between the normal and suppressed responses. Note that there is a modest, but persistent representation of lower frequency components in this difference tracing beginning at approximately 7 msec and extending to the latest portions of the response.

ined changes like those in Figure 4–9. They found that they could detect enhancement in the changes due to contralateral stimulation by restricting the analysis of the TEOAE to periods beginning at 8 ms after the stimulus. With proper controls, it has been demonstrated that the alteration of emissions in the presence of contralateral stimulation can be mediated by action of the efferent auditory system (Kujawa, Glattke, Fallon, & Bobbin, 1992, 1993, 1994). The systematic study of these effects offers the opportunity of viewing the influence of the central nervous system on mechanical activity of the cochlea.

Summary and Conclusions

TEOAEs offer investigators the tools to examine the integrity of the peripheral auditory system; the stimulus and recording techniques have a rich history of their applications to the auditory periphery. It is thought that the responses are caused by action of the hair cells, that they reflect the stimulus spectral characteristics, and that they saturate at moderate levels of stimulation. The characteristics are similar to those of cochlear microphonics, which have been the object of scrutiny for more than 65 years. The process of extracting average TEOAEs from background noise borrows heavily from other small-signal averaging techniques that have been employed in human electrocochleography and auditory brain stem response recordings for more than 30 years. Like electrophysiological responses, the emissions are *epiphenomena*. They occur in the presence of normal peripheral function, but they do not constitute the basis for hearing.

Most of the clinical records summarized in the literature have been based on recordings obtained using ILO 88 equipment and the so-called nonlinear stimulus mode. Under the default stimulus and recording conditions, the ILO 88 apparatus detects TEOAEs that are greater than 20 dB SPL in newborns. Responses that are obtained from older children and adults tend to range from 10 to 15 dB SPL. Normal TEOAE responses mirror the spectral properties of the stimulus used to elicit them. Clicks elicit broad-spectrum responses that are most robust in the mid-frequency region, probably owing to the fact that the middle ear transfer is most favorable in the region between 1000 and 3000 Hz. Responses obtained for tone bursts have narrow band spectra that are predicted by the stimulus properties. There appears to be an interaction between SOAEs and TEOAEs: If an SOAE can be recorded from an ear, the TEOAE obtained from that ear is likely to be more robust than from an ear without an SOAE. SOAEs are more prevalent in women than in men and occur more in right ears than in left ears. The prevalence of SOAEs may be correlated with the finding that TEOAEs recorded from children and adults are larger in women than in men and are larger in the right ear than in the left.

These complex, powerful tools have provided clinicians with many opportunities to explore details of cochlear function that heretofore were hidden in the shadows of the most dense bone of the skull. They have contributed to tremendous advances in the understanding of how normal and disordered systems function, and they will likely address problems of hearing impairment for long time.

Acknowledgments

This work was supported in part by NIH grant DC01409 (TJG).

References

Berlin, C. I., Hood, L. J., Wen, H., Szabo, P., Cecola, R. P., Rigby, P., & Jackson, D. R. (1993). Contralateral suppression of non-linear click-evoked otoacoustic emissions. *Hearing Research, 71*, 1–11.

Bonfils, P., & Uziel, A. (1989). Clinical applications of evoked otoacoustic emissions: Results in normally hearing and hearing impaired subjects. *Annals of Otorhinolaryngology, 98*, 326–331.

Bonfils, P., Bertrand, Y., & Uziel, A. (1988). Evoked otoacoustic emissions: Normative data and presbycusis. *Audiology, 27*, 27–35.

Brown, A. M. (1988). Continuous low level sound alters cochlear mechanics: An efferent effect? *Hearing Research, 34*, 27–38.

Collet, L., Gartner, M., Moulin, A., & Morgon, A. (1990). Age-related changes in evoked otoacoustic emissions. *Annals of Otology, Rhinology and Laryngology, 99*, 993–997.

Collet, L., Gartner, M., Veuillet, E., Moulin, A., & Morgon, A. (1993). Evoked and spontaneous otoacoustic emissions: A comparison of neonates and adults. *Brain Development, 15*, 249–252.

Collet, L., Kemp, D. T., Veuillet, E., Duclaux, R., Moulin, A., & Morgon, A. (1990). Effect of contralateral auditory stimuli on active cochlear micromechanical properties in human subjects. *Hearing Research, 43*, 252–262.

Davis, H. (1983). An active process in cochlear mechanics. *Hearing Research, 9*, 79–90.

Elberling, C., Parbo, J., Johnsen, N.J., and Bagi, P. (1985). Evoked acoustic emissions: Clinical application. *Acta Oto-Laryngologica, 421* (Suppl.), 77–85.

Glattke, T. J. (1983). *Short latency auditory evoked potentials.* Baltimore: University Park Press.

Glattke, T. J., Pafitis, I. A., Cummiskey, C., & Herer, G. R. (1995). Identification of hearing loss in children using measures of transient otoacoustic emission reproducibility. *American Journal of Audiology, 4,* 71–86.

Glattke, T. J., Robinette, M. S., Pafitis, I.A., Cummiskey, C., & Herer, G. R. (1994, July). TEOAEs and age. Paper presented at the XXII International Congress of Audiology, Halifax, Nova Scotia.

Grandori, F., and Ravazzani, P. (1993). Non-linearities of click-evoked otoacoustic emissions and the derived non-linear response. *British Journal of Audiology, 27,* 97–102.

Harris, F. P., & Glattke, T. J. (1992). The use of suppression to determine the characteristics of otoacoustic emissions. *Seminars in Hearing, 13,* 67–80.

Harris, F. P., & Probst, R. (1991). Reporting click-evoked and distortion-product otoacoustic emission results with respect to the pure tone audiogram. *Ear and Hearing, 12*(6), 399–405.

Hills, D. A., & Glattke, T. J. (1996, April). The effect of reducing the analysis window on TEOAE reproducibility scores. Paper presented at the annual meeting of the American Academy of Audiology, Salt Lake City, UT.

Johnsen, N.J., Bagi, P., Parbo, J. & Elberling, C. (1988). Evoked otoacoustic emissions from the human ear. IV: Final results in 100 neonates. *Scandinavian Audiology, 17,* 27–34.

Johnsen, N. J., & Elberling, C. (1982). Evoked acoustic emissions from the human ear: II. Normative data in young adults and influence of posture. *Scandinavian Audiology, 11,* 68–77.

Johnsen, N. J. & Elberling, C. (1983). Evoked acoustic emissions from the human ear: III. Findings in neonates. *Scandinavian Audiology, 12,* 17–24.

Johnstone, B., Patuzzi, & Yates (1986). Basilar membrane measurements and the traveling wave. *Hearing Research, 22,* 147–153.

Jung, M. D., & Smurzynski, J. (1991). Otoacoustic emissions in normal and hearing-impaired children and normal adults. *Laryngoscope, 101,* 965–976.

Kemp, D. T. (1978). Stimulated acoustic emissions from within the human auditory system. *Journal of the Acoustical Society of America, 64,* 1386–1391.

Kemp, D. T. (1979a). Evidence of mechanical nonlinearity and frequency selective wave amplification in the cochlea. *Archives of Otorhinolaryngology, 224,* 37–46.

Kemp, D. T. (1979b). The evoked cochlear mechanical response and the auditory microstructure. *Scandinavian Audiology, 9* (Suppl.), 35–46.

Kemp, D. T., Bray, P., Alexander, L., & Brown, A. M. (1986). Acoustic emission cochleography—practical aspects. *Scandinavian Audiology, 15* (Suppl.), 71–95.

Kemp, D. T., & Ryan, S. (1993). The use of transient evoked otoacoustic emissions in neonatal hearing screening programs. *Seminars in Hearing, 14,* 30–45.

Kemp, D. T., Ryan, S., & Bray, P. (1990). A guide to the effective use of otoacoustic emissions. *Ear and Hearing, 11,* 93–105.

Kok, M. R., van Zanten, G. A., & Brocaar, M. P. (1992). Growth of evoked otoacoustic emissions during the first few days of postpartum. *Audiology, 31,* 140–149.

Kok, M. R., van Zanten, G. A., Brocaar, M. P., & Jongejan, H.T.M. (1994). Click-evoked oto-acoustic emissions in very-low-birthweight infants: A cross-sectional data analysis. *Audiology, 33,* 152–164.

Kok, M. R., van Zanten, G. A., Brocaar, M. P., & Wallenburg, H.C.S. (1993). Click-evoked oto-acoustic emissions in 1036 ears of healthy newborns. *Audiology, 32,* 213–223.

Kujawa, S. G., & Glattke, T. J. (1989). Influence of contralateral acoustic stimulation on spontaneous otoacoustic emissions. *Asha, 31,* 123.

Kujawa, S. G., Glattke, T. J., Fallon, M., & Bobbin, R. P. (1992). Intracochlear application of acetylcholine alters sound-induced mechanical events within the cochlear partition. *Hearing Research, 61,* 106–116.

Kujawa, S. G., Glattke, T. J., Fallon, M., & Bobbin, R. P. (1993). Contralateral sound suppresses distortion product otoacoustic emissions through cholinergic mechanisms. *Hearing Research, 68,* 97–106.

Kujawa, S. G., Glattke, T. J., Fallon, M., & Bobbin, R. P. (1994). A nicotinic-like receptor mediates suppression of distortion product otoacoustic emissions by contralateral sound. *Hearing Research, 74,* 122–134.

Kulawiec, J. T., and Orlando. M. S. (1995). The contribution to spontaneous otoacoustic emissions to the click evoked otoacoustic emissions. *Ear and Hearing, 16,* 515–520.

Lafreniere, D., Jung, M.D., Smurzynski, J., Leonard, G., Kim, D. O., & Sasek, J. (1991). Distortion-product and click-evoked otoacoustic emissions in healthy newborns. *Archives of Otolaryngology—Head and Neck Surgery, 117,* 1382–1389.

Morlet, T., Collet, L., Duclaux, R., Lapillonne, A., Salle, B., Putet, G., & Morgon, A. (1995). Spontaneous and evoked otoacoustic emissions in pre-term and full-term neonates: Is there a clinical application. *International Journal of Pediatric Otorhinolaryngology, 33,* 207–212.

Mott, J. B., Norton, S. J., Neely, S. T., & Warr, W. B. (1989). Changes in spontaneous otoacoustic emissions produce by acoustic stimulation of the contralateral ear. *Hearing Research, 38,* 229–242.

Norton, S. J., & Neely, S. T. (1987). Tone-burst-evoked otoacoustic emissions from normal-hearing subjects. *Journal of the Acoustical Society of America, 81,* 1860–1872.

Norton, S., & Widen, J. E. (1990). Evoked otoacoustic emissions in normal-hearing infants and children: Emerging data and issues. *Ear and Hearing, 11,* 121–127.

Prieve, BA., (1993). Otoacoustic emissions in infants and children. *Seminars in Hearing, 13,* 37–52.

Prieve, B. A., & Falter, S. R. (1995). COAEs and SSOAEs in adults with increased age. *Ear and Hearing, 16,* 521–528.

Prieve, B. A., Gorga, M. P., Schmidt, A., Neely, S., Peters, J., Schultes, L., and Jesteadt, W. (1993). Analysis of transient-evoked otoacoustic emissions in normal-hearing and hearing-impaired ears. *Journal of the Acoustical Society of America, 93,* 3308–3319.

Probst, R., Coats, A. C., & Martin, G. K., and Lonsbury-Martin, B. L. (1986). Spontaneous, click- and toneburst-evoked otoacoustic emissions from normal ears. *Hearing Research, 21,* 261–275.

Robinette, M. (1992). Clinical observations with transient evoked otoacoustic emissions with adults. *Seminars in Hearing, 13,* 23–36.

Smurzynski, J. (1994). Longitudinal measure of distortion-product and click-evoked otoacoustic emissions of preterm infants: Preliminary Results. *Ear and Hearing, 15,* 210–223.

Smurzynski, J., Jung, M. D., Lafreniere, D., Kim, D. O., Kamath, M. V., Rowe, J. C., Holman, M. C., & Leonard, G. (1993). Distortion-product and click-evoked otoacoustic emissions of preterm and full-term infants. *Ear and Hearing, 13,* 258–274.

Smurzynski, J., Jung, M., Leonard, G., & Kim, D. O. (1993). Otoacoustic emissions in full-term newborns at risk for hearing loss. *Laryngoscope, 103,* 1334–1341.

Stover, L., & Norton, S. J. (1993). The effects of aging on otoacoustic emissions. *Journal of the Acoustical Society of America, 94,* 2670–2681.

Thornton, A. R. D., Kimm, L., Kennedy, C. R., & Cafarelli-Dees, D. (1994). A comparison of neonatal evoked otoacoustic emissions obtained using two types of apparatus. *British Journal of Audiology, 28,* 99–109.

Uziel, A., & Piron, J. P. (1991). Evoked oto-acoustic emissions from normal newborns and babies admitted to an intensive care baby unit. *Acta Oto-Laryngologica, 482* (Suppl.) 85–91.

van Zanten, B. G. A., Kok, M.R., Brocaar, M. P., & Sauer, P. J. J. (1995). The click-evoked oto-acoustic emission, C-EOAE, in preterm-born infants in the post conceptional age range between 30 and 688 weeks. *International Journal of Pediatric Otorhinolaryngology, 32* (Suppl.), S187–S197.

Wever, E.G ., & Bray, C. W. (1930). Action currents in the auditory nerve in response to acoustical stimulation. *Proceedings of the National Academy of Sciences, 16,* 344–350.

Whitehead, M. L., Jimenez, A. M., Stagner, B. B., McCoy, M.J., Lonsbury-Martin, B. L., & Martin G. K. (1995). Time-windowing of click-evoked otoacoustic emissions to increase signal-to-noise ratio. *Ear and Hearing, 16,* 599–611.

Wilson, J. P. (1980). Recording the Kemp echo and tinnitus from the ear canal without averaging. *Journal of Physiology, 298,* 8–9.

Wilson, J. P. (1980a). Evidence for a cochlear origin for acoustic re-emissions, threshold fine-structure and tonal tinnitus. *Hearing Research, 2,* 233–252.

Wit, H. P., & Ritsma, R. J. (1979). Stimulated acoustic emissions from the human ear. *Journal of the Acoustical Society of America, 66,* 911–913.

Xu, L., Probst, R., Harris, F. P., & Roede, J. (1994). Peripheral analysis of frequency in human ears revealed by tone burst evoked otoacoustic emissions. *Hearing Research, 74,* 173–180.

Zorowka, P., Schmitt, H. J., Eckel, H. E., Lippert, K. L., Schönberger, W., & Merz, E. (1993). Serial measurements of transient evoked otoacoustic emissions (TEOAEs) in healthy newborns and in newborns with perinatal infection. *International Journal of Pediatric Otorhinolaryngology, 27,* 245–254.

5

Distortion Product Otoacoustic Emissions

BRENDA L. LONSBURY-MARTIN
GLEN K. MARTIN
MARTIN L. WHITEHEAD

Introduction

Evoked otoacoustic emissions (OAEs) are low-level audio-frequency sounds that are produced by the cochlea as part of the normal-hearing process. The most outstanding features of evoked OAEs with respect to their suitability as a clinical test are that they can be measured simply, noninvasively, and readily in the outer-ear canal by a sensitive microphone. The two types of OAEs, which are currently undergoing intensive development for clinical applications, are the transient evoked OAEs (TEOAEs) and the distortion-product OAEs (DPOAEs).

Kemp (1978), the English biophysicist who discovered otoacoustic emissions and published the first scientific description of TEOAEs (Kemp, 1978), introduced DPOAEs shortly thereafter (Kemp, 1979). The DPOAEs are an intermodulation-distortion response produced by the ear in response to two simultaneous, pure-tone stimuli referred to as the *primary tones*. Such a response is described as being *distorted* because it originates from the cochlea as a tonal signal that is not present in the eliciting pure-tone stimuli. By convention, the lower-frequency pure tone is referred to as the f_1 *primary*, and its level, as L_1; and the higher-frequency pure-tone is referred to as the f_2 *primary*, and its level, as L_2. The primaries are related in frequency in that the frequency separation of f_2 from f_1, commonly called the f_2/f_1 *ratio*, is typically around $f_1 \times 1.2$ (i.e., the primary tones are within one-third octave of each other). The most frequently measured acoustic intermodulation-distortion product is at the frequency $2f_1 - f_2$ (i.e., the cubic-difference tone), although the cochlea also produces concurrently DPOAEs at other frequencies (e.g., $f_2 - f_1$, $2f_2 - f_1$, $3f_1 - 2f_2$) in response to such bitonal stimulation (Pickles, 1988). Indeed, the only emitted distortion component utilized for clinical purposes has been the $2f_1 - f_2$

because it is the largest DPOAE in all mammals. Although $2f_1 - f_2$ DPOAEs can be detected in essentially all normal human ears, they are typically extremely small (i.e., 5–15 dB SPL), even at high primary-tone levels. In fact, DPOAEs are usually from about 60 to 70 dB below the moderate levels of the stimulus tones routinely employed to evoke them.

The DPOAEs appear not to be produced by a simple cochlear analogue of an overloading type of non-linearity that is usually associated with, e.g., over-driving an amplifier. Rather, the DPOAE generator operates even at very low stimulus levels, and is a normal aspect of cochlear functioning. In general, the intermodulation distortion that produces DPOAEs is thought to arise from fundamental processes within the cochlea, particularly those associated with the nonlinearity of outer–hair-cell motion. Such processes respond to low-sound levels by using metabolic energy to increase the sound-induced motion of the basilar membrane near the characteristic-frequency place. Thus, like the other types of OAEs, DPOAEs are thought to be generated by the active cochlear process responsible for enhancing basilar-membrane vibration. The general process responsible for the enhancement of basilar-membrane motion is commonly referred to as the *cochlear amplifier* (Davis, 1983).

DPOAE Measurement

Equipment

Figure 5–1 shows a schematic of the basic components of a standard computer-based DPOAE-measurement device. Like the other evoked OAEs, DPOAEs are elicited and measured by an acoustic speculum that is sealed snugly into the ear canal using a removable soft-rubber or foam eartip. To measure DPOAEs, the probe assembly usually incorporates several miniature microphones, whose averaged output minimizes the noise level of the probe pickup. Most commonly these are Knowles subminiature transducers developed for hearing-aid use. The probe also contains either two miniature speakers, or short lengths of plastic tubing (called *sound-delivery tubes*), which are routed through the probe from external speakers typically attached to the subject's shoulder, headband, or garment collar and are open to the ear canal. Two speakers are required to elicit DPOAEs, so that the f_1 and f_2 primary tones are mixed acoustically, rather than electrically, to prevent the generation of artifactual intermodulation-distortion products by a single speaker when driven simultaneously by two tones.

Stimuli are digitally synthesized, and the responses collected and processed either by a digital signal-processing (DSP) board mounted within a flexible and relatively inexpensive personal computer (PC), or directly by the PC's central-processing unit (CPU). Depending upon the device used, the inclusion of attenuators or impedance-matching components between the stimulus output of the DSP board and the speakers is necessary. Additionally, the microphone preamplifier may necessarily be followed by an amplifier in some systems. Because of the small amplitudes of DPOAEs, a critical constraint on the microphone and DSP board is low intrinsic noise levels.

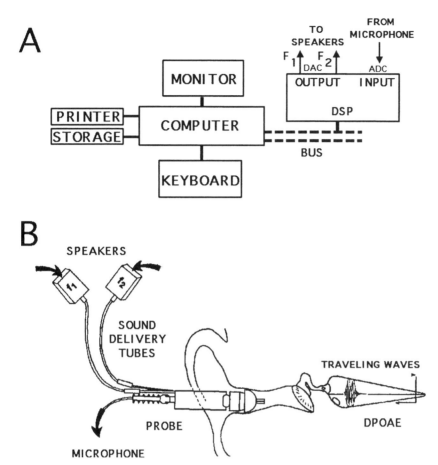

Figure 5–1. Schematic of basic components of a typical DPOAE-measurement device. *A*: Computer-based elements. All commercial instruments are based upon inexpensive computers fitted with plug-in boards for signal generation and response measurement. Signals are digitally synthesized and go through a digital-to-analogue converter (DAC) to the speakers, and the microphone is sampled with an analogue-to-digital converter (ADC). *B*: Typical speaker-microphone arrangement for DPOAE measurement. The microphone is housed in a probe that is inserted into the ear canal. To reduce artifactual intermodulation distortion, the two speakers are typically located externally to the microphone housing, and the two simultaneously presented stimulus tones (f_1 and f_2) are delivered separately to the ear canal by tubes that pass through the probe. To reduce the level of external noise at the microphone and to prevent leakage of stimulus and DPOAE energy, the probe is tightly sealed into the ear canal with a flexible rubber tip. The evoking stimuli vibrate the eardrum and middle-ear ossicles, which in turn produce a pressure wave in the cochlear fluids, initiating a traveling wave of basilar-membrane displacement. Audio-frequency vibratory energy generated within the cochlea follows this pathway in reverse. This results in vibration of the ear drum, which acts as a speaker to produce the faint sounds that are recorded as DPOAEs by the ear-canal microphone assembly.

In contrast to TEOAEs, DPOAEs are measured in the presence of the stimulating tones. However, they can easily be detected using narrowband filtering, typically spectral using Fourier analysis, because they are separated in frequency from the much larger eliciting stimuli. Figure 5–2 illustrates an example of a spectrum of sound pressure in a human ear canal at the $2f_1 - f_2$ frequency during stimulation with the f_1 and f_2 primaries.

Several companies offer devices designed to measure DPOAEs. Models currently available include the ILO 92 (Otodynamics), the model 330 (Virtual), the GSI 60 (Grason-Stadler), the Celesta 503 (Madsen Electronics), the CUBeDIS (Mimosa Acoustics), and the Scout (Bio-Logic). The commercial systems are all based on narrowband-spectral analysis. Most of the devices use a custom-built plug-in board for IBM-compatible PCs. However, both the Virtual Corporation and Mimosa Acoustics devices utilize commercially available DSP boards adapted for Apple (model 330) or IBM (model 330, CUBeDIS) computer. The model 330 instrument is the only commercial system that can be operated by either an IBM or Apple computer. Because of the large dynamic range needed to measure these low-level acoustic signals in the presence of much higher-level stimuli, 16-bit analogue-to-digital converters (ADCs) have typically been utilized in the measurement instru-

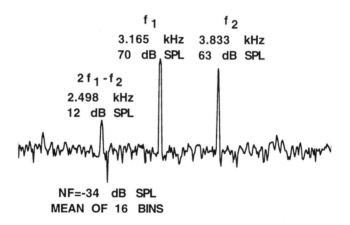

Figure 5–2. The DPOAE response is shown in the frequency spectrum of the sound field in the sealed-ear canal of a normal human upon stimulation by two pure tones of frequencies f_1 = 3.165 and f_2 = 3.833 kHz at L_1 = 70 and L_2 = 63 dB SPL (f_2/f_1 = 1.21). The small, (12 dB SPL) sharp peak at 2.498 kHz is the $2f_1 - f_2$ DPOAE. The noise floor (NF) was estimated by taking the mean level of eight spectral bins above and below the DPOAE frequency bin. This DPOAE was obtained utilizing a customized laboratory system (Otoscan), which uses a commercially available microphone system (Etymotic Research 10-B) and dual earphones (Etymotic Research 2), and a relatively inexpensive audio DSP board (DigiDesign, Audiomedia) designed for a microcomputer (Macintosh). The f_1 and f_2 stimuli were presented for 100 ms, and the microphone output was sampled for 93 ms, i.e., 4,096 points at a sample rate of 44.1 kHz. The spectrum displayed is the result of a fast Fourier transform (FFT) analysis of the synchronous average of 32 samples, which were obtained in about 3 s. It is evident from this record that the DPOAE at about 2.5 kHz is clearly above the background noise level.

mentation. For the commercially available devices, the f_1 and f_2 primary tones are digitally synthesized and presented to the ear canal either continuously or as simultaneous long-duration tone pulses. Either presentation method is satisfactory if the timing of response sampling is locked to the DPOAE phase, i.e., time-locked, in order to reduce noise in the synchronous average, while preserving the DPOAE signal.

Various sampling frequencies have been utilized in the commercially available equipment. It is common to measure DPOAE frequencies as low as about $2f_1 - f_2 = 300$ Hz, although both acoustic noise from the environment and physiological noise from the subject make DPOAE frequencies less than about 1 kHz difficult to measure. At high frequencies, DPOAEs can provide useful information above $2f_1 - f_2 = 6$ kHz, and most available equipment records to this frequency limit, which is constrained primarily by the technical limitations of the loud speakers.

Response Forms

When illustrated in a graphics format, the DPOAE is typically plotted as a function of the primary-tone frequencies, rather than the DPOAE frequency, because research findings indicate that the $2f_1 - f_2$ DPOAE is generated in the region of the cochlea that maximally responds to the primary tones, and, thus, best reflects cochlear status in this region (Brown & Kemp, 1984; Martin, Probst, Scheinin, Coats, & Lonsbury-Martin, 1990). The reference frequency typically used has been the geometric mean of the primary tones, i.e., $(f_1 \times f_2)^{.5}$; however, f_2 is also used. Current thinking concerning which frequency most accurately reflects the $2f_1 - f_2$ generation site is that the relation may be level-dependent, with lower-level tones best activating the frequency region nearest to f_2 and moderate-level to higher-level primaries optimally stimulating the geometric-mean region.

The DPOAE magnitude is taken as the level of the DPOAE-frequency FFT bin that contains both the DPOAE and some background noise. To determine whether this measure reflects the presence of a DPOAE, the level of the bin is compared to the level of closely adjacent-frequency bins, which contain only background noise. Because most contaminating noises are relatively broadband, the noise levels in the adjacent-frequency bins are well-correlated to that in the DPOAE-frequency bin. Typically, a DPOAE is assumed to be present if the level of the DPOAE-frequency bin is greater than that of the noise-level estimate derived from the adjacent bins by some criterion-based amount. For example, in our laboratory, the background noise at each frequency is estimated as the mean level of eight FFT bins (i.e., an 86-Hz interval) above and eight bins below the DPOAE-frequency bin, and the criterion adopted is commonly 3 dB above this level. Other systems utilize a different number of noise bins and different criteria for combining the levels of these bins to form the noise-level estimate (e.g., the 90th percentile of the levels of the noise bins).

The amplitude of the DPOAE depends systematically upon the parameters of the stimulus tones, i.e., frequencies, levels, frequency separation, and level difference. Except for a slight drop off of a few dB for frequencies less than 1 kHz and greater than 6 kHz and a slightly more pronounced dip around 2 to 3 kHz,

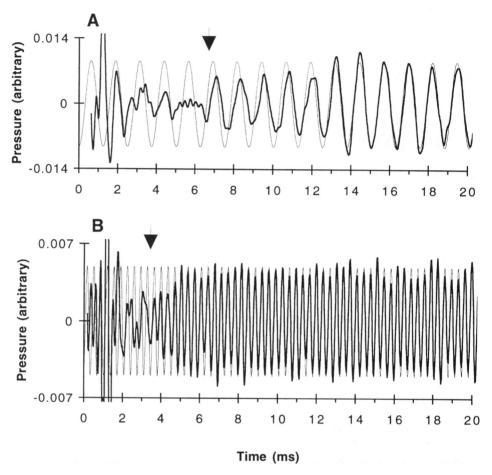

Figure 5–3. Visualization of the onset latency for $2f_1 - f_2$ DPOAEs measured from a normal human ear using direct measures based on cancellation methods. *A*: A low-frequency DPOAE (onset latency at arrow = 6.2 ms) elicited by primary tones at $f_1 = 0.947$, $f_2 = 1.098$, $L_1 = L_2 = 75$ dB SPL [DPOAE = 0.8 kHz; geometric mean (GM) = 1 kHz]. *Heavy line*: The DPOAE waveform after low-pass and high-pass filtering; *Faint line*: Sinusoid synthesized for comparison at the DPOAE frequency with the same amplitude and phase as the DPOAE at a steady state. Note the stimulus-onset artifact around 1–2 ms. Also note that for the initial five cycles after the onset, the DPOAE amplitude was smaller than at steady-state, and the DPOAE phase lagged that at steady-state. *B*: Same as *A*, except the high-frequency DPOAE (latency at arrow = 2.4 ms) was elicited by primary tones at $f_1 = 3.639$, $f_2 = 4.404$, $L_1 = L_2 = 75$ dB SPL (DPOAE = 2.9 kHz; GM = 4 kHz).

DPOAE level is fairly constant as a function of frequency (Figure 5–6) in response to moderate primary tones that are equal in level ($L_1 = L_2$). The amplitude of the DPOAE is also systematically dependent on the relative levels of the stimulus tones and can be increased slightly for suprathreshold stimuli by decreasing L_2 below L_1 (Gaskill & Brown, 1990; Hauser & Probst, 1991; Whitehead, Stagner, McCoy, & Lonsbury-Martin, 1995b). Finally, DPOAE level is strongly dependent on the frequency separation of the stimulus tones, being largest when f_2/f_1 is around 1.21 to 1.22 (Gaskill & Brown, 1990; Harris, Lonsbury-Martin, Stagner, Coats, & Martin, 1989).

In order for DPOAEs to be clinically useful, it is necessary to devise a systematic means by which such responses from a patient can be judged to be normal or pathological. The most objective approach is to compare the value of some property of the patient's DPOAEs to its distribution in normal ears. In this manner, cochlear impairment is indicated when responses in the test ear are below the range of responses in the normal population.

For example, a commonly measured DPOAE feature is amplitude, which is typically plotted as a function of frequency of the primary tones, across a range of frequencies (Lonsbury-Martin, Harris, Hawkins, Stagner, & Martin, 1990; Spektor, Leonard, Kim, Jung, & Smurzynski, 1991; Smurzynski & Kim, 1992; Gorga et al, 1993). In earlier work, this plot was often called the *DPOAE audiogram*. However, because it does not represent a true sensitivity measure like a clinical audiogram the terms *DP-gram* or *DPOAE-frequency-level function* are more preferred. The advantage of the DP-gram is that it describes the detailed frequency pattern of a cochlear impairment. Figure 5–6 illustrates the average DP-gram for a set of normal ears and Figure 5–14 shows several examples of DP-grams.

Another response form that is less commonly used to assess DPOAE amplitude is the response/growth or input/output (I/O) function (Figures 15–14B, D). The I/O function plots DPOAE amplitude as a function of the level of the primary tones, for a number of progressively increasing stimulus levels, typically for a set of discrete frequencies, which are selected to complement the conventional audiometric-test frequencies. A major benefit of the I/O response measure is that the detection *threshold*, i.e., a user-selected criterion level (typically 3 dB) above the related noise floor, can be determined in addition to suprathreshold levels of DPOAEs. Although there is no information from systematic investigations that supports the possibility that DPOAE thresholds are more clinically useful than the more commonly used DPOAE-amplitude measure, preliminary data suggest that threshold may be a better indicator of hearing sensitivity than of its magnitude, particularly when high-level primaries are used to elicit the DPOAEs (Stover & Norton, 1993; Stover, Monyoya, Gorga, & Neely, 1995).

Recently, there has been a concerted effort to develop an algorithm based on the slope of DPOAE-I/O function data for the objective estimation of detection threshold (Nelson & Kimberly, 1992; Whitehead, Lonsbury-Martin, & Martin, 1993). Because DPOAE growth is not always monotonic and detection threshold depends primarily on the unpredictably variable noise floor, automated algorithms to identify the DPOAE-detection threshold would be useful in the clinical application of DPOAEs. However, problems associated with the greater variability of noise floors associated with time-locked averaging, which is the current method of choice for DPOAE measurement in clinical settings, rather than spectral averaging, make such objective methods difficult to implement. It is likely that alternative strategies for estimating DPOAE threshold based on a criterion absolute amplitude (i.e., requiring threshold DPOAEs to be 2 SDs above the mean noise floor) would be less affected by the influence of noise on DPOAE growth near the noise floor (Whitehead, Lonsbury-Martin, & Martin, 1993).

In addition to detection threshold, the growth of the response can be simply

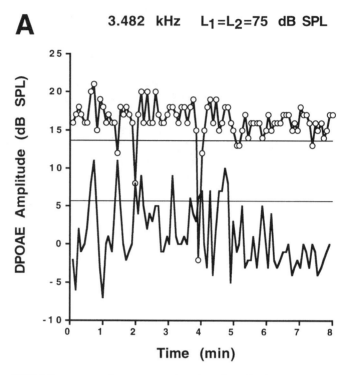

Figure 5–4. DPOAEs measured as temporal-series plots during an 8-min segment of an acoustic-neuroma surgery on a 32-year old female patient. *A*: The effects of operating-room noise on DPOAE amplitudes (GM = 3.482 kHz). Computer-based determinations selected the most robust DPOAE out of every four samples permitting the DPOAE to be measured every 1.6 sec. During this time, DPOAE amplitudes varied around an average of 16.2 dB SPL (± 2.7 dB). Open circles = DPOAE amplitudes; set of two thin lines parallel to the abscissa = ±1-SD range of DPOAEs at 3.5 kHz (GM) in a population of normal ears; heavy dark line without symbols = noise floor. *B*: Phase angle of DPOAE shown in *A*. DPOAE phase was measured relative to the primary tones that were initiated at the same phase for each time average. Note the relatively stable phase-angle activity at an average of 314° (± 14°) during the recording interval.

derived from the slope of the I/O function. With increasing $L_1 = L_2$ stimulus tones, DPOAEs increase in amplitude on average at a growth rate of around 1 dB/dB, and saturate above stimulus levels of about 75 dB SPL (Lonsbury-Martin et al., 1990; Nelson & Kimberly, 1992; Popelka, Osterhammel, Nielson, & Rasmussen, 1993). Other DPOAE features that can be extracted from the I/O function include the maximum emission generated at distinct frequencies, and the general shape of the function. None of the latter properties associated with the DPOAE I/O function have been studied systematically as a potentially useful clinical measure. However, an initial attempt was recently made to examine the utility of information provided by the form of the DPOAE I/O by determining the prevalence of various shapes in normal ears in terms of amount of saturation (Stover & Norton, 1993). In

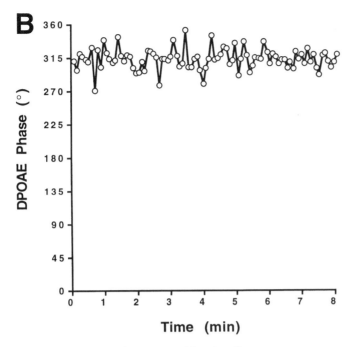

Figure 5.4. (*Continued*)

this study, some six DPOAE-I/O patterns were distinguished, including "no saturation" (i.e., monotonic) and ones with varying degrees of saturation or growth
irregularity, ranging from functions exhibiting simple nonmonotonic growth (i.e.,
bent-over at the highest stimulation levels) to patterns involving more complicated
shapes that included notching and more complicated combinations of both monotonic and nonmonotonic components. Although it is likely that irregular I/O
shapes occur less frequently with primary tones having level differences (Gaskill &
Brown, 1990), the clinical implications of the shape of the DPOAE I/O function
remain unclear.

Other far less-studied measures of normal DPOAE activity include onset latency,
phase, suppression, and tuning. For example, DPOAEs have latencies that presumably reflect the delay due to the processes that govern mechanical transmission
within the cochlea associated with the traveling wave and the development of
resonance (O Mahoney & Kemp, 1995). Such latencies are measurable in either the
frequency domain (Mahoney & Kemp, 1995) using FFT analyses or in the time
domain (Kemp & Brown, 1983). A typical method of measuring DPOAE latency is
the phase-gradient method (also called the group-delay method [Kimberly, Braun,
& Eggermont, 1993] in which f_2 is held constant while f_1 is swept in frequency). The
rate of phase change of the DPOAE, i.e., the slope of the phase change of the
DPOAE with frequency, is used to calculate latency (O Mahoney & Kemp, 1995).
With this approach, phase increases rapidly and monotonically with increasing f_1.
Given the short distances involved, group-delay analyses have shown that DPOAEs

have remarkably long latencies that increase from less than 3 ms at frequencies above 6 kHz to more than 10 ms below 1 kHz (O Mahoney & Kemp, 1995; Kimberley et al., 1993; Brown, Kimberley & Eggermont, 1995).

Other latency-measuring methods involve the cancellation of almost all of the components of the time-averaged DPOAE waveform, except for the $2f_1 - f_2$ DPOAE sinusoidal signal (Whitehead, Stagner, Martin, & Lonsbury-Martin, 1996). In this manner, following additional digital filtering of the time record, the DPOAE latency can be directly measured. The plots of Figure 5–3 show such visualization of the $2f_1 - f_2$ DPOAE for a low-frequency (geometric mean = 1 kHz, DPOAE = 0.8 kHz [Figure 5–3A]) and for a higher-frequency (geometric mean = 4 kHz, DPOAE = 2.9 kHz [Figure 5–3B]) emission. These data indicate that for moderately high-level stimuli (i.e., 75 dB SPL), the higher-frequency DPOAE had a shorter latency at about 2.4 ms than the lower-frequency DPOAE at about 6.2 ms. The DPOAE onset latencies also increased systematically at any specific frequency as the levels of the stimulating tones decrease, and they were faster in laboratory mammals than in human beings, presumably because of the shorter cochleas of the smaller animals (Whitehead et al. 1996).

The relatively long latencies noted in the literature (O Mahoney & Kemp, 1995; Brown, Kimberly, & Eggermont, 1994; Whitehead et al., 1996) may have resulted from the low velocity of the traveling wave or displacement wave by which low to moderate levels of acoustic energy propagate along the basilar membrane, from the basal end to the more apical sites at which DPOAEs are generated. Additional temporal delays are presumably added by the sharp filtering or resonance that occurs for each frequency around its characteristic place along the basilar membrane and by the travel time of the emission energy back along the basilar membrane to the middle ear and pick-up microphone in the outer-ear canal. Regardless of their eventual usefulness in distinguishing normal from abnormal cochlear functioning, DPOAE latencies are important in clinical applications because they can be used to identify genuine physiological responses, i.e., potential artifacts that may be mistaken for DPOAEs are unlikely to have such long latencies.

Direct information from measures of DPOAE phase relative to the input stimuli have not been studied systematically. Therefore, there are little data available concerning DPOAE phase in normal ears. However, experimental clinical evidence indicates that changes in DPOAE-phase angle from a baseline condition may be an early indicator of cochlear compromise that is more sensitive than corresponding DPOAE amplitudes. Figure 5–3 shows an 8-min sample of an intraoperative record that depicts the stability of DPOAE amplitude compared to the phase during surgery for removing an acoustic neuroma from the cerebellopontine-angle region of a patient. It is clear from these recordings that DPOAE-phase angle is reasonably stable under operating-room conditions associated with normal cochlear function. Future work will determine the benefits of monitoring DPOAE phase compared to amplitude in detecting subtle changes in cochlear functioning.

Other features of DPOAEs include their suppression. Suppression is a well-known phenomenon of cochlear non-linearity in which one tone has the ability to interfere with the response of another. In the case of DPOAEs, the suppression process has been studied less as a phenomenon in itself and more as a means to produce suppression-tuning curves (Brown & Kemp, 1984) as a measure of the

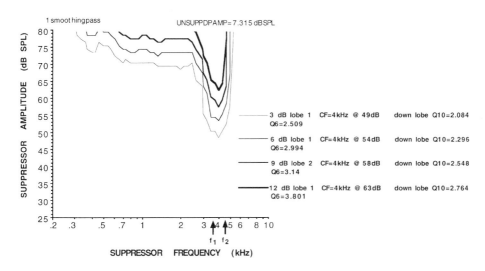

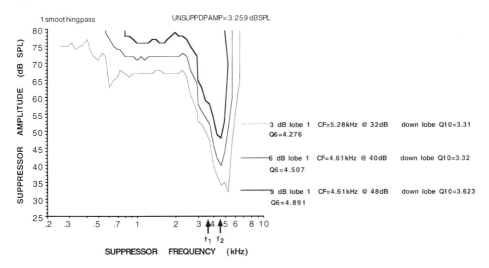

Figure 5–5. Iso-suppression tuning curves at 4 kHz (GM) for suppression criteria of 3, 6, 9, and 12 dB using equilevel $L_1 = L_2$ *vs* L_1-L_2 difference primaries measured from a 20-yr-old woman with normal hearing. A: Iso-suppression tuning curves elicited by primaries at $L_1 = L_2 = 55$ dB. Note that the suppression threshold for the minimum suppression criterion at 3 dB is 49 dB SPL, and the related Q_{10dB} factor is 2.1. B: Iso-suppression tuning curves elicited by primaries at L_1-$L_2 = 25$ dB ($L_1 = 55$ and $L_2 = 30$ dB SPL). Note that the threshold for the 3-dB suppression criterion is 32 dB SPL, and the Q_{10dB} factor = 3.31. For both plots, the unsuppressed DPOAE amplitude is noted at the top of the tuning curve, suppression thresholds and Q (6 and 10 dB) factors for the other suppression criteria (i.e., 6, 9, 12 dB) are noted at the bottom right, and the primary-tone frequencies are indicated at along the abscissa (f_1, f_2).

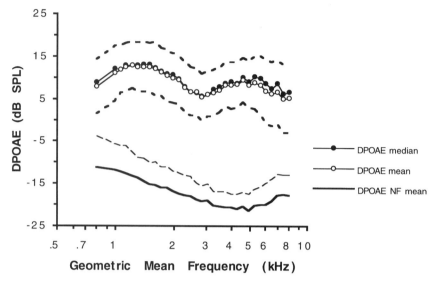

Figure 5–6. Average DPOAE amplitudes (*solid circles*: median, *open circles*: mean) as a function of frequency in 0.1-octave bands in response to 75-dB SPL primaries for 149 normal ears. The *bold dashed lines* around the average DPOAE data indicate the ±1-SD range. The *heavy line* along the bottom of the plot represents the mean noise floor (NF), and the *dashed line* above it indicates the +1-SD limits of the average NF.

frequency selectivity of the emission-generation process. However, studies have described the rate of suppression using suppression-growth functions, and they showed that the function was steeper for lower-frequency DPOAEs than for higher-frequency DPOAEs when the suppressor was centered at the geometric mean of the primary tones (Harris, Probst, & Xu, 1992; Harris, Probst, Plinkert, & Xu, 1993).

There is also little systematic information available regarding DPOAE tuning using suppression methods. However, a recent study by Kummer, Janssen, and Arnold (1995) indicated that DPOAE iso-suppression curves from normal human ears showed tuning capability that was comparable to that of single cochlear-nerve fibers in experimental animal models. The DPOAE-tuning curves displayed in Figure 5–5 indicate that using substantial L_1-L_2 differences of around 25 dB make the responses more sensitive and sharper than those elicited with $L_1 = L_2$ primary tones. In addition, experimental evidence suggests that extending the frequency-measurement range to frequency regions that are one to two octaves above the DPOAE-generation site, in order to describe more complete suppression-response areas, may also provide greater insight into cochlear functioning (Martin, White-head, Stagner, & Lonsbury-Martin, 1995). Clearly, a database of DPOAE suppression contours from normal ears is needed before the sensitivity of the measures to hearing abnormalities in impaired ears can be determined.

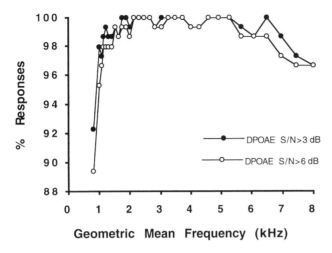

Figure 5–7. Prevalence of DPOAEs with respect to signal-to-noise ratio (S/N) as a function of frequency in 0.1-octave intervals. Percentage of ears showing responses with S/Ns >3 (*solid circles*) or >6 dB (*open circles*) is plotted for each 0.1-octave frequency step. S/Ns were >6 dB in 95% of ears at all frequencies, except the lowest at 0.8 kHz.

DPOAEs in Normal Ears

The most common application of clinical tests with DPOAEs is for detecting an abnormal reduction of DPOAE amplitude with a DP-gram. Therefore, a database of DPOAE amplitudes of normal human ears is needed. The following description of the normative properties of DPOAEs provides some details about the distribution of DPOAE level across a population of normal ears. This data set was obtained from 149 clinically normal ears of 94 subjects, with a mean [±1 standard deviation (SD)] age of 29.2 plus or minus 8.6 yrs (range 15–64 years). In cases in which statistical analyses were performed to illustrate a trend in the data, only one ear from each subject was included. Findings in individual reports may contrast with some of the following results, but reports that use large databases will likely uncover similar results.

All ears had normal tympanograms and 1-kHz contralateral and ipsilateral acoustic-reflex thresholds, no history of hearing disorders, and behavioral thresholds of ≤20 dB HL, measured by routine pure-tone audiometry at octave intervals between 250 Hz and 8 kHz and also at 3 and 6 kHz in the majority of ears. The DPOAEs were obtained using primary levels of 75 dB SPL at the geometric-mean frequencies of the primaries in 0.1-octave steps from 0.8–8 kHz, with $f_2/f_1 = 1.21$.

DPOAE Amplitude as a Function of Frequency

In 0.1-octave steps, the mean DPOAE amplitudes peaked at about 1.2 kHz (12.9 ± 5.4 dB SPL) and 5.7 kHz (8.31 ± 6.9 dB SPL) separated by a minimum at about 2.8 kHz (5.5 ± 5.6 dB SPL). Median DPOAE amplitudes (solid circles) were within

± 1 dB of the means up to 5.3 kHz, and were 1 to 1.8 dB higher than the means above 5.3 kHz (Figure 5–6). Over the frequency range in which DPOAEs were measured, SDs varied around 5.5 dB (range 5.1–6.5 dB).

All ears demonstrated DPOAE responses over a wide frequency range. Specifically, DPOAE S/N ratios were >6 dB, which was the highest S/N ratio measured, for over 95% of ears at all frequencies, except for the lowest frequency, which was at 0.8 kHz (Figure 5–7). The mean DPOAE S/N ratio varied between 19 and 30 dB. Thus, DPOAEs are typically present in all clinically normal ears, demonstrate large S/N ratios, and exhibit moderate variability. Moreover, it is clear that DPOAE testing can be extended to both lower and higher frequencies than those used.

Distribution of DPOAE Amplitudes

Distributions of DPOAE amplitudes for each 0.1-octave frequency were also examined for their goodness of fit to a Gaussian (i.e., normal) distribution using the Chi² test. Some representative distributions using 3-dB bins are shown in Figure 5–8. In general, below 4 kHz, the distributions of DPOAEs were typically not significantly different from Gaussian and demonstrated significant but minor deviations from Gaussian at only two frequencies (1 and 1.41 kHz). However, at most frequencies above 4 kHz, DPOAE-amplitude distributions deviated significantly from Gaussian in that they were skewed toward low DPOAE levels. However, at all frequencies, the observed deviations from Gaussian were minor as indicated by the similarity of the median and mean DPOAE amplitudes (Figure 5–6). Thus, DPOAE amplitude distributions in clinically normal ears are approximately Gaussian, although there are small deviations from Gaussian for DPOAEs at most frequencies above 4 kHz. This finding holds promise for the direct application of simple parametric statistical analyses (e.g., z-scores) to emission-amplitude data in order to determine the likelihood that any measured DPOAE amplitude is from the normal population. At frequencies greater than 4 kHz, a simple, minor pre-analysis transform of DPOAE amplitude could be used to further normalize the distributions.

Influence of Ear Side, Gender, and Age on DPOAE Amplitudes

The plots of Figure 5–9 through Figure 5–11 illustrate the variation in DPOAE amplitude with respect to ear, gender, and age.

EAR SIDE

The analysis outcome for ears (Figure 5–9) was based on only the 55 subjects for whom both ears were tested. The mean behavioral thresholds were lower (i.e., better) in right ears than in left ears for the mid-frequencies. The difference was significant only at 1 kHz (p <0.005). However, the corresponding DPOAE amplitudes did not show any clear differences between right and left ears.

GENDER

The analysis of outcome based on gender (Figure 5–10) was based on 79 female ears and 70 male ears. Behavioral thresholds were significantly lower (i.e., better)

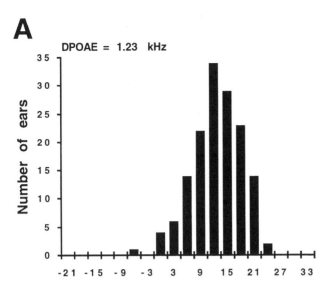

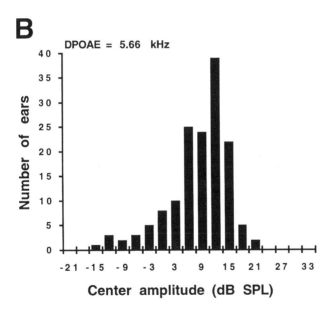

Figure 5–8. Typical distributions of DPOAE amplitudes in 3-dB bins for low and high frequencies. *A*: Amplitudes for low frequencies, e.g., 1.23 kHz, tended to be Gaussian or normal like. *B*: For frequencies >4 kHz, e.g., 5.66 kHz, amplitudes tended to be skewed toward lower values.

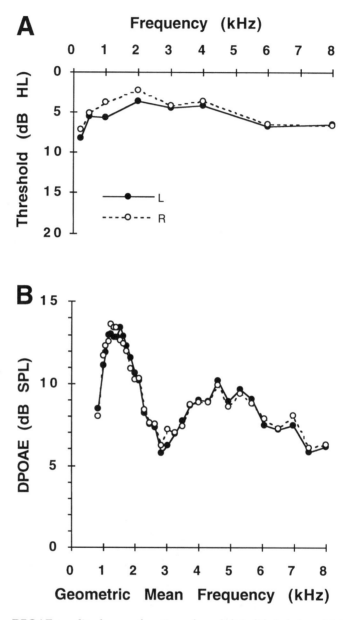

Figure 5–9. DPOAE amplitudes as a function of ear: left (*solid circles*) *vs* right (*open circles*) ears. *A*: Mean behavioral thresholds were slightly better for the right than for the left ear, particularly for the middle frequencies. *B*: Mean DPOAE amplitudes in 0.1-octave steps showing insignificant differences between right and left ears. To determine the statistical significance ($p < 0.05$) of the observed differences, analyses of variance (ANOVA) and t-tests were used.

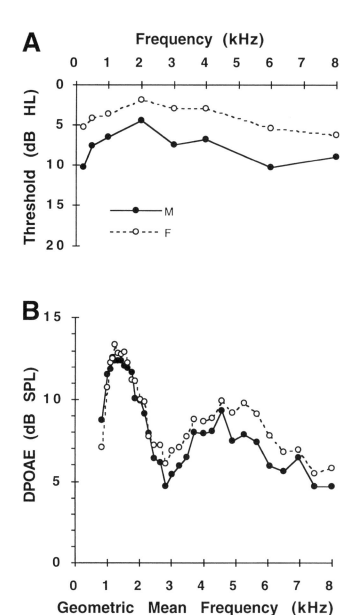

Figure 5–10. DPOAE amplitudes as a function of gender: male (*solid circles*) versus female (*open circles*) ears. *A*: Mean behavioral thresholds were better in women than in men at all frequencies. *B*: Mean DPOAE amplitudes in 0.1-octave steps were greater for women, particularly for frequencies above about 2.5 kHz. To determine the statistical significance ($p < 0.05$) of the observed differences, analyses of variance (ANOVA) and t-tests were used.

for women than for men at all frequencies. For DPOAEs, amplitudes were greater for women at most frequencies, although the differences were negligible, below a geometric-mean frequency of 2 kHz, and were significant only for the three geometric-mean frequencies in the 5-kHz range (i.e., at 5, 5.3, and 5.7 kHz).

AGE

For analyzing the influence of age (Figure 5–11) on DPOAE amplitude, ears were divided into three groups: 15 to 24 years (n = 47), 25 to 34 yrs (n = 66), and 35 years or older (n = 36, with only two ears >50 years). Behavioral thresholds increased significantly with age at and above 3 kHz. The DPOAE amplitudes decreased with increasing age at most frequencies, particularly for geometric-mean frequencies greater than 2 kHz. The differences were significant for most frequencies.

DPOAEs tend to be larger in woman than in men, and decreased with increasing age, particularly at high frequencies. In all cases, the variations in DPOAE amplitudes reflected variations of the corresponding behavioral thresholds. Whereas gender and ear differences were usually small, variations between age groups were large. Thus, separate population norms may be required for different age groups in clinical tests. This suggestion contrasts to that of Stover and Norton (1993) who examined the effects of age on DPOAE amplitudes in a smaller group of similar normal-hearing subjects and used statistical methods that permitted the influence of age and hearing level on DPOAEs to be analyzed separately. However, related findings from a preliminary study in our laboratory (Arnold, Lonsbury-Martin, & Martin, 1996) using comparable statistical techniques (i.e., multiple-regression analyses) with a larger subject population than that used by Stover and Norton showed that age influences DPOAE amplitude more than hearing level. Our findings support the adoption of age-adjusted norms for the clinical application of DPOAEs.

Advantages of DPOAE Testing

Finally, a potential advantage of DPOAE testing may be the systematic relation of some feature with hearing threshold. An example of the feasibility of this possibility is illustrated in Figure 5–12.

For each behavioral-threshold test frequency, the correlation coefficient (r) between the corresponding 0.1-octave band DPOAE amplitude and hearing threshold was also calculated. The resulting r values are plotted as a function of frequency (Figure 5–13). The absolute *r* values should be treated with caution because the behavioral thresholds are not distributed along a continuous variable, but are constrained to 5-dB steps within a relatively narrow range (i.e., all behavioral thresholds were < 20 dB HL). For each hearing-test frequency, the amplitudes of the DPOAE at that frequency were negatively correlated with behavioral threshold (Figure 5–13). That is, DPOAE amplitude decreased as hearing threshold increased. The correlation coefficients were significant (p <0.01), above 3 kHz, and the values were small (−0.01 to −0.29), reflecting the extremely large variability (Figure 5–12). Thus, DPOAE amplitudes are negatively correlated with hearing thresholds in clinically normal ears, but the correlations are weak, such that less than 10% of the variance in hearing threshold was predicted by the 0.1-octave band

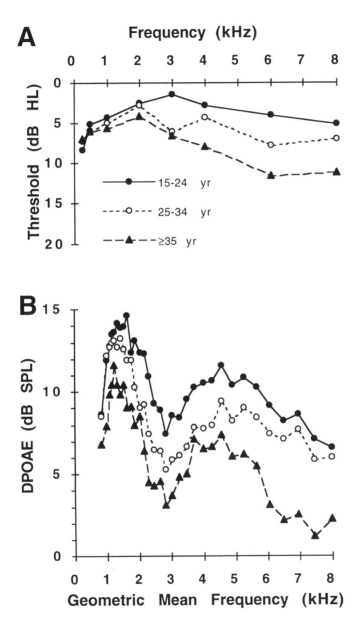

Figure 5–11. DPOAE amplitudes as a function of age: 15–24 (*solid circles*), 25–34 (*open circles*), and 35 (*solid triangles*) years. *A*: Mean behavioral thresholds increased with age above 2 kHz. *B*: Mean DPOAE amplitudes in 0.1-octave steps were smaller with increasing age, particularly for frequencies above 2 kHz. To determine the statistical significance ($p < 0.05$) of the observed differences, analyses of variance (ANOVA) and t-tests were used.

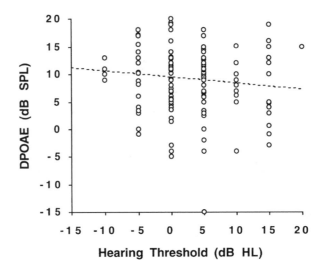

Figure 5–12.   Scatter plot of DPOAE amplitudes as a function of hearing level at 2 kHz. The great variability of DPOAE amplitudes is apparent. The *dashed line* represents a least-squares regression fit to the data indicating that for every increase of 1 dB in hearing level, DPOAE amplitude decreased by 0.3 dB.

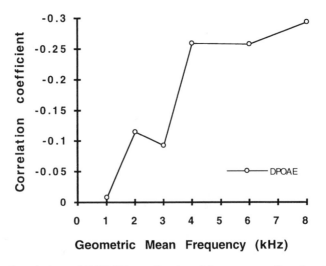

Figure 5–13.   Correlation of DPOAE amplitude with corresponding hearing level as a function of audiometric frequencies from 1–8 kHz.

DPOAE amplitude at the same frequency. It is possible that DPOAE levels over a wider frequency band (i.e., averaging DPOAE amplitude over several 0.1-octave bands around the related audiometric-threshold frequency) may have better reflected the corresponding hearing sensitivity for a particular frequency region.

The merits of having available a reliable database of DPOAE amplitudes from normal ears against which to judge the status of an unknown test ear are illustrated in Figure 5–14.

Current Controversies

There are several controversies at present in the DPOAE field that are clearly relevant to the clinical application of this type of emitted response. These issues include the optimal L_1-L_2 difference and stimulus calibration.

L_1-L_2 Difference

One controversy concerns the levels of the primary tones that optimally evaluate the functional status of the cochlear amplifier. Evidence from experimental studies in rabbits and various rodent species indicates that the $2f_1 - f_2$ DPOAE is produced by partially discrete mechanisms below and above stimulus levels of 60 to 70 dB SPL. Thus, this DPOAE shows differential parametric properties below and above these stimulus levels (Whitehead, Lonsbury-Martin, & Martin, 1992a). Additionally, in laboratory mammals, sharp notches are present in some DPOAE I/O functions at stimulus levels of between 55 and 70 dB SPL. Such DPOAE amplitude notches are associated with rapid DPOAE phase reversals, suggesting a cancellation of two distinct components of approximately equal amplitude that are about 180 degrees out of phase with each other, at the stimulus level of the notch (Whitehead et al. 1992a; Brown, 1987; Whitehead, Lonsbury-Martin, & Martin, 1990; Whitehead, Lonsbury-Martin, & Martin, 1992b). Moreover, DPOAEs elicited by primary tones below 60 to 70 dB SPL have been considerably more vulnerable to a variety of physiological insults than DPOAEs elicited by stimuli above these levels (Whitehead et al., 1992b; Schmeidt & Adams, 1981; Kemp & Brown, 1984; Schmiedt, 1986; Brown, McDowell, & Forge, 1989; Norton & Rubel, 1990) supporting the notion that the $2f_1 - f_2$ DPOAE is dominated by different generator mechanisms below and above 60 to 70 dB SPL in rabbits and rodents.

However, there are significant differences in the properties of DPOAEs between primate and nonprimate mammalian species. DPOAEs are smaller in primates than in nonprimate mammals, but the other evoked OAEs (i.e., the TEOAEs and stimulus-frequency OAEs) tend to be larger and spontaneous OAEs are more common in primates than in other mammals. In addition, DPOAE growth with increasing stimulus levels tends to saturate at lower stimulus levels in animals than in humans beings, and the maximum DPOAE amplitude occurs at a greater frequency separation of the stimulus tones in animals than in human beings. These differences suggest that caution is needed when generalizing from nonprimate animal models to the human applications. Thus, although there appear to be discrete mechanisms producing DPOAEs above and below 60 to 70 dB SPL in rabbits and rodents, it should not be assumed that there are corresponding discrete

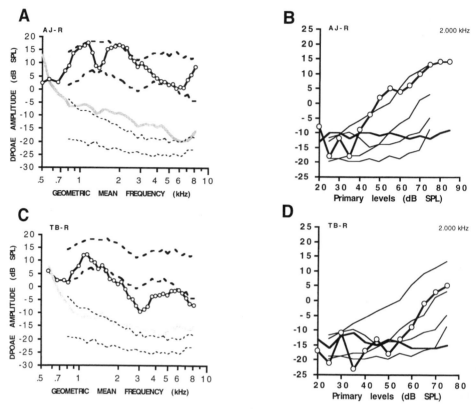

Figure 5–14. Examples of several types of DPOAE-amplitude functions (*open circles*) for the right ear of a 25-yr-old normal-hearing woman (*A, B*), and the right ear of a 48-yr-old man (*C, D*) with noise-induced hearing loss. DP-grams (*A, C*) were elicited with 75-dB primaries, and DPOAE I/O functions (*B, D*) tested with primary tones from 20–75 dB SPL are illustrated for 2 kHz. For the DP-gram plots, the *bold dashed lines* represent the ±1 SD of average DPOAE amplitudes for normal ears, and the *thin dashed lines* in the bottom portion of each plot indicate this range for the related noise floors. The *stippled line* in each DP-gram plot represents each subject's noise floor. On the I/O plots, the thin lines without symbols indicate the average levels of DPOAEs (*top portion of plot*) and noise floors (*bottom portion of plot*), and the *bold line without symbols* parallel to the abscissa represents the noise floor for each subject. *A*: Note the normal amplitudes of the DP-gram, in the presence of relatively high noise-floor levels. *B*: Normal 2-kHz I/O. *C*: Note the low-normal DPOAE amplitudes up to about 2 kHz, and the lower than normal amplitudes of DPOAEs for frequencies above ~2 kHz. *D*: Note the elevated threshold, low-normal amplitudes for suprathreshold primary tones >60 dB SPL, and steeper than normal growth slope exhibited by the 2-kHz I/O.

Follow-up pure-tone audiometry indicated that the woman's hearing was better than 15 dB HL at the conventional behavioral-test frequencies. In contrast, the man had worked as a well-driller during high school and college and complained of a loss in hearing sensitivity and tinnitus. Routine audiometric testing indicated that this ear, indeed, exhibited a mild to moderate high-frequency hearing loss that began around 2 kHz and showed a clear notch around 3 kHz.

low-level and high-level DPOAE generators in humans or, if there are such discrete mechanisms in humans, that they contribute to the ear-canal DPOAE over the same stimulus ranges as in nonprimate species. Although it is not clear at what stimulus level the DPOAEs in human ears become independent of outer–hair-cell status, in the clinical application of DP-grams, moderate stimulus levels of 65 to 75 dB SPL are typically used when $L_1 = L_2$ (Lonsbury-Martin et al., 1990; Smurzynski & Kim, 1992).

Whereas DPOAEs measured with $L_1 = L_2$ at moderate stimulus levels have demonstrated considerable clinical potential, the vulnerability of DPOAEs to cochlear trauma have appeared to increase as stimulus level decreases, both in animal models and in patients with sensorineural hearing loss (Martin et al., 1990; Lonsbury-Martin & Martin, 1990; Lonsbury-Martin, Whitehead, & Martin, 1991). Studies of the effects of level difference (L_1-L_2) between the primary tones on DPOAE amplitude in humans (Gaskill & Brown, 1990; Hauser & Probst, 1991) and laboratory mammals (Whitehead et al., 1992a; Whitehead et al., 1990; Brown & Gaskill, 1990; Mills & Rubel, 1994) have indicated that the maximum DPOAE amplitude occurs when $L_2 < L_1$. From the human studies, however, the increase of mean DPOAE amplitude obtained by decreasing L_2 below $L_1 = L_2$ was small (Hauser & Probst, 1990; Rasmussen, Popelka, Osterhammel, & Nielsen, 1993; Whitehead, McCoy, Lonsbury-Martin, & Martin, 1995a). Thus, such small increases in normative DPOAE amplitudes of typically less than 3 dB, over the range of stimulus frequencies and levels used in collecting DP-grams and I/O functions for clinical purposes, would unlikely substantially enhance the performance of clinical tests using DPOAEs.

However, other human data (Gaskill & Brown, 1990; Whitehead et al., 1995a; Gorga et al., 1993) have indicated that L_2 could be decreased considerably below $L_1 = L_2$ (i.e., up to 10–15 dB) without reducing DPOAE amplitude. Furthermore, decreasing L_2 below $L_1 = L_2$ by 25 dB (i.e., L_1-L_2 = 25 dB) enhanced the temporary reduction of DPOAEs by a brief exposure to a moderately intense pure tone (Sutton, Lonsbury-Martin, Martin, & Whitehead, 1994). Indeed, recent work showed that decreasing L_2 below $L_1 = L_2$ increased the reduction of DPOAEs associated with permanent cochlear trauma without reducing normative DPOAE amplitudes (Whitehead et al., 1995a). Consequently, this ability to increase the vulnerability of DPOAEs to traumas producing permanent sensorineural hearing loss has the potential to enhance the performance of clinical tests utilizing DPOAEs, which may be important in the longitudinal monitoring of persons at risk for hearing loss (e.g., patients administered ototoxic drugs, persons working in noisy environments).

However, for clinical tests based on detecting a reduction of DPOAE amplitude below population norms, test performance likely depends on factors in addition to mean DPOAE amplitudes in normal ears and the vulnerability of the DPOAE to trauma. Thus, it appears that DPOAEs in humans are quite vulnerable to cochlear trauma even at relatively high stimulus levels. For example, for primaries as high as $L_1 = L_2 = 75$ dB SPL, the highest levels commonly used in studies of the clinical applications of DPOAEs, emission level is often substantially reduced, relative to norms, at hearing levels of 20 to 30 dB HL, and is typically within the noise floor at hearing levels of greater than 50 dB HL (Lonsbury-Martin, Whitehead, & Martin,

1991). Thus, whereas decreasing stimulus levels in order to increase the vulnerability of DPOAEs to trauma may potentially improve the ability of DPOAEs to detect mild hearing losses, it may have little effect on the detection of moderate or severe hearing losses. Future research will determine the usefulness of adopting different stimulus levels of f_1 and f_2 for unique clinical applications, which will probably depend on the degree of cochlear dysfunction to be detected.

Sound Calibration

Another controversy is over stimulus calibration for DPOAE measurement. The stimulus-presentation strategy used by most investigators studying DPOAEs in humans (e.g., Gaskill & Brown, 1990; Smurzynski & Kim, 1992; Gorga et al., 1993; Rasmussen et al., 1993), and by the DPOAE-measurement devices commercially available adjusts the speaker command-voltage levels as a function of frequency to produce a constant SPL as measured at the DPOAE-measurement microphone. Siegel (1994) noted that, because of the presence of standing waves in the ear canal, the use of this in-the-ear adjustment strategy imposes large, systematic but idiosyncratic variations of stimulus level at the ear drum as a function of frequency. In particular, there are substantial increases of stimulus SPL at the eardrum in the 3- to 7-kHz–frequency region in which quarter-wave cancellations of stimulus energy occur at the microphone (Siegel, 1994; Whitehead, Stagner, Lonsbury-Martin, & Martin, 1995c).

To minimize the stimulus-calibration problem, in our laboratory we use an iso-voltage stimulus-presentation strategy based on the knowledge provided by the manufacturer (Etymotic Research literature) that the ER-2 speakers were designed to produce a flat response in a Zwislocki coupler. Thus, it is assumed that the frequency response of these speakers, used in conjunction with the ER-10 microphone probe, is approximately flat at the eardrum. Therefore, the level of the voltage command applied to the speakers to produce a given SPL at the eardrum is held constant across frequency. That is, for each ear, the voltage applied to the speakers to produce a given SPL at any frequency is the voltage that produces that SPL at 1 kHz, as measured at the microphone. Because the frequency response of the ER-10 microphone is flat in the frequency range of interest, its output is not adjusted.

Even with the iso-voltage approach, idiosyncratic variations of eardrum-stimulus level as a function of frequency occur, because the frequency response of the speakers in individual ears differs from that of a Zwislocki coupler. However, these variations are expected to be largely restricted to the 7 to 9 kHz region in which half-wave enhancement of stimulus levels at the eardrum occurs. In addition to being restricted to higher frequencies (>6 kHz rather than >3 kHz, approximately), the variations in stimulus level for the iso-voltage strategy are expected to be smaller than for the in-the-ear adjustment strategy (Siegel, 1994; Whitehead et al., 1995c).

Another approach to the stimulus-calibration problem for measuring DPOAEs is to utilize the strategy adopted by the ILO92 system (Otodynamics). Essentially, this DPOAE-measurement device exhibits a compromise between the in-the-ear adjustment and the iso-voltage stimulus-presentation strategies. In this manner, the adjustment of the speaker-command voltage across frequency is limited to not more that $+6$ or -9 dB relative to the voltage that produces the desired stimulus SPL at the DPOAE-measurement microphone at 2 kHz.

Certainly, the sound-calibration issue is most problematic for clinical applications that involve the determination as to whether a test ear is impaired based on the value of some DPOAE property that can be compared to the distribution of the feature in normal ears. Clearly, this concern is less important in serial-monitoring uses in which the goal is to identify simple change in some DPOAE characteristic from a baseline condition. For example, in monitoring for potential ototoxicity, only a change that is relative to the pre-treatment value needs to be determined. However, for many clinical applications it is certain that some agreement must be reached by investigators and clinicians who measure DPOAEs, and the manufacturers who devise DPOAE-testing equipment concerning the best method to combat the difficulties associated with calibrating high-frequency stimuli.

Summary and Conclusions

Both controversies involving the optimal combination of stimulus levels and the most accurate method of calibrating evoking stimuli are relevant to a complete understanding of DPOAE generation. It is clear that the field is still in the early stages of gathering information relevant to these issues. However, such controversies need to be settled in order to identify the best means of applying DPOAEs clinically. Regardless, the major expectation concerning the clinical efficacy of OAEs is that emitted responses will eventually be useful as predictors of hearing level. Such capability would permit hearing capacity in patient populations that have been traditionally difficult to test, such as newborns, to be more accurately estimated than is currently possible. In addition, OAEs would provide the tester with an objective and, thus, more rigorous estimation of the contributions that the peripheral ear makes to a particular individual's hearing status. Because of the ability of tonal stimuli to deliberately deliver a moderate amount of sound energy to a focused frequency region of the cochlea, DPOAEs have the best promise of predicting behavioral threshold at a specific frequency, within a timely manner that is compatible with clinical testing. However, whether DPOAE amplitude and threshold or some other form of response measure, such as onset latency, is the better predictor of hearing is still unknown. Because the evidence to date suggests that DPOAE-amplitude behavior sets broad constraints on related hearing thresholds, properties other than magnitude and threshold deserve consideration. There is no question that DPOAE amplitudes have been the most intensely studied aspect of this class of emission in both normal and pathological ears. However, a more complete description of the other features of the DPOAE response in normal ears is needed, before the effectiveness of these analyses in the clinical setting can be fully appreciated.

Acknowledgments

Portions of this work were supported by grants from the Deafness Research Foundation, and the Public Health Service (DC00613, DC01668, ES03500).

References

Arnold, D. J., Lonsbury-Martin, B. L, & Martin, G. K. (1996). Influence of ultra-high frequency hearing on distortion-product otoacoustic emission levels in humans. *Abstracts of the nineteenth midwinter meeting: Association for Research in Otolaryngology, 19,* 25.

Brass, D., & Kemp, D. T. (1993). Suppression of stimulus frequency otoacoustic emissions. *Journal of the Acoustical Society of America, 93,* 920–939.

Brown, A. M. (1987). Acoustic distortion from rodent ears: A comparison of responses from rats, guinea pigs and gerbils. *Hearing Research, 31,* 25–38.

Brown, A. M., & Gaskill, S. A. (1990). Measurement of acoustic distortion reveals underlying similarities between human and rodent mechanical responses. *Journal of the Acoustical Society of America, 88,* 840–849.

Brown, A. M., & Kemp, D. T. (1984). Suppressibility of the $2f_1 - f_2$ stimulated acoustic emissions in gerbil and man. *Hearing Research, 13,* 29–37.

Brown, D. K., Kimberley, B. P., & Eggermont, J. J. (1994). Cochlear traveling-wave delays estimated by distortion-product emissions in normal hearing adults and term-born neonates. *Journal of Otolaryngology, 23,* 234–237.

Brown, A. M., McDowell, B., & Forge, A. (1989). Acoustic distortion products can be used to monitor the effects of chronic gentamicin treatment. *Hearing Research, 42,* 143–156.

Davis, H. (1983). An active process in cochlear mechanics. *Hearing Research, 9,* 79–90.

Gaskill, S. A., Brown, A. M. (1990). The behavior of the acoustic distortion product, $2f_1$-f_2, from the human ear and its relation to auditory sensitivity. *Journal of the Acoustical Society of America, 88,* 821–839.

Gorga, M. P., Neely, S. T., Bergman, B. M., Beauchaine, K. L., Kaminski, J. R., Peters, J., & Jesteadt, W. (1993). Otoacoustic emissions from normal-hearing and hearing-impaired subjects: Distortion product responses. *Journal of the Acoustical Society of America, 93,* 2050–2060.

Harris, F. P, Lonsbury-Martin, B. L., Stagner, B. B., Coats, C. A., & Martin, G. K. (1989). Acoustic distortion products in humans: Systematic changes in amplitude as a function of f_2/f_1 ratio. *Journal of the Acoustical Society of America, 85,* 220–229.

Harris, F.P., Probst, R., & Xu, L. (1992). Suppression of the $2f_1 - f_2$ otoacoustic emission in humans. *Hearing Research, 64,* 133–141.

Harris, F. P., Probst, R., Plinkert, P., & Xu, L. (1993). Influence of interference tones on $2f_1 - f_2$ acoustic distortion products. In H. Duifhuis, J. W. Horst, P. van Dijk, et al. (eds.): *Proceedings from the Internation Symposium on Biophysics of Hair Cell Sensory Systems* (pp. 87–93). London: World Scientific.

Hauser, R., & Probst, R. (1991). The influence of systematic primary-tone level variation L_2-L_1 on the acoustic distortion product emission $2f_1 - f_2$ in normal human ears. *Journal of the Acoustical Society of America, 89,* 280–286.

Kemp, D. T. (1978). Stimulated acoustic emissions from within the human auditory system. *Journal of the Acoustical Society of America, 64,* 1386–1391.

Kemp, D. T. (1979). Evidence of mechanical nonlinearity and frequency selective wave amplification in the cochlea. *Archives of Otorhinolaryngology—Head and Neck Surgery, 224,* 37–45.

Kemp, D. T., & Brown, A. M. (1983). A comparison of mechanical nonlinearities in the cochleae of man and gerbil from ear canal measurements. In R. Klinke & R. Hartmann (eds.): *Hearing: Physiological bases and psychophysics* (pp. 82–88). Berlin: Springer-Verlag.

Kemp, D. T., & Brown, A. M. (1984). Ear canal acoustic and round window correlates of $2f_1 - f_2$ distortion generated in the cochlea. *Hearing Research, 13,* 39–46.

Kimberley, B. P, Brown, D. K., & Eggermont, J. J. (1993). Measuring human cochlear traveling wave delay using distortion product emission phase responses. *Journal of the Acoustical Society of America, 94,* 1343–1350.

Kummer, P., Janssen, T., & Arnold, W. (1995). Suppression tuning characteristics of the $2f_1 - f_2$ distortion-product emissions in humans. *Journal of the Acoustical Society of America, 98,* 197–210.

Lonsbury-Martin, B. L., Harris, F. P., Hawkins, M. D., Stagner B. B., & Martin G. K. (1990). Distortion-product emissions in humans: I. Basic properties in normally hearing subjects. *Annuals of Otology, Rhinology, and Laryngology, 99* (Suppl. 147), 3–13.

Lonsbury-Martin, B. L., & Martin, G. K. (1990). The clinical utility of distortion-product otoacoustic emissions. *Ear and Hearing, 11,* 144–154.

Lonsbury-Martin, B. L., Whitehead, M. L., & Martin, G. K. (1991). Clinical applications of otoacoustic emissions. *Journal of Speech and Hearing Research, 34,* 964–981.

Martin, G. K., Ohlms, L. A., Franklin, D. J., Harris, F. P., & Lonsbury-Martin, B. L. (1990). Distortion-product emissions in humans: III. Influence of sensorineural hearing loss. *Annuals of Otology, Rhinology, and Laryngology, 99* (Suppl. 147), 29–44.

Martin, G. K., Probst, R., Scheinin, S. A., Coats, A. C., & Lonsbury-Martin, B. L. (1987). Acoustic distortion products in rabbits. II. Sites of origin revealed by suppression and pure-tone exposures. *Hearing Resarch, 28,* 29–44.

Martin, G. K., Whitehead, M. L., Stagner, B. B., & Lonsbury-Martin, B. L. (1995). Suppression and enhancement of DPOAEs by interference tones above f_2 in rabbits. *Abstracts of the eighteenth midwinter meeting: Association for Research in Otolaryngology, 18*, 124.

Mills, D. M., & Rubel, E. W. (1994). Variation of distortion product otoacoustic emissions with furosemide injection. *Hearing Research, 77*, 183–199.

Nelson, D. A., & Kimberley B. P. (1992). Distortion-product emissions and auditory sensitivity in human ears with normal hearing and cochlear hearing loss. *Journal of Speech and Hearing Research, 35*, 1142–1159.

Norton, S. J., & Rubel, E. W. (1990). Active and passive ADP components in mammalian and avian ears. In P. Dallos, C. D. Geisler, J. W. Matthews, et al. (eds.): *Mechanics and biophysics of hearing* (pp. 219–226). New York: Springer-Verlag.

O Mahoney, C. F., & Kemp, D. T. (1995). Distortion product otoacoustic emission delay measurement in human ears. *Journal of the Acoustical Society of America, 97*, 3721–3735.

Pickles, J. O. (1988). Active mechanical processes in the cochlea: Cochlear emissions. In *An Introduction to the Physiology of Hearing* (2nd ed., pp. 141–145). London: Academic.

Popelka, G. R., Osterhammel, P. A., Nielsen, L. H., & Rasmussen, A. N. (1993). Growth of distortion product otoacoustic emission with primary-tone level in humans. *Hearing Research, 71*, 12–22.

Rasmussen, A. N., Popelka, G. R., Osterhammel, P. A., & Nielsen, L. H. (1993). Clinical significance of relative probe-tone levels on distortion-product otoacoustic emissions. *Scandinavian Audiology, 22*, 223–229.

Schmiedt, R. A. (1986). Acoustic distortion in the ear canal: I. Cubic difference tones: Effects of acute noise injury. *Journal of the Acoustical Society of America, 79*, 1481–1490.

Schmiedt, R. A., & Adams, J. C. (1981). Stimulated acoustic emissions in the ear canal of the gerbil. *Hearing Research, 5*, 295–305.

Siegel, J. H. (1994). Ear-canal standing waves and high-frequency sound calibration using otoacoustic emission probes. *Journal of the Acoustical Society of America, 95*, 2589–2597.

Smurzynski, J., & Kim, D. O. (1992). Distortion-product and click-evoked otoacoustic emissions of normally-hearing adults. *Hearing Research, 58*, 227–240.

Spektor, Z., Leonard, G., Kim, D. O., Jung, M. D., & Smurzynski J. (1991). Otoacoustic emissions in normal and hearing-impaired children and normal adults. *Laryngoscope, 101*, 965–976.

Stover, L. J., Montoya, D., Gorga, M. P., & Neely, S. T. (1995). Clinical efficacy of distortion product otoacoustic emission input/output functions. *Abstracts of the eighteenth midwinter meeting: Association for Research in Otolaryngology, 18*, 125.

Stover, L., & Norton, S. J. (1993). The effects of aging on otoacoustic emissions. *Journal of the Acoustical Society of America, 94*, 2670–2681.

Sutton, L. A., Lonsbury-Martin, B. L., Martin, G. K., & Whitehead, M. L. (1994). Sensitivity of distortion-product otoacoustic emissions in humans to tonal over-exposure: Time course of recovery and effects of lowering L_2. *Hearing Research, 75*, 161–174.

Whitehead, M. L., Lonsbury-Martin, B. L., & Martin, G. K. (1990). Actively and passively generated acoustic distortion at $2f_1 - f_2$ in rabbits. In P. Dallos, C. D. Geisler, J. W. Matthews, et al. (eds.): *Mechanics and biophysics of hearing* (pp. 243–250). New York: Springer-Verlag.

Whitehead, M. L., Lonsbury-Martin, B. L., & Martin, G. K. (1992a). Evidence for two discrete sources of $2f_1 - f_2$ distortion-product otoacoustic emission in rabbit: I. Differential dependence on stimulus parameters. *Journal of the Acoustical Society of America, 91*, 1587–1607.

Whitehead, M. L., Lonsbury-Martin, B. L., & Martin, G.K. (1992b). Evidence for two discrete sources of $2f_1 - f_2$ distortion-product otoacoustic emission in rabbit: II. Differential physiological vulnerability. *Journal of the Acoustical Society of America, 92*, 2662–2682.

Whitehead, M. L., Lonsbury-Martin, B. L., & Martin, G. K. (1993). The influence of noise on the measured amplitudes of distortion-product otoacoustic emissions. *Journal of Speech and Hearing Research, 36*, 1097–1102.

Whitehead, M. L., McCoy, M. J., Lonsbury-Martin, B. L., & Martin, G. K. (1995a). Dependence of distortion-product otoacoustic emissions on primary levels in normal and impaired ears: I. Effects of decreasing L_2 below L_1. *Journal of the Acoustical Society of America, 97*, 2346–2358.

Whitehead, M. L., Stagner, B. B., McCoy, M. J., & Lonsbury-Martin, B. L., (1995b). Dependence of distortion-product otoacoustic emissions on primary levels in normal and impaired ears: II. Asymmetry in L1,L2 space. *Journal of the Acoustical Society of America, 97*, 2359–2377.

Whitehead, M. L., Stagner, B. B, Lonsbury-Martin, B. L., & Martin G. K. (1995c). Effects of ear-canal standing waves on measurements of distortion-product otoacoustic emissions. *Journal of the Acoustical Society of America, 98*, 3200–3214.

Whitehead, M. L., Stagner, B. B., Martin, G. K., & Lonsbury-Martin B. L. (1996). Visualization of the onset of distortion-product otoacoustic emissions, and measurement of their latency. *Journal of the Acoustical Society of America, 100*, 1663–1679.

6

Ipsilateral Suppression of Transient Evoked Otoacoustic Emissions

George A. Tavartkiladze
Gregory I. Frolenkov
Alexandr V. Kruglov
Serge V. Artamasov

Introduction

Recently, many studies have been devoted to the suppression of transient evoked otoacoustic emissions (TEOAEs) by contralateral acoustic stimulation (Collet, 1993). This effect is believed to be mediated by the medial olivocochlear system (Veuillet, Collet, & Duclaux, 1991), and it is relatively small. Typically, the TEOAE suppression associated with contralateral stimuli of 70 to 75 dB SPL is about 1 to 2 dB (Veuillet, Collet, & Duclaux, 1991). In contrast to contralateral stimulation, ipsilateral masking can result in more pronounced suppression of TEOAEs (Kemp & Chum, 1980; Tavartkiladze, Frolenkov, & Kruglov, 1993; Wilson, 1980). The mechanisms underlying this effect seem to be twofold. From one view, the suppression results from intracochlear masking processes; from another view, it appears to be mediated through the olivocochlear system. The chapter describes various aspects of TEOAE masking properties under simultaneous and forward masking conditions which have been investigated for several years (Frolenkov, Artamasov, Kruglov, & Tavartkiladze, 1995; Tavartkiladze, Frolenkov, & Kruglov, 1991; Tavartkiladze, Frolenkov & Artamasov, 1996).

Ipsilateral Simultaneous Masking of TEOAEs

Since the first description by Kemp (1978), the measurements of TEOAEs have progressed from laboratory research to clinical application. Today it is universally accepted that OAE phenomena are of cochlear origin (Probst, 1991; Zurek, 1985).

Nonetheless, the particular segments of the cochlear partition that generate TEOAEs in response to a stimulus with given frequency composition remain unresolved (Hilger, Furness & Wilson,1995; Kemp, 1986; Tavartkiladze, Frolenkov & Kruglov, 1993). This situation is due to the very complex structure of the TEOAE frequency spectrums and to the fact that not all frequencies evoke TEOAEs (Probst, Coats, Martin & Lonsbury-Martin, Martin,1986). Information about the location of the cochlear partition vibration maximum can be revealed by constructing TEOAE tuning curves under simultaneous tonal masking conditions. Unfortunately, only a few researchers have described the results of TEOAE simultaneous-masking investigations (Kemp & Chum, 1980; Wilson, 1980).

Simultaneous-Masking Procedures

All our simultaneous-masking experiments were performed with subjects who were 21 to 33 years of age, with audiometric thresholds less than 20 dB HL within the frequency range of 125 to 8000 Hz, with type A tympanograms, and with no signs of otologic diseases during the investigation. Because spontaneous otoacoustic emissions (SOAEs) could modify TEOAE responses (Probst, Coats, Martin, & Lonsbury-Martin, 1986), the existence of either SOAE or (synchronized) quasi-SOAEs was tested using the ILO 88 system (Otodynamics).

TEOAEs were recorded with a custom-designed acoustic probe, consisting of a microphone (EA-1842) and two Knowles electroacoustic transducers (ED-1913) (Figure 6–1). The free field calibration of the probe microphone was carried out by short broadband clicks with initial rarefaction wave. The probe under calibration was placed close to the measuring microphone (4676, Bruel & Kjaer) connected to a measuring amplifier (2235 noisemeter, Bruel & Kjaer). The output of the measuring amplifier was used for calibration of the probe. (The frequency response of the probe-microphone channel is presented in the left bottom panel of Figure 6–1.)

During the experiments, probe-microphone output was amplified and fed to a Medelec "Sensor-3" Clinical Averager using an effective filter bandwidth of 300 Hz (6 dB per octave) to 6000 Hz (12 dB per octave). One of the electroacoustical transducers was used to deliver test stimuli, which were 60 and 500 μs clicks, and tone bursts of different frequencies with trapezoidal envelope: 1 cycle rise per fall, 1 cycle plateau for frequencies less than 1 kHz, and 2 cycles rise per fall, 3 cycles plateau for frequencies more than 1 kHz. To reduce the intersubject variability of TEOAE amplitude, the stimulus intensity was related to the subject's sensation level and set at 20 dB SL to provide selective excitation of the limited segment of cochlear partition. The stimulus repetition rate was 20 Hz.

TEOAE-response waveforms were obtained with synchronous averaging of 2000 consecutive responses to test stimuli. The signal was then routed into two independent channels of the averaging system. Thus, averaged responses to even and odd stimuli were obtained. The sum of the curves formed the TEOAE record, and the difference between them was used for noise-level estimation. The second electroacoustical transducer was employed to deliver masking tones of different frequencies. First, the subjective threshold of tone perception was determined for each frequency. After that, masking was continued with constant intensity during the averaging process. Any intensity changes were performed at least 1 to 2 min

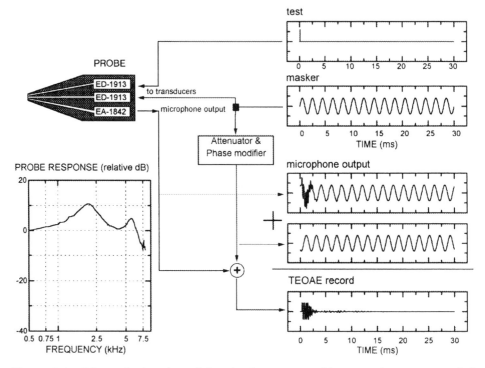

Figure 6–1. Schematic drawing of the simultaneous masking experiments setup. Left bottom panel represents the probe-microphone frequency response.

before the start of averaging. For masker-artifact cancellation, the reference masker was attenuated, phase-corrected, and electrically added to the probe-microphone output (Figure 6–1) before leading it to the averager. The degree of attenuation and phase correction angle were manually adjusted in such a way as to minimize amplitude of the signal at the averager input. The adjustment was necessary each time when the frequency or intensity of the masker tone were changed.

The results obtained were used for the construction of iso-suppression tuning curves. For each frequency of masking tone, the relation between the masker intensity (5–60 dB SL) and TEOAE amplitude was determined. Then the masking tone intensity necessary for 50% reduction of TEOAE amplitude was approximated from this relation. If the TEOAE attenuation was less than 50%, even under the highest levels of masking tone (50–60 dB SL), the masking tone of this frequency was not considered to produce TEOAE reduction and this intensity was marked by the arbitrary value of 180 dB.

TEOAE-Amplitude Calculation

Linear component cancellation (Bray & Kemp, 1987; Kemp, Bray, Alexander, & Brown, 1986) was not suitable for these experiments, because the method dramatically reduced the amplitude of TEOAE evoked by stimuli of a relatively low intensity (Frolenkov, Artamasov, Kruglov, & Tavartkiladze, 1995; Grandori & Ravazzani, 1993; Tavartkiladze, Frolenkov, Kruglov & Artamasov, 1994). Instead, TEOAEs were recorded by ordinary averaging. However, linear component cancellation was used for the determination of time window of analysis. For this purpose, the control TEOAE recordings were made at different click intensities (0–46 dB SL), and for each subject the difference was obtained between TEOAE records to 30 dB SL click and to 20 dB SL click after multiplying the latter record by a 10 dB correction coefficient (Figure 6–2). The difference consisted of non-linear TEOAE components only and was used to determine the analysis window (Figure 6–2). Additionally, the appropriateness of the time window estimate was determined by the construction of input/output curves for the RMS amplitude of TEOAE in time intervals shorter than the window chosen. Any time intervals that did not include non-linear TEOAE components were excluded from consideration. Then TEOAE recordings in the determined time window were multiplied to Hamming window function and fast Fourier transform (FFT) analysis was performed. The amplitude of the TEOAE was calculated as the square root of the difference between the signal power and noise power in the frequency range where the spectrum of signal exceeded that of noise more than 3 dB SL.

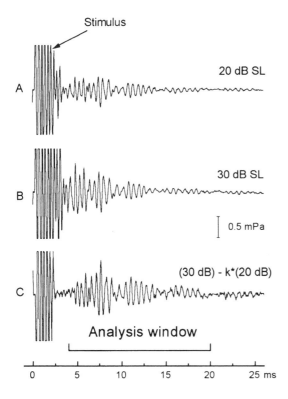

Figure 6–2. Analysis time determination. *A, B*: TEOAE responses evoked by 50 µs clicks with intensity of 30 dB SL and 20 dB SL correspondingly. *C*: The difference of the above recordings after multiplying of the record *B* by the 10 dB correction coefficient. This difference consists of non-linear TEOAE components only and was used to determine the analysis window (indicated by horizontal line). The zero point on the time scale corresponds to the stimuli onsets. Stimulus artifact on record C was not completely canceled due to the signal limitation by the ADC converter.

Properties Of Click-Evoked and Tone-Burst–Evoked OAEs

TEOAEs were found in all subjects tested. Click-evoked OAE pattern and durations differed in various subjects. The maximum duration was observed in the persons with SOAE. TEOAE amplitude increased with the rise of test stimulus intensity and tended to saturate at higher intensities, which is close to previous data (Bray & Kemp; Grandori, 1985; Grandori & Ravazzani, 1993; Kemp, Bray, Alexander, & Brown). Nevertheless, some peculiarities in input/output functions of different click-evoked OAE time components were revealed. Figure 6–3 illustrates normal input/output functions in linear scale (i.e., in the scale where input/output function of the passive linear system is a straight line) obtained in a subject

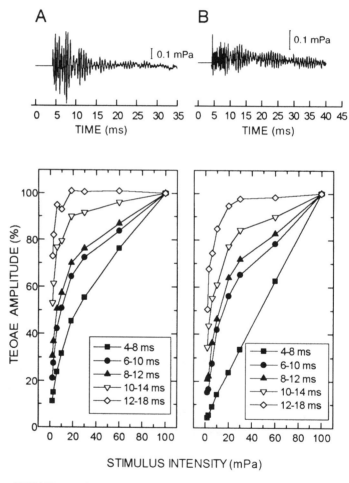

Figure 6–3. TEOAE samples (top) and their input/output curves (*bottom*) for different TEOAE time components (their latency indicated by different legends) in the subjects without (*A*) and with SOAE (*B*). TEOAE responses were evoked by 50 µs clicks with a stimulus amplitude of 20 dB SL. Stimuli artifacts were zeroed.

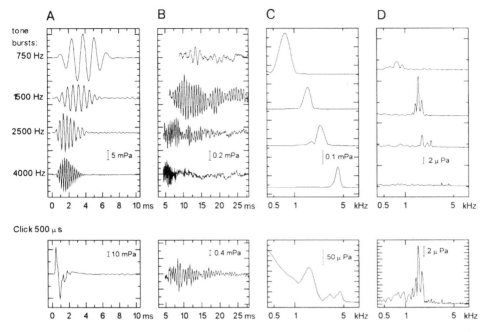

Figure 6–4. TEOAE samples (*B*) evoked by different stimuli (*A*) and the corresponding frequency spectra of stimuli (*C*) and of TEOAE (*D*). Stimuli amplitude was 20 dB SL; other parameters are indicated in the left column of the figure.

without SOAEs. For the subject, there was a clear relation between latency and input/output curve shape: With the longer latency of TEOAE components, the input/output function became more nonlinear and saturated. The minimal latency of TEOAE components with significant non-linearity varied in different subjects from 4 to 6 ms. The relation between the latency and the degree of non-linearity of TEOAE time components was observed in all the subjects tested, even in the persons with SOAEs.

Tone-burst evoked OAE duration and spectra differed in various subjects. Nevertheless, the following TEOAE properties common for all the subjects were observed (Figure 6–4):

1. TEOAE amplitude in response to tone bursts of different frequencies interacted with stimulus frequency. Maximum amplitude and duration were generally found with the stimulus frequencies from 1 to 1.5 kHz (Figure 6–4). When the stimulus frequency increases above 1.5 kHz, the TEOAE duration decreases significantly.

2. The TEOAE in response to broadband stimulation had the amplitude and duration similar to those of the TEOAE elicited by the most effective tone burst (Figure 6–4).

3. The TEOAE spectrum consisted of a number of separate frequency components (Figure 6–4). Narrowband stimuli generated only the components located

within the frequency range that corresponded to the stimulus spectrum (Figure 6–4), and broadband stimulation could elicit the TEOAE components practically within the entire frequency-interval tested (0.25–6 kHz).

4. All the frequency components produced with broadband stimulation could be found in the spectra of the TEOAE caused by narrow-band stimuli. The latter property was particularly prominent when the spectra were plotted using a linear frequency scale (Figure 6–4).

TEOAE Tuning Properties

The TEOAEs were suppressed in all the experiments with simultaneous tonal masking. Figure 6–5 shows typical TEOAEs recorded in response to 1.5-kHz tone bursts without masking and with masking tone of various intensities. In the experiments, the masking effect increased directly with the sensation level of the masking tone. With the tone at 40 dB SL, almost total suppression of TEOAE was observed. The response suppression was found only at the masking-tone frequency equal or close to that of the TEOAE stimulus (Figure 6–5). Figure 6–6 shows typical iso-suppression tuning curves of tone-burst and click-evoked OAEs. In all subjects and for all stimuli the tuning curve corresponded to the TEOAE frequency spectrum. In the case of tone-burst stimulation, locations of the maxima of the TEOAE stimulus spectrum and tuning-curve tip were the same. The tuning

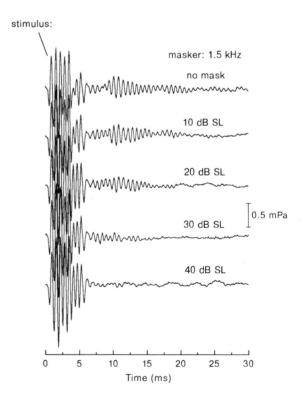

Figure 6–5. TEOAE reduction under simultaneous masking by 1.5 kHz tone of increasing intensity (indicated on the records). OAE were evoked by 1.5 kHz, 20 dB SL tone bursts. The *straight line* in the bottom left corner indicates the stimulus artifact.

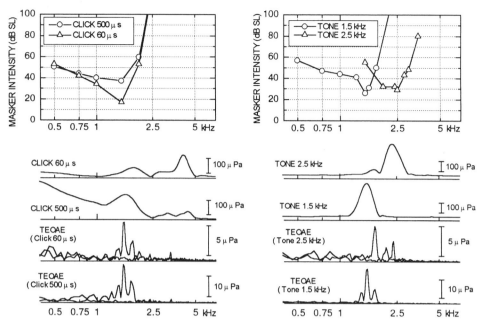

Figure 6–6. Iso-suppression tuning curves (*top*) of OAEs evoked by clicks of different durations (*A*) and by tone bursts of different frequencies (*B*). Bottom records show from top to bottom: the spectra of stimuli and the spectra of corresponding TEOAEs. Stimuli intensity was 20 dB SL. *Dashed lines* indicate noise level.

properties of click-evoked OAE were different, and TEOAE spectral maxima, as well as TEOAE tuning-curves tips, did not correspond to the stimulus spectra. Indeed, clicks of various duration (60 μs and 500 μs) had quite different spectra (Figure 6–6). Irrespective of the click-stimuli spectra, the spectra of TEOAE were practically identical, and correspondingly similar TEOAE tuning-curves were obtained. In addition, the smaller difference between the tip and the low-frequency segment of the tuning curve with the 500 μs stimulus closely correlated to the existence of low-frequency TEOAE components which were not observed for the 60 s-click stimulation. In this subject tone burst stimulation with a frequency of 1.5 kHz was the most effective for the TEOAE excitation (compare Figure 6–4). The TEOAE evoked by this stimulus had in its spectrum essentially the same peaks that dominated the spectra of TEOAE to broad-band stimulation (Figure 6–5). As a result, the tuning curve of the TEOAE to the 1.5 kHz tone burst was similar to the tuning curves of click-evoked OAEs (Figure 6–6). TEOAE spectra of all the test subjects were characterized by the dominant peaks within the 1 to 2 kHz range, and the peaks strictly determined the tuning curves of both OAEs evoked by clicks of different duration and by TEOAEs to the tone burst of the most effective frequency. Nevertheless, the apparent independence of TEOAE-frequency composition and iso-suppression tuning curves from the stimuli spectra was only relative. When the stimulus energy was concentrated within the frequency range that did not comprise the frequencies of the dominant peaks of TEOAE to broad-band stimulation, the TEOAE with different frequency composition was observed (Figure 6–4). For example, OAEs evoked by 2.5 kHz tone bursts had the spectral peaks within the range of 1.8 to 2.6 kHz and the tuning curve with the tip located around 2.5 kHz (Figure 6–6). Comparison of the tone-evoked OAE tuning curves showed that OAEs evoked with 2.5 kHz tone burst were characterized by a somewhat wider tuning curve than the TEOAEs to 1.5 kHz stimulation. This difference was not surprising considering the wider spectrum of TEOAE to the 2.5 kHz tone burst (Figure 6–6). The tuning-curve shape was a typically flat, low frequency "plateau" in all subjects; and a steep, high frequency rise (Figure 6–6) was observed in all subjects.

The relation of TEOAE simultaneous-masking properties to the TEOAE-frequency composition was further explored by construction of tuning curves of the separate TEOAE frequency components (Figure 6–7). It was found that the components were suppressed independently and had individual tuning curves with the typical shape (Figure 6–6). The tips of the tuning curves were closely related to the frequency of separate components (Figure 6–7). The intensities of masking tones that corresponded to the tuning curves tips tended to be higher for dominant peaks

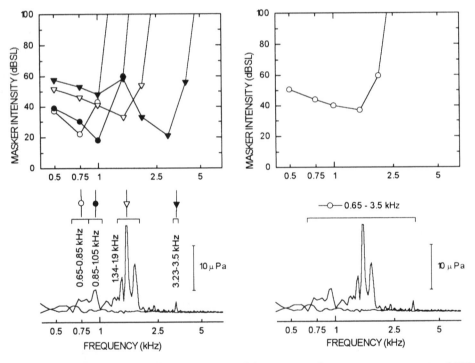

Figure 6–7. Iso-suppression tuning curves of the separate frequency components of 500 μs-click evoked OAE (*left*) and of the overall TEOAE response (*right*). The tuning curves were constructed for the frequency ranges indicated above the TEOAE spectrum (bottom records). Dashed lines indicate noise level.

(Figure 6–7). Usually the amplitudes of the TEOAE frequency components differed, and the tuning curve constructed from the total TEOAE spectrum was determined by the contribution of TEOAE dominant spectral peaks (Figure 6–7). Finally, the independent suppression of the TEOAE frequency components was observed in all the subjects. Unfortunately, neither subjects had SOAEs, and it could not be determined how the presence of SOAEs could modify the suppression of TEOAE spectral constituents.

TEOAE Generation Sources

The findings indicate that the main contributions to the TEOAE generation most probably originated from a number of local sources individually distributed along the cochlea. Indeed, frequency locations of TEOAE spectral peaks and their amplitude distribution were peculiar to each subject. Locations of the TEOAE spectral peaks were independent of the stimuli frequency composition, but each spectral peak was excited only when the stimulus energy was concentrated within the frequency range that covered the frequency of the particular peak (Figure 6–4). Moreover, each spectral component was suppressed independently under simultaneous-masking conditions (Figure 6–7).

All the data suggested that the major TEOAE spectral peaks reflected the vibratory activity of the independent emission sources. The total TEOAE response was likely to represent the superposition of the emissions generated by these independent sources. Their power could have been different, which could the explain relative independence of the TEOAE spectra and tuning curves from the stimuli frequency composition (Figure 6–4 & Figure 6–6). Indeed, in all subjects peaks of a 1- to 2-kHz frequency dominated in the spectra of OAEs evoked by different clicks, even by tone bursts with the frequency of 1 to 2 kHz. This fact was reflected in the corresponding tuning curves, as well (Figure 6–6). Thus, one possibility was that the main contribution to the TEOAE generation was made by the 1- to 2-kHz region of cochlear partition. This possibility was suggested by Avan, Bonfils, Loth, Narcy, and Trotoux (1991) who studied the properties of click-evoked OAEs. Nevertheless, their suggestion only explained cases of broad-band stimuli (for example, clicks) and tonal stimulation with the most effective frequencies. Frequency- specific stimulation have produced TEOAEs with different frequency composition that correspond to the stimulus spectrum (Figure 6–6) (Elberling, Parbo, Johnsen, & Bagi, 1985; Hauser, Probst, & Lohle, 1991; Norton & Neely, 1987; Probst, Coats, Martin & Lonsbury-Martin). The tuning curves of these tone-burst–evoked OAEs have reflected their frequency-specific generation. The predominance of the peaks with 1- to 2-kHz frequencies in the click-evoked TEOAE spectra, was partly explained by the spectral characteristic distortion due to reverse middle-ear transmission of sound (Kemp, 1980).

The "true" frequency-specific TEOAEs was thought to exist in a small percentage of normal-hearing subjects (Probst, 1990). At the same time, the short-latency TEOAE components were also suggested to contain this type of TEOAE (Kubo, Sakashita, Hachikawa, Minowa, & Nakai, 1991). This chapter's data are not sufficient to exclude both possibilities; nevertheless, we did not observe the TEOAE spectra partially or totally "mirroring" the stimulus frequency composition.

Hence, the contribution of the "true" frequency-specific TEOAE (if it existed) to the total TEOAE response was negligible in these investigations. The hypothesis about the existence of local individually distributed OAE generators was first suggested for the description of SOAE properties (Zurek, 1981). Moreover, morphological indications were found showing that SOAE generation was likely to be related to local irregularities of outer–hair-cell distribution along the organ of Corti (Lonsbury-Martin, Martin, Probst, & Coats, 1988; Martin, Lonsbury-Martin, Probst & Coats, 1988). It was shown that the sources responsible for SOAE generation also contributed to the generation of both stimuli following OAEs and TEOAEs. Finally, the comparison of the latter types of OAEs, obtained from the same ear revealed their frequency peaks' similarities (Martin, Lonsbury-Martin, Probst, & Coats) (Figure 6–3 and Figure 6–9), which could indicate possible identity of their generators. Thus, the hypothesis of the existence of OAE local generators previously proposed for SOAEs (Lonsbury-Martin, Martin, Probst & Coats; Martin, Lonsbury-Martin, Probst & Coats) and supported for TEOAEs by investigations presented in this chapter seems true for all types of OAEs: spontaneous, stimulus-following, and transient evoked. Validity of this speculation and the nature of proposed generators still need to be investigated. Additional study concerning this question (Hilger, Furness, & Wilson 1995) revealed equivocal results. On one hand, no relation between outer–hair-cell irregularities and the fine structure of the TEOAE spectra was found. On the other hand, the total TEOAE intensity was found to be proportional to the number of irregularities of the outer hair cells in the cochlea (Hilger, Furness, & Wilson).

This chapter's data support the earlier observations (Kemp & Chum; Wilson) of the frequency selective reduction of TEOAE under simultaneous masking conditions. The TEOAE tuning-curve shape (Figure 6–6 & Figure 6–7) was similar to that of the outer–hair-cell AC response (Dallos, 1985; Kossl & Russell, 1992). These findings suggested the existence of some common mechanisms underlying the phenomena. Nevertheless, the tuning curves were wider in TEOAE experiments. This fact could be explained by the short duration of stimuli and, accordingly, the increased spectral width of the stimuli. However, it was found that the TEOAE tuning-curve shape was more closely related to the spectrum of TEOAE, but not to that of the stimulus (Figure 6–6). Furthermore, when the TEOAE spectrum had prominent, sharp peaks, a much sharper tuning could be observed, even for OAEs evoked by a relatively broad-band stimulus (Figure 6–6). This property makes the simultaneous masking of TEOAE similar to that of SOAE (Wilson & Sutton, 1981; Zurek, 1981).

Ipsilateral Forward-Masking of TEOAEs

Neurons of the medial olivocochlear system (MOCS) can be effectively activated with both contralateral and ipsilateral sound (Liberman & Brown, 1986). Direct electrical stimulation of the crossed olivocochlear bundle (the subsystem of the MOCS presumably consisting of the ipsilaterally activating efferent fibers [Warren & Liberman, 1989] at the floor of the fourth ventricle) has resulted in bilateral desensitization of the cochleas (Rajan, 1988, 1990), as well as in the suppression of the DPOAEs (Mountain, 1980). Therefore, it is reasonable to suggest some functional significance of the ipsilaterally activated olivocochlear feedback. Nevertheless, the latter reflex arc has received little attention in the literature. Evidence was presented for the involvement of efferent system in the ipsilateral forward-masking of the compound-action potential (Bonfils & Puel, 1987), and there is a recently reported comparisons between ipsilateral, contralateral, and binaural forward-masking of TEOAEs (Berlin, Hood, Hurley, Wen, & Kemp, in press). Nevertheless, the majority of the data related to the cochlear efferent physiology were obtained in experiments on the anesthetized animals, which may have changed reflex properties of the efferent neurons (Liberman & Brown). As a result, in an awake human being even the question about the latency of the contralateral activation of MOCS is still disputable (Lind, 1994). There are indications for the existence of the ipsilaterally activated efferent suppression of TEOAE in normal hearing subjects (Tavartkiladze, Frolenkov, & Artamasov, 1996). Comparison of the ipsilateral and contralateral efferent-mediated TEOAE suppressions in the same subject could be useful for the clinical testing of MOCS functioning.

Forward-Masking Experiments

As in the simultaneous-masking studies, persons investigated were normal-hearing subjects with no history of otologic disease, with audiometric thresholds less than 20 dB within the frequency range of 125-8000 Hz, and type-A tympano-grams. Absence of the spontaneous OAEs was proved by the ILO 88 analyzer (Otodynamics). Suppression of TEOAE by the continuous contralateral-noise stimulation is known to be of the same order of magnitude as the TEOAE spontaneous changes (Berlin, Hood, Wen, et al., 1993) and slightly more than the TEOAE changes with directed attention (Froehlich, Collet, & Morgon, 1993). The TEOAE suppression by relatively short acoustic stimuli (clicks or broad-band noise no more than 30 ms duration) was investigated. This effect was expected to be somewhat smaller than the suppression associated with continuous noise presented contralaterally. To minimize baseline changes all TEOAE recordings were performed in one lengthy recording session without change of the probe's position in the test ear.

The ILO 88 system (with software version 3.94L) was set up with uniform (80-μs) linear clicks as stimulus 1 and quad-spaced clicks as stimulus 2. Stimulus 1 was routed to channel A as the ipsilateral acoustic stimulus. Stimulus 2 was fed to channel B. In click-to-click forward-masking experiments, the latter stimulus was delivered ipsilaterally through the second electroacoustic transducer of the ILO probe and was used as a masker. In noise-to-click forward-masking experiments, output of the channel B triggered the general-purpose digital generator (HP33120A, Hewlett Packard). After appropriate attenuation (output attenuator of the Midi-mate 602 audiometer, Madsen Electronics) digitally generated broad-band (50K– 8000 Hz) noise bursts of 10 or 30 ms duration were delivered ipsilaterally to the second electroacoustic transducer of the ILO probe or contralaterally to the TDH-39 headphone. Canceling of masking-signal artifact was observed in the course of averaging because the ILO system alternates the phase of every accepted stimulus and response. Before the execution of forward masking experiments, the TEOAE was also masked by continuous broad-band noise delivered contra-

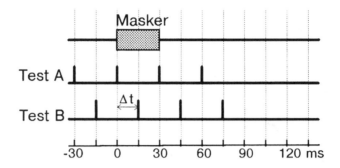

Figure 6–8.   Time patterns used in forward masking studies. For the picture clarity only the case of noise-to-click masking was illustrated. Test clicks were separated by the 30 ms interval. Test sequences were delivered with the rate of 3 Hz. Time delay (Δt) between the masker onset and the second click in the test sequence varied from 1 to 30 ms in click-to-click masking experiments and was equal to 0 (test A) or 15 ms (test B) in noise-to-click masking experiments.

laterally. In all forward masking experiments test clicks were delivered in sequence (inter-click interval 30 ms) with the repetition rate of 3 Hz (Figure 6–8). Such a low stimulation rate was used in order to guarantee a 200 ms pause between the test series. This time was probably essential for the excitation decay in the olivo-cochlear reflex arc (Warren & Liberman, 1989). Emission to each test click was stored separately. At least 1000 TEOAE responses were recorded without window-ing. After averaging TEOAE responses in each software buffer (to different test clicks) were time-windowed (4–15 ms) and their RMS amplitudes were calculated using ILO 88 software. To trace baseline variations in response amplitude (Berlin, Hood, Wen, et al., 1993), TEOAE records were obtained alternatively: with and without contralateral or ipsilateral masking stimulation. Each TEOAE record in the presence of noise preceded the record without a masker. The mean differences (and their standard errors) of TEOAE amplitudes from these pairs (5 pairs per each point) were calculated. The time delay (Δt) between the onset of masker and the second test click in sequence was adjusted to be 1 to 30 ms (Figure 6–1). In noise-to-click forward-masking experiments it was fixed at two predetermined values: 0 ms (test A) or 15 ms (test B). A tone-tailed test (*t-test*) was applied to determine the statistical significance of the TEOAE amplitude changes under masking conditions.

Contralateral Masking With Continuous Broad-Band Noise

Contralateral noise remarkably reduced the TEOAE amplitude. In one subject OAE evoked by the clicks of moderate intensity of 65.5 dB SPL (relating to subjec-tive threshold it was 30 dB SL) were diminished by as much as 2.3 dB with the use of 60 dB SL contralateral noise. The effect was observed at the masker intensities up to 30 dB SL (Figure 6–9).

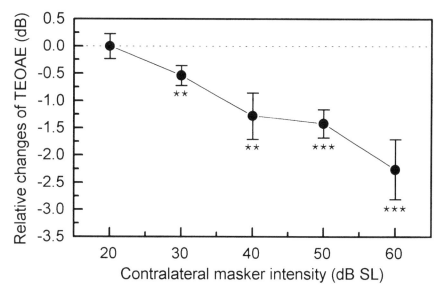

Figure 6–9. TEOAE suppression produced by continuous contralateral broad-band noise of different intensities. Noise intensities were related to the subjective threshold (SL). TEOAE was elicited by 65.5 dB SPL (30 dB SL) clicks.

Ipsilateral Click-to-Click Forward Masking

TEOAEs were dramatically suppressed during the first ms after masking click delivery (Figure 6–10). This suppression consisted in the overall decrease of emission-time components and maybe a more prominent reduction of long-latency emission. The amplitude of emission recovered to 90% of the control value in 5 ms. Changes of emission amplitude at longer interstimulus intervals were not significant.

Contralateral Versus Ipsilateral Noise-To-Click Forward Masking

Contralateral broad-band noise burst stimulation with the intensity of 50 dB SL (65 dB nHL) evoked statistically significant reduction of TEOAE amplitude 15 ms after masker onset (Figure 6–11). This effect became more prominent with the increase of noise duration up to 30 ms. The same noise stimulation presented ipsilaterally evoked similar effect at the intervals between the masker and the test of more than 30 ms (Figure 6–11). These effects could not be related to the efferent feedback activation by the test sequence because there were no statistically significant changes in the amplitude of OAE evoked by different clicks in test sequence without masking (Figure 6–11). The time course of ipsilateral and contralateral suppressions was practically identical. Nevertheless, the prominent ipsilateral suppression at the masker-stimulus onset delay of 15 ms was also found. It corresponded to the 5 ms difference between the masker end and the stimulus delivery,

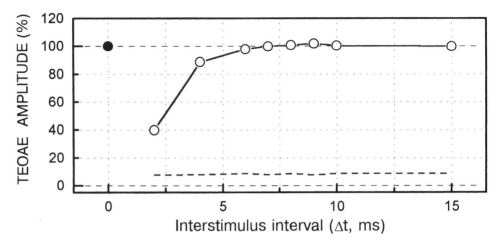

Figure 6–10. Changes of TEOAE amplitude with interstimulus time interval (Δt) under click-to-click forward masking conditions. *Filled circle* indicates the control TEOAE amplitude (TEOAE amplitude to the first click in test sequence). *Dashed line* indicates noise level. Test click amplitude = 20 dB SL; masking click amplitude = 46 dB SL.

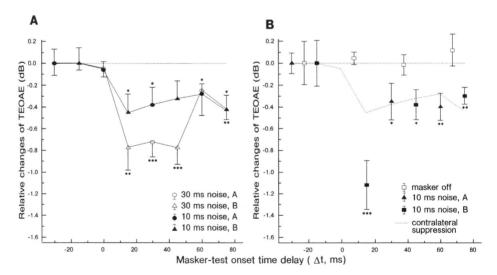

Figure 6–11. Temporal dynamics of contralateral (A) and ipsilateral (B) suppression of TEOAE. Each point represents the mean difference of TEOAE amplitudes (5 pairs) recorded in masker-on and masker-off conditions. *Open squares* on B show the mean TEOAE amplitudes without masker. The latter amplitudes were related to the mean amplitude of TEOAE evoked by the first click in test sequence. Error bars indicate standard errors.

and obviously related to the dramatic TEOAE suppression revealed in click-to-click forward masking experiment (Figure 6–10).

Middle-Ear Reflexes

In the noise-to-click forward-masking experiments noise intensities as high as 50 dB SL were used. With the noise presented continuously, this value was found to be only slightly below the threshold of stapedial muscle reflex in one subject (Figure 6–12). Nevertheless, the middle-ear reflex threshold using short-noise bursts of the maximum for our experiments duration (30 ms), was determined to be as much as 80 dB SL, which is 30 dB higher than the intensity used in the masking experiments (Figure 6–12). To eliminate the possibility of the middle-ear reflexes that cannot be recorded with conventional impedance measurements, the sound pressure in the outer-ear canal during alternative presentation of contralateral noise was evaluated. There was no pressure excursion at the 40 to 110 ms poststimulus time when the stapedial reflex could be observed (Figure 6–12) (Fisch & Schulthess, 1963; Metz, 1951). The observation could not rule out the theoretical possibility of slowly developing reflex tension in the middle-ear muscles. In order to exclude this possibility, the TEOAE amplitudes were compared without masker and just before masker onset (it is a response to the first click in test sequence). No statistically significant differences were found (Figure 6–12).

Efferent-Mediated Effects in Ipsilateral-TEOAE Suppression

The magnitudes of the TEOAE suppression caused by contralateral continuous noise (e.g., 0.6 dB with the contralateral noise at 30 dB SL in one subject (Figure 6–9) were only slightly less than the previously reported mean values for normal-hearing subjects (0.7 dB with the masker intensity of 20 dB SL) (Collet, Kemp, Veuillet, Duclaux, Moulin, & Morgon, 1990). Hence, the excitability of the olivo-cochlear reflex arc (at least from contralateral side) was unlikely to differ significantly from the typical one. The dramatic decrease of the TEOAE under click-to-click forward-masking conditions at the interstimulus intervals smaller than 5 ms (Figure 6–10) could be attributed exclusively to the intracochlear processes due to the longer minimal latency of the medial olivo-cochlear neuron responses to the external sound. This latency was found to be at least 6 to 8 ms in cats (Liberman & Brown, 1986) and 7 ms in guinea pigs (Brown, 1989), and there is no reason to expect the significant reduction of this time in human beings. Moreover, practically complete TEOAE inhibition observed within the first 5 ms poststimulus (Figure 6–10) correlated well with the degree of the TEOAE suppression that was reported previously for the ipsilateral simultaneous TEOAE masking (Tavartkiladze, Frolenkov, Kruglov, & Artamasov, 1994). Hence, the TEOAE suppression observed 5 ms after the end of ipsilateral masking noise burst (Figure 6–11, B) may have been mainly of cochlear origin.

It is known that short acoustic clicks with relatively low repetition rate are quite ineffective in eliciting efferent response (Liberman & Brown, 1986). Longer stimuli (e.g., tone bursts of 50 ms) are capable of exciting the MOCS neurons (Brown, 1989). Accordingly, noise bursts presented contralaterally or ipsilaterally elicited a statistically significant TEOAE reduction 30 ms and more after the end of noise stimula-

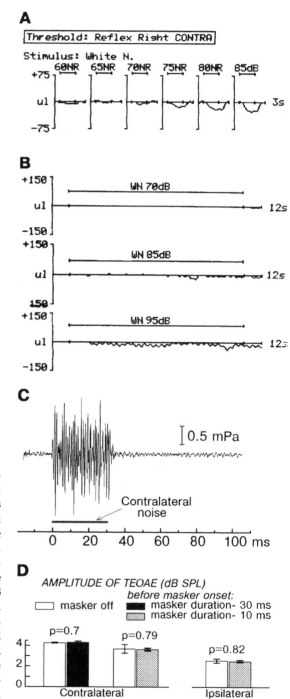

Figure 6–12. Absence of the middle ear reflexes. *A*: Acoustic reflex measurements with continuous white noise. *B*: Acoustic reflex measurements with 30 ms noise bursts used in masking studies. *C*: Sound pressure in the outer-ear canal during contralateral noise stimulation (65 dB nHL /50 dB SL/, indicated by horizontal bar). *D*: Absence of the static changes of the TEOAE during contralateral or ipsilateral noise stimulation. Noise intensities on *A* and *B* are marked in dB HL. Hearing threshold of subject tested was 15 dB HL.

tion (Figure 6–11). The latency of this effect from the contralateral side was found to be less than 15 ms (Figure 6–11). This value differs somewhat from the previously reported estimate of the contralateral TEOAE-suppression latency (<40–140 ms) (Lind, 1994) and from the latency of the efferent-mediated ipsilateral suppression of the compound-action potential in guinea pigs (30–40 ms [Bonfils & Puel, 1987]). But, so far, no systematic studies of this question have been performed. Moreover, at the 15 ms intervals between contralateral noise and test click the possibility that additional TEOAE suppression related to the intracochlear processes on the ipsilateral side cannot be excluded. The degree of acoustic isolation between the two ears was not greater than 40 dB, and attenuated noise could stimulate ipsilateral cochlea owing to crosstalk. Nevertheless, the effect at longer noise-to-click intervals appeared to result from MOCS activation because (a) its duration was not explained by intracochlear suppression (Figure 6–10 and Figure 6–11) and (b) the suppression magnitude was similar from ipsi-lateral and contralateral sides. The long duration of the efferent-mediated inhibition of TEOAEs (>80 ms [Figure 6–11]) did not contradict previously reported TEOAE forward-masking data (Lind, 1994; Gobsch, Kevanishvilli, Gamebeli, & Gvelesiani, 1992) and other studies of ipsilateral effects (Berlin, Hood, Hurley, Wen, & Kemp, 1995).

The most striking result of these experiments was the close resemblance of the magnitudes and time courses of the efferent-mediated effects elicited from contralateral and ipsilateral sides (Figure 6–11). Recently Berlin, Hood, Hurley, Wen, and Kemp (1995) compared forward masking of TEOAE by ipsilateral, contralateral, and binaural noise. In full accordance the data presented in this chapter, they found TEOAE suppression of approximately the same magnitude (about 0.5 dB) for both ipsi-lateral and contralateral noise stimulation. Binaural noise stimulation caused more prominent reduction of TEOAE amplitude (about 1–1.5 dB). Differences between ipsi-lateral and contralateral effects were not significant 20 to 100 ms after noise stimulation (Berlin et al., 1995). These results appear to contradict the results of Liberman and Brown (1986) who reported that 59% of MOCS neurons are most sensitive to the ipsilateral stimuli, 29%, to the contralateral ones, and 11%, from both sides. Consequently one could expect some difference in the magnitude of the efferent-mediated TEOAE suppression evoked by contralateral and ipsilateral stimulation. This discrepancy may can be related to the fact that the MOCS neuron excitability pattern depends on the level of general anesthesia. Indeed, it was speculated that percent of binaurally responding MOCS neurons can be higher in less anesthetized animals (Liberman & Brown, 1986). Moreover, in unanesthetized decerebrated cats, 60% of efferent units were reported to respond to both contralateral acoustic stimulation and ipsilateral electrical stimulation (Fex, 1962, 1965). Thus, in awake human beings, a significant portion of MOCS neurons can be expected to be bilaterally activated. This could explain the similar magnitudes of the efferent-mediated TEOAE suppressions evoked by contralateral and ipsilateral stimuli.

Summary and Conclusions

Today, TEOAE registration is a valuable clinical tool in audiology. Along with the registration of TEOAE itself, diagnostic significance has also been reported for the contralateral efferent-mediated TEOAE-suppression effects (Aran, 1995; Berlin,

Hood, Cecloa, Jackson, & Szabo, 1993). Clinical investigations of ipsilateral TEOAE suppression could provide valuable insight to both intracochlear two-tone interaction processes and efferent-mediated processes.

References

Aran, J.-M. (1995) Current perspectives on inner ear toxicity. *Otolaryngology—Head and Neck Surgery, 112*, 133–144.

Avan, P., Bonfils, P., Loth, D., Narcy, P., & Trotoux J. (1991) Quantitative assessment of human cochlear function by evoked otoacoustic emissions. *Hearing Research, 52*, 99–112.

Berlin, C. I., Hood, L. J., Cecola, R. P., Jackson, D. F., & Szabo P. (1993). Does type I afferent neuron dysfunction reveal itself through lack of efferent suppression? *Hearing Research, 65*, 40–50.

Berlin, C. I., Hood, L. J., Wen, H., Szabo, P., Cecola, R. P., Rigby, P., & Jackson, D. F. (1993). Contralateral suppression of non-linear click-evoked otoacoustic emissions. *Hearing Research, 71*, 1–11.

Berlin, C. I., Hood, L. J., Hurley, A. E., Wen, H., & Kemp, D. T. (1995). Binaural noise suppresses linear click-evoked otoacoustic emissions more than ipsilateral or contralateral noise. *Hearing Research, 87*, 96–103.

Bonfils, P., & Puel, J.-L. (1987). Functional properties of the crossed part of the medial olivo-cochlear bundle. *Hearing Research, 28*, 125–130.

Bray, P., & Kemp, D. T. (1987). An advanced cochlear echo suitable for infant screening. *British Journal of Audiology, 21*, 191–204.

Brown, M. C. (1989). Morphology and response properties of single olivocochlear fibers in the guinea pig. *Hearing Research, 40*, 93–110.

Collet, L. (1993). Use of otoacoustic emissions to explore the medial olivocochlear system in humans. *British Journal of Audiology, 27*, 155–159.

Collet, L., Kemp, D., Veuillet, E., Duclaux, R., Moulin, A., & Morgon, A. (1990). Effect of contralateral auditory stimuli on active cochlear micromechanical properties in human subjects. *Hearing Research, 3*, 251–262.

Dallos, P. (1985). Response characteristics of mammalian cochlear hair cells. *Journal of Neuroscience, 5*, 1591–1608.

Elberling, C., Parbo, J., Johnsen N. J., Bagi, P. (1985). Evoked acoustic emissions: Clinical application. *Acta Oto-Laryngologica, 421* (Suppl.), 77–85.

Fex, J. (1962). Auditory activity in centrifugal and centripetal cochlear fibers in cat. *Acta Physiologica Scandinavia, 189* (Suppl.), 2–68.

Fex, J. (1965). Auditory activity in uncrossed centrifugal cochlear fibers in cat. *Acta Physiologica Scandinavia, 64*, 43–57.

Fisch, U., & Schulthess, G. (1963). Electromyographic studies on the human stapedial muscle. *Acta Oto-Laryngologica, 56*, 287–297.

Froehlich, P., Collet, L., & Morgon, A. (1993). Transient evoked otoacoustic emission amplitudes change with changes of directed attention. *Physiology and Behavior, 53*, 679–682.

Frolenkov, G. I., Artamasov, S. V., Kruglov, A. V., & Tavartkiladze, G. A. (1995). Time and frequency components of transient evoked otoacoustic emission: The input/output functions. *Abstracts of the eighteenth midwinter meeting: Association for Research in Otolaryngology* (p. 21), St. Petersburg, FL.

Gobsch, H., Kevanishvili, Z., Gamgebeli, Z., & Gvelesiani, T. (1992). Behaviour of delayed evoked otoacoustic emission under forward masking paradigm. *Scandinavian Audiology, 21*, 143-–148.

Grandori, F. (1985) Non-linear phenomena in click- and tone-burst-evoked otoacoustic emissions. *Audiology, 24*, 71–80.

Grandori, F., & Ravazzani, P. (1993) Non-linearities of click-evoked otoacoustic emissions and the derived non-linear technique. *British Journal of Audiology, 27*, 97–102.

Hauser, R., Probst, R., & Lohle, E. (1991). Click- and tone-burst-evoked otoacoustic emissions in normally hearing ears and in ears with high-frequency sensorineural hearing loss. *European Archives of Oto-Rhino-Laryngology, 248*, 345–352.

Hilger, A. W., Furness, D. N., & Wilson, J. P. (1995). The possible relationship between transient evoked otoacoustic emission and organ of Corti irregularities in the guinea pig. *Hearing Research, 84*, 1–11.

Kemp, D. T. (1978). Stimulated acoustic emissions from within the human auditory system. *Journal of the Acoustical Society of America, 64*, 1368–1391.

Kemp, D. T. (1980). Towards a model for the origin of cochlear echoes. *Hearing Research, 2*, 533–548.

Kemp, D. T. (1986). Otoacoustic emissions, traveling waves and cochlear mechanisms. *Hearing Research, 22*, 95–104.

Kemp, D. T. (1988). Developments in cochlear mechanics and techniques for noninvasive evaluation. *Advances in Audiology, 5*, 27–45.

Kemp, D. T., & Chum, R. A. (1980). Properties of the generator of stimulated acoustic emissions. *Hearing Research, 2*, 213–232.

Kemp, D. T., Bray, P., Alexander, L., & Brown, A. M. (1986). Acoustic emission cochleography: Practical aspects. *Scandinavian Audiology, 25* (Suppl.), 71–95.

Kossl, M., & Russell, I. J. (1992) The phase and magnitude of hair cell receptor potentials and frequency tuning in guinea pig cochlea. *Journal of Neuroscience, 12*, 1575–1586.

Kubo, T., Sakashita, T., Hachikawa, K., Minowa, Y., & Nakai, Y. (1991). Frequency analysis of evoked otoacoustic emissions. *Acta Oto-Laryngologica, 486* (Suppl.), 73–77.

Liberman, M. C., & Brown, M. C. (1986). Physiology and anatomy of single olivocochlear neurons in the cat. *Hearing Research, 24*, 17–36.

Lind, O. (1994). Contralateral suppression of TEOAE. Attempts to find a latency. *British Journal of Audiology, 28*, 219–225.

Lonsbury-Martin, B. L., Martin, G. K., Probst, R., & Coats, A. C. (1988). Spontaneous otoacoustic emissions in nonhuman primate: II. Cochlear anatomy. *Hearing Research, 33*, 69–94.

Martin, G. K., Lonsbury-Martin, B. L., Probst, R., & Coats, A. C. (1988). Spontaneous otoacoustic emissions in a nonhuman primate: I. Basic features and relations to other emissions. *Hearing Research, 33*, 49–68.

Metz, O. (1951). Studies on the contraction of the tympanic muscles as indicated by changes in the impedance of the ear. *Acta Oto-Laryngologica, 39*, 397–405.

Mountain, D. C. (1980). Changes in endolymphatic potential and crossed olivocochlear bundle stimulation alter cochlear mechanics. *Science, 210*, 71–72.

Norton, S. J., & Neely, S. T. (1987). Tone-burst-evoked otoacoustic emissions from normal-hearing subjects. *Journal of the Acoustical Society of America, 81*, 1860–1872.

Probst, R., Coats, A. C., Martin, G. K., & Lonsbury-Martin, B. L. (1986). Spontaneous, click-, and toneburst-evoked otoacoustic emissions from normal ears. *Hearing Research, 21*, 261–275.

Probst, R. (1990). Otoacoustic emissions: An overview. *Advances in Oto-Rhino-Laryngology, 44*, 1–91.

Probst, R. (1991). A review of otoacoustic emissions. *Journal of the Acoustical Society of America, 89*, 2027–2067.

Rajan, R. (1988). Effect of electrical stimulation of the crossed olivocochlear bundle on temporary threshold shifts in auditory sensitivity: I. Dependence on electrical stimulation parameters. *Journal of Neurophysiology, 60*, 549–567.

Rajan, R. (1990). Functions of the efferent pathways to the mammalian cochlea. In M. Rowe & L. Aitkin (eds)., *Information processing in mammalian auditory and tactile systems* (pp. 81–96). New York: Wiley.

Tavartkiladze, G. A., Frolenkov, G. I., & Kruglov, A. V. (1991, September). On the site of the evoked otoacoustic emission generation. *Proceedings from the XII biennial symposium of the International Electric Response Audiometry Study Group* (p. 58), Terme di Comano, Italy.

Tavartkiladze, G. A., Frolenkov, G. I., & Kruglov, A. V. (1993) Delayed evoked otoacoustic emission and mechanisms of its generation. *Sensory Systems, 7*, 85–99.

Tavartkiladze, G. A., Frolenkov, G. I., Kruglov A. V., & Artamasov, S. V. (1994). Ipsilateral suppression effects on transient evoked otoacoustic emission. *British Journal of Audiology, 28*, 193–204.

Tavartkiladze, G. A., Frolenkov, G. I., & Kruglov A. V. (1995). Ipsilateral suppression of transient evoked otoacoustic emission. In *Abstracts of the eighteenth midwinter meeting: Association for Research in Otolaryngology* (p. 122). St. Petersburg, FL.

Tavartkiladze G. A., Frolenkov, G. I. & Artamasov, S. V. (1996). Ipsilateral suppression of transient evoked otoacoustic emission: role of the medial olivocochlear system. *Acta Oto-Laryngologica, 116*, 213–218.

Veuillet, E., Collet, L., & Duclaux, R. (1991). Effect of contralateral acoustic stimulation on active cochlear micromechanical properties in human subjects: Dependence on stimulus variables. *Journal of Neurophysiology, 65*, 724–735.

Veuillet, E., Collet, L., & Morgon, A. (1992).Differential effects of ear-canal pressure and contralateral acoustic stimulation on evoked otoacoustic emissions in humans. *Hearing Research, 61*, 47–55.

Warren, E. H., & Liberman, M. C. (1989). Effects of contralateral sound on auditory-nerve responses: I. Contributions of cochlear efferents. *Hearing Research, 37*, 89–104.

Wilson, J. P. (1980). Evidence for a cochlear origin for acoustic re-emissions, threshold fine-structure and tonal tinnitus. *Hearing Research, 2*, 233–252.

Wilson, J. P. & Sutton, G. J. (1981). Acoustic correlates of tonal tinnitus. In *Tinnitus: Ciba Foundation symposium* (pp. 82–107). London: Pitman Books.

Zurek, P. M. (1981). Spontaneous narrowband acoustic signals emitted by human ears. *Journal of the Acoustical Society of America, 69*, 514–523.

Zurek, P. M. (1985). Acoustic emissions from the ear: A summary of results from humans and animals. *Journal of the Acoustical Society of America, 78*, 340–344.

Zwicker, E. (1983). On peripheral processing in human hearing. In R. Klinke, R. Hartmann (eds): *Hearing: Physiological bases and psychophysics* (pp. 104–110). Berlin: Springer.

7

Influence of Middle-Ear Disease on Otoacoustic Emissions

ROBERT H. MARGOLIS
MARY BETH TRINE

Introduction

Because otoacoustic emissions (OAE) are transmitted from the cochlea to the ear canal via the middle ear, the transmission properties of the middle ear directly influence OAE characteristics. The effectiveness of the stimulus used to evoke OAEs is also influenced by middle-ear transmission characteristics. Although the middle ear can transmit sound bidirectionally, the forward transmission (toward the cochlea) characteristics and backward transmission characteristics are different. In addition, the simultaneous forward and backward transmission of the stimulus and the response in certain OAE types, such as distortion-product emissions (DPOAEs), results in interactions between the stimulus and response.

The effects of middle-ear dysfunctions on OAEs are complex. In general, middle-ear dysfunctions reduce measured emission amplitudes and sometimes eliminate the response entirely. Changes in OAE characteristics due to middle-ear dysfunction result from changes in both forward and backward transmission. Various middle-ear disorders affect forward and backward transmission differently; one condition (e.g., small eardrum perforation) may influence primarily forward transmission and another condition (e.g., scarred eardrum) may have a greater effect on backward transmission. Therefore, for clinical applications it is important to evaluate middle-ear functioning to distinguish between middle-ear abnormalities and cochlear dysfunction. Conditions of the external and middle ear are thought to significantly impact on the outcomes of infant hearing screening programs. The success or failure of such programs may hinge on the ability to minimize false positive screening outcomes that are caused by transient, external, and middle-ear conditions.

Middle-Ear Transmission System

Models of Middle-Ear Function

Electrical analogue models of the middle ear provide a means for understanding and predicting the response of the middle ear to a wide range of acoustic stimuli in normal and pathological ears. These models represent the anatomical structures of the ear by electrical components that quantitatively express the effects of mass, compliance (springiness), and resistance of each structure. The ossicles are represented as mass elements; the tympanic membrane, muscles, tendons, ligaments, and enclosed air spaces are spring elements; and friction encountered between ossicles, within the tympanic membrane, and at the stapes-labyrinthine fluid interface are resistive elements. A block diagram of such a model is presented in Figure 7–1.

To understand the role of the middle ear in OAEs, a few important features of middle-ear functioning should be noted. First, the ear is a complex network with multiple pathways for the flow of energy. Energy that flows through the shunt

MIDDLE EAR MODEL

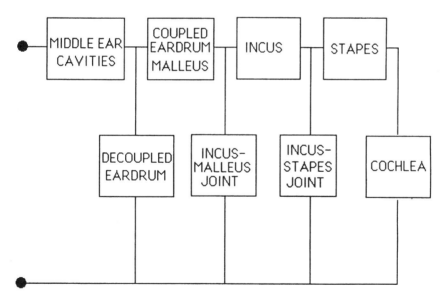

Figure 7–1.   Network model of the middle ear. The diagram represents models of the type developed by Zwislocki (1962) and Kringlebotn (1988). Each block in the model represents one or more structures and in the more complete form of the model, would include a network of resistors, capacitors, and inductors (representing friction, spring elements, and mass elements, respectively). Note that energy that flows through the shunt elements (Blocks 2, 4, & 6) does not reach the inner ear (Block 8).

elements does not reach the inner ear. This indicates that there is vibratory energy in the system that is not transmitted to the inner ear. Second, the system has an input impedance that represents the opposition offered by the total system to the flow of energy through the system. The *input impedance* is the quantity that is measured by tympanometry. Because the input impedance is influenced by components that are in the pathway to the inner ear, and also by components that are not in the pathway to the cochlea, the input impedance is a poor predictor of hearing sensitivity. An ear with middle-ear fluid can have a flat tympanogram (high input impedance) and clinically normal hearing. An ear with otosclerosis can have a normal tympanogram (normal input impedance) and a large conductive hearing loss. Third, the system is capable of bidirectional transmission. Without this property, it would not be possible to measure OAEs in the ear canal. However, the forward and the backward transmission properties of the middle ear are not the same. Finally, both the forward transmission and the backward transmission characteristics are frequency-dependent. OAE characteristics are subject to the effects of forward transmission on the spectral content of the effective stimulus reaching the inner ear and the effect of the frequency response of the middle ear on OAE spectral characteristics. Wada et al. (1993) demonstrated a close relation between middle-ear resonance and spectral peaks in the TEOAE.

Forward Transmission Through the Middle Ear

The importance of forward transmission through the middle ear is that this characteristic determines the effectiveness of the evoking stimulus that reaches the cochlea. In a purely conductive hearing loss, the magnitude of the loss is a measure of the reduction in forward transmission. The effect is to attenuate the effective stimulus by the amount of the hearing loss. Because the amount of the hearing loss varies with the frequency, the attenuation of the stimulus is also frequency-selective. To determine the effect of attenuating the stimulus we can examine input-output functions (growth curves) for various emission types. Figure 7–2

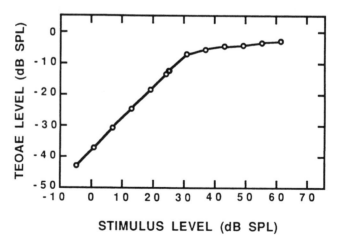

Figure 7–2. TEOAE input-output function. (Data from Zwicker, 1983.)

presents a typical transient-evoked emission (TEOAE) input-output function from a normal-hearing subject (Zwicker, 1983). In general, TEOAE input-output functions from normal subjects are steep for low-intensity stimuli and become nearly flat at higher stimulus levels. Naeve, Margolis, Levine, and Fournier (1992) reported slopes of 0.2 dB/dB in the flat portion of the click-evoked TEOAE input-output function. Thus, a 10-dB change in stimulus level would produce only a 2 dB change in overall emission level. Furthermore, the forward-transmission effect of a conductive hearing loss would be to reduce the emission level in a manner that is similar to reducing the stimulus level by the amount of the hearing loss. If the stimulus level was high so that the response growth is in the flat portion of the input-output function, a 10-dB conductive hearing loss would cause a 2 dB decrease in response amplitude. Increasing the stimulus level by 10 dB would fully compensate for the loss of forward transmission.

Input-output functions for DPOAEs have different characteristics than those for TEOAEs. Nelson and Kimberly (1992) described five types of DPOAE growth curves that occur in normal-hearing subjects. Figure 7–3 presents examples of each type of growth curve with the proportion of occurrences of each type in their normal hearing subjects. The variety of shapes of input-output functions indicates that the forward transmission effect of middle-ear disease can influence DPOAE recordings in several ways. For example, the forward-transmission effect of a 10-dB conductive loss on DPOAEs evoked by 80-dB SPL primaries could be to decrease the emission level (linear, flat-steep, or diphasic), to increase the emission level (nonmonotonic), or to have no effect (saturating). When the growth curve increases with stimulus level (linear, flat-steep, diphasic), the slopes tend to be substantially larger than the slopes of TEOAE growth curves. Therefore, a conductive loss and consequent change in forward transmission could have a greater influence on DPOAEs than on TEOAEs; increasing the stimulus level by the amount of the conductive hearing loss would compensate for the loss in forward transmission.

The effect of ear-canal volume between the probe and the tympanic membrane also influences forward transmission. A smaller volume results in a higher stimulus sound pressure and a higher ear-canal resonant frequency.

Backward Transmission Through the Middle Ear

In transmission of OAE energy from the cochlea to the outer ear, the eardrum acts like the cone of a loudspeaker by transducing the mechanical energy of the ossicles into airborne acoustic energy. Backward transmission is less efficient than forward transmission by 12 to 16 dB according to Kemp's (1980) calculations. An emission that is 10 dB SPL in the ear canal could be audible to others if it weren't for the 12 to 16 dB loss that results from backward transmission.

Just as ear canal volume affects the intensity and spectrum of the stimulus, it also influences the characteristics of the response and contributes to the backward-transmission characteristic. The sound pressure that is produced in the ear canal is inversely proportional to the ear-canal volume (Kemp, 1980). Figure 7–4 illustrates the effect of ear-canal volume on TEOAE amplitude and indicates that a deep insertion is desirable to maximize the amplitude of the response. Kemp, Ryan, and Bray (1990) presented a good discussion of the importance of probe fit. A loss in backward transmission due to middle-ear dysfunction would reduce the emission

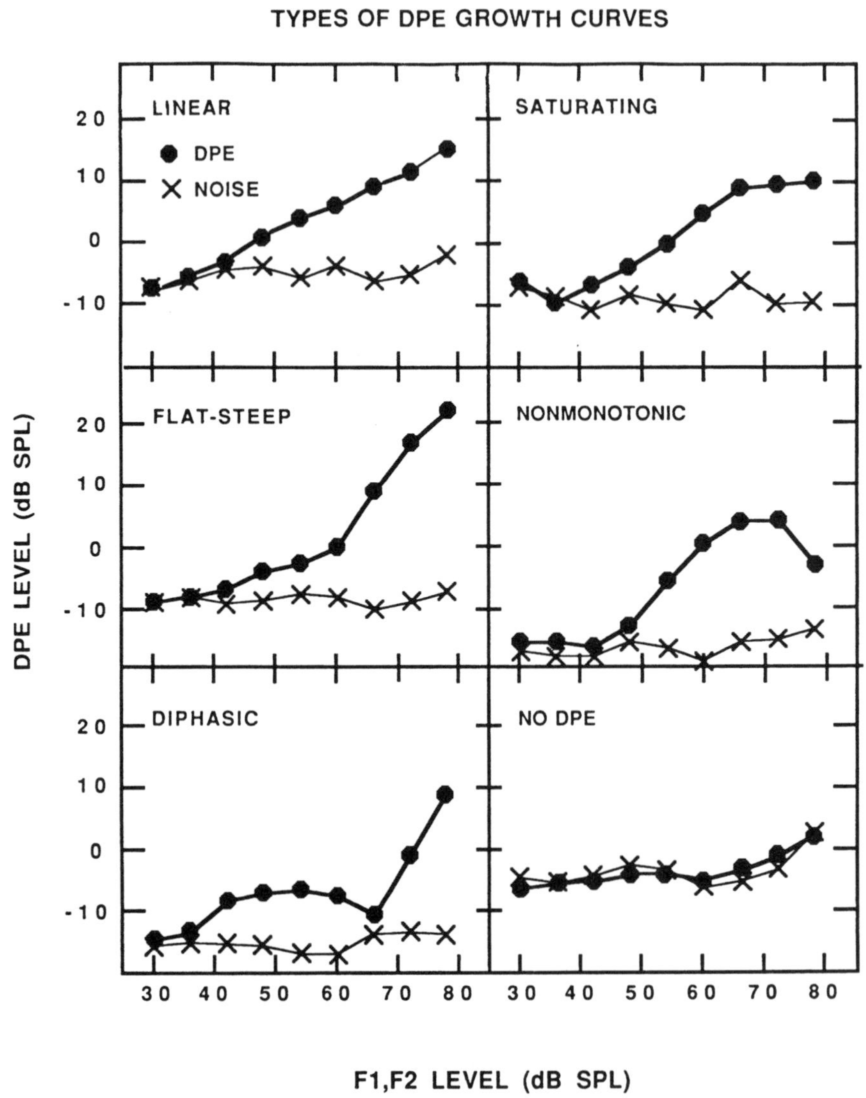

TYPES OF DPE GROWTH CURVES

Figure 7–3. Types of DPOAE input-output functions. The percentages are the prevalances of each type among normal-hearing subjects. (Adapted from Nelson & Kimberly, 1992. Used with permission.)

level measured in the ear canal. Because emission levels are often just barely above the noise floor (even after filtering, spectral averaging, and time-domain averaging), the loss in backward transmission due to middle-ear dysfunction is often sufficient to eliminate the response entirely (i.e., to drop the response level below the noise floor). Thus, patients with mild hearing losses due to otitis media may have no measurable emission, although the effect of the hearing loss on forward transmission would not be expected to eliminate the response.

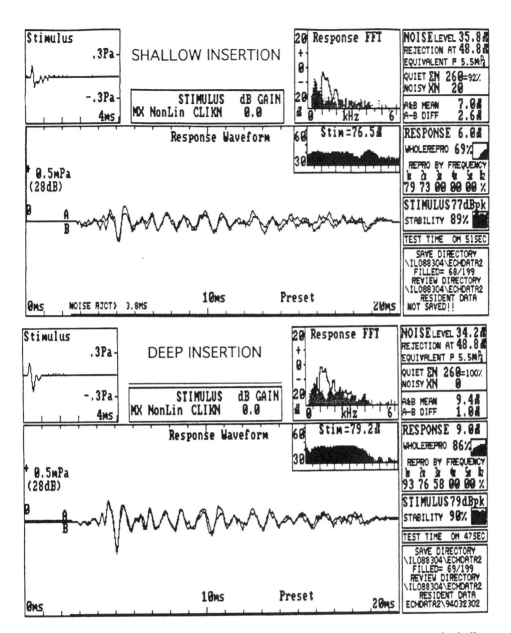

Figure 7–4. Effect of probe insertion depth on TEOAEs. Using a large tip with shallow insertion (*top*) the TEOAE response amplitude was 6 dB. Using a smaller tip with deeper insertion, the emission amplitude increased to 9 dB. Note the effect of stimulus level (76.5 and 79.2 dB for shallow and deep insertion, respectively.) The recordings were made on the same ear with probe tips of different sizes. The smaller tip was inserted as deeply as possible; the larger tip as shallow as possible while achieving a seal. Three effects are notable. First, the stimulus spectrum changed due to differences in the resonant characteristics of the ear canal. Second, the stimulus intensity differed by 2.7 dB in the two conditions because the smaller ear-canal volume resulted in a higher sound pressure. Based on the slope of the normal input-output function (0.2 dB/dB), the change in stimulus level would be expected to produce a change in TEOAE amplitude of 0.54 dB. Third, the TEOAE level changed by 3 dB, a larger change than the expected effect of the change in stimulus level. The change in TEOAE level results primarily from the effect of ear-canal volume on the sound pressure of the TEOAE in the ear canal.

Effects of Air Pressure on Otoacoustic Emissions

The determination of the effects of air pressure applied either to the external ear or middle ear has been useful for studying OAEs for a number of reasons. First, air pressure is a convenient method for changing middle-ear transmission properties in a controlled fashion. Second, because there is much information regarding the effects of air pressure on the input impedance of the ear (tympanometry), changes in OAEs due to air pressure changes can be related to middle-ear impedance characteristics. Third, because middle-ear air pressure results from the normal gas-exchange mechanism of the middle ear and many normal ears have pressure in the middle-ear space, it is important to know the effect of middle-ear pressure on normal OAE characteristics. Fourth, because abnormal middle-ear pressure is thought to be related to otitis media, an understanding of its effects on OAEs may provide a basis for evaluating middle-ear function.

Effects of Ear-Canal Air Pressure on OAEs

Ear-canal air pressure effects have been measured for three emission types: spontaneous emissions (SOAEs), TEOAEs, and DPOAEs.

Ear-canal pressure has been found to change both the amplitude and frequency of SOAEs (Kemp, 1981; Schloth & Zwicker, 1983; Wilson & Sutton, 1981). In general, positive or negative ear-canal pressure (relative to middle-ear pressure) increases the frequency and decreases the amplitude of spontaneous emissions. Although changes in SOAE amplitude can be attributed to the effect of pressure on forward and backward transmission, changes in SOAE frequency cannot. Frequency changes are probably the result of interactions between the middle ear and the cochlear generator of the SOAE.

Ear-canal air pressure changes the amplitude, spectrum, and reproducibility of TEOAEs. Figure 7–5 shows that both positive and negative ear-canal pressure reduce TEOAE amplitude in a symmetrical fashion; a positive or negative pressure of 100 daPa reduces the emission amplitude by about 2.5 dB. Other investigators have obtained similar results (Bray, 1989; Robinson & Haughton, 1991; Veuillet, Collet, & Morgon, 1992). Although ear-canal air pressure can influence stimulus characteristics, the reduction in TEOAE amplitude due to ear-canal air pressure is almost entirely due to a reduction in backward transmission efficiency. The reduction in TEOAE amplitude results from an attenuation of the low-frequency components of the emission (Figure 7–6). Figure 7–6 shows the change in the TEOAE spectrum that results from an ear-canal pressure of 200 daPa. The preferential effect on low-frequency transmission is the expected result of increasing the stiffness of the spring elements of the ear. Because the impedance of a spring decreases with frequency (Margolis, 1981), the increase in the stiffness of the eardrum has its greatest effect on low frequency transmission.

Because the amplitude of the emission is decreased, also reducing the signal-to-noise level of the emission, a reduction in the reproducibility occurs. Using the commonly-employed reproducibility criterion of 0.5, Naeve et al. (1992) reported that a substantial proportion of responses were reduced to below that criterion by negative ear-canal pressure. The implication is that middle-ear air pressure, which is frequently encountered in clinical populations, may cause the emission amplitude to be reduced to the point of being undetectable.

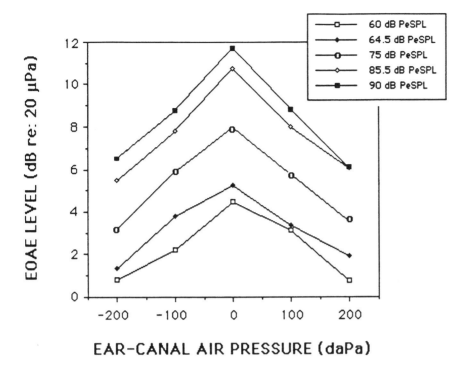

Figure 7–5. Effect of ear-canal air pressure on TEOAE response amplitudes for click stimuli presented at the indicated levels (*insert*). (From Naeve et al., 1992. Used with permission.)

Effects of ear-canal air pressure on DPOAEs has also been studied. Because the input-output functions for DPOAEs are usually steeper than those for TEOAEs for stimulus levels typically employed, a larger forward transmission effect is expected. That is, the change in the effective stimulus level due to ear-canal pressure has a greater influence on DPOAE amplitude than on TEOAE amplitude. Consequently, ear-canal pressure changes DPOAE amplitude more than TEOAE amplitude. Osterhammel, Nielsen, and Rasmussen (1993) recorded DPOAEs for f_1 -f_2 combinations that range in frequency from 1 to 8 kHz. At 1 kHz, the effect of positive and negative pressure symmetrically reduced DPOAE amplitude by about 8 dB for 100 daPa and 11 dB for 200 daPa. These changes are several times larger than the effects on TEOAEs. Similar to the effect on TEOAEs, the effect of ear-canal pressure on DPOAEs is the smallest around 2 kHz. At higher frequencies the effect becomes more complex. Above 4 kHz, negative pressure decreases DPOAE amplitude, and positive pressure causes slight increases in amplitude. The effect on low-frequency emission is consistent with the increase in stiffness caused by ear-canal pressure, which preferentially affects the low frequencies in both forward and backward transmission. The complex effect of ear-canal pressure on high-frequency DPOAEs has not been explained.

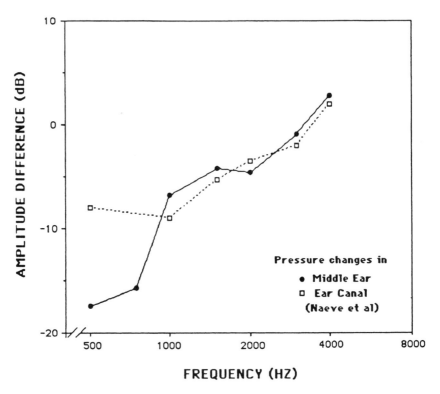

Figure 7–6.   Effect of ear-canal and middle-ear pressure on TEOAE spectrum. (From Trine et al., 1993. Used with permission.)

Effects of Middle-Ear Air Pressure on OAEs

Middle-ear pressure and ear-canal pressure have similar effects on middle-ear function. A positive pressure applied to the ear canal influences middle-ear transmission in the same way as a negative pressure of equal magnitude applied to the middle ear. The effects of middle-ear pressure, then, should be predictable from the studies of ear-canal pressure. However, middle-ear pressure is not as easy to control experimentally. Air pressure can easily be applied to the ear canal. Middle-ear pressure can be produced by enclosing the subject in a pressure chamber, or it can be created by the gas-exchange dynamics of the subject's ear.

In a discussion of the effects of middle-ear disease on OAEs, Owens, McCoy, Lonsbury-Martin, and Martin (1992) presented data from two cases in which the tympanograms indicated various amounts of intratympanic pressure. They suggested that even a mild degree of middle-ear pressure can significantly reduce measured TEOAE and DPOAE amplitudes.

A systematic study of middle-ear pressure effects on TEOAEs was reported by Trine, Hirsch, and Margolis (1993). We tested a series of patients with negative tympanometric peak pressures ranging from −100 to −310 daPa. TEOAEs were recorded with ambient ear-canal air pressure and with the ear-canal pressure

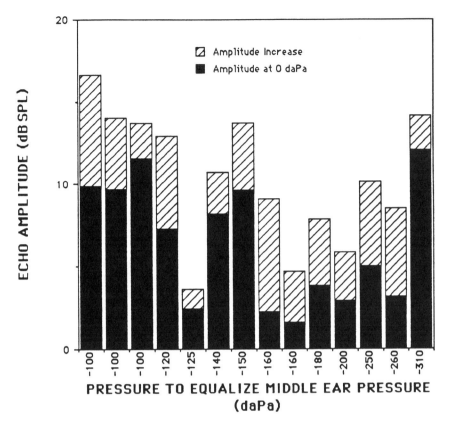

Figure 7–7.   Effect of compensating for middle-ear pressure on TEOAE amplitudes from 14 patients with significant negative middle-ear pressure. The *solid* portion of the bar indicates the emission amplitude with ambient ear-canal air pressure. The *striped* portion indicates the amplitude increase that occurred when the ear-canal pressure was set to compensate for the middle-ear pressure. Through most of the spectrum, the effect of ear-canal and middle-ear pressure is identical. Both act as a high-pass filter, attenuating low-frequency energy. (From Trine et al., 1993. Used with permission.)

adjusted to compensate for the negative middle-ear pressure. Figure 7–7 demonstrates that in all cases, compensation for middle-ear pressure increased the emission amplitude. Although the correlation between the change in TEOAE amplitude and tympanometric peak pressure was weak, the magnitudes of the change (1–7 dB) were similar to the effects of ear-canal pressure. In 12 of the 14 cases, the increase in TEOAE amplitude resulting from middle-ear pressure compensation was accompanied by an increase in reproducibility. The effect of middle-ear pressure (−100 daPa) on TEOAE spectrum is shown in Figure 7–6.

Except for the cases reported by Owens et al. (1992), the effects of middle-ear pressure on DPOAEs have not been studied. However, based on the steeper input-output functions that characterize DPOAEs and the resulting effect of changes in forward transmission, the effect of middle-ear pressure on distortion-product emissions is probably greater than the effect on TEOAEs.

EFFECTS OF OTITIS MEDIA ON OTOACOUSTIC EMISSIONS

Because of the high prevalence of otitis media in populations that are of interest for OAE testing, such as infants and children, it is important to understand the potential effects of otitis media on OAE measurements. The presence of middle-ear effusion affects both forward and backward transmission through the middle ear. The effect on forward transmission can be at least partially compensated by an increase in stimulus level. A reduction in backward transmission may reduce the emission amplitude to a level that is below the noise floor. The only compensation for that effect would be to reduce the noise floor by improved noise-reduction techniques. Improvement in noise-reduction methods may make it possible to detect emissions in patients with middle-ear disorders for whom OAEs are not detectable with the current equipment.

Owens et al. (1992) recorded TEOAEs and DPOAEs in patients with various amounts of middle-ear effusion. They were unable to record TEOAEs in any cases where there was effusion, even in a patient with a small volume of fluid. In that case, DPOAEs were observed only in the low frequencies. DPOAEs were not observed in patients with large volumes of middle-ear fluid.

Van Cauwenberge, Vinck, De Vel, and Dhooge (1995) recorded TEOAEs from 85 ears of 61 children with otitis media. All had flat tympanograms at the time of testing. Emissions were present in seven ears (8%). They reported that the emissions were characterized by a small overall wave reproducibility and were confined to a narrow spectral region between 2 and 4 kHz.

Although otitis media often eliminates OAE responses, it is possible to record emissions in some patients with middle-ear effusion. In normal ears, it is not uncommon to encounter TEOAE amplitudes with signal-to-noise ratios of 10 to 15 dB. Because the hearing loss in children with otitis media ranges from 0 to 50 dB (Hunter, Margolis, & Giebink, 1994), it is not surprising that some patients with otitis media have measurable emissions. Case 2 is an example of a small reproducible emission that was recorded from a patient with fluid in the middle ear.

Effects of Other Middle-Ear Pathologies on Otoacoustic Emissions

Any condition that alters the mechanical characteristics of the middle ear will influence OAE measurements. However, various abnormalities influence forward and backward transmission differently. This was demonstrated by Wiederhold (1990, 1993) who measured DPOAEs in anesthetized cats before and after middle-ear abnormalities were created. Two types of middle-ear conditions were studied— mass loading of the tympanic membrane and eardrum perforations. To create mass loading, weights (7 or 14 mg) were placed on the tympanic membrane over the umbo. By measuring the amplitude of the eighth cranial nerve action potential, the effect of the eardrum abnormality on forward transmission was assessed. DPOAEs in the mid-frequency region (~3 kHz) were reduced far more than was expected by the effect of forward transmission. Thus, the weight applied to the eardrum affected the transmission of the emission from the inner ear to the ear canal more than the transmission of the stimulus from the ear canal to the inner ear. The difference in forward and backward transmission, estimated by Kemp (1980) to be 12 to 16 dB, was increased by the eardrum abnormality. Wiederhold suggested that a scarred tympanic membrane could have a similar effect.

Small eardrum perforations affected DPOAEs differently than mass loading. The change in DPOAE amplitude was essentially identical to that predicted by the change in forward transmission. Thus, the change appeared to be due entirely to a change in the effective stimulus reaching the inner ear and not to a change in the transmission of the emission from the inner ear to the ear canal. The reduced response amplitude could be fully compensated by increasing the stimulus level. Because effects of perforations of different sizes and different locations were not explored, caution must be used in generalizing the results to patients with eardrum perforations.

The effect of otosclerosis on tone-burst evoked OAEs was studied by Rossi, Solero, Rolando, and Olina (1988). They recorded OAEs from eight patients with unilateral otosclerosis for air-conducted and bone-conducted 1-kHz tone bursts. Air-conducted stimuli presented at 30–dB HL did not evoke measurable emissions. Bone-conducted stimuli, however, did elicit measurable responses. Because bone-conduction stimulation avoids most of the reduction in forward transmission, the effective stimulus reaches the cochlea at a higher intensity than the air-conduction stimulus. Had the investigators used a higher intensity air-conduction stimulus, they may have observed a response. From their data, it is not possible to estimate forward and backward transmission effects of otosclerosis.

Developmental Effects

Developmental changes of the ear canal and middle ear are of critical importance in the application of OAE measurement to infant hearing screening. Substantial changes in the structure of both the ear canal and middle ear occur during the first year of life with more modest developmental changes occurring into adolescence (Eby & Nadol, 1986). The changes have great influence on the vibratory response of the ear canal and on the input impedance the middle ear (Holte, Margolis, & Cavanagh, 1991; Keefe, Bulen, Arehart, & Burns, 1993).

Studies of temporal bones of infants indicate that, unlike inner-ear development (which is virtually complete at birth), the middle ear and external ear continue to change. There are four development changes that may influence OAE measurement: resorption of mesenchyme, pneumatization of the middle ear and mastoid, change in the position of the eardrum, and development of the osseous portion of the ear canal.

Mesenchyme is embryonic connective tissue that is formed during development and is resorbed or transformed by the time development is complete. Mesenchyme has been observed in the temporal bones of infants by several investigators (De Sa, 1973; Eavey, 1993; Paparella, Shea, Meyerhoff, & Goycoolea, 1980). This observation is important because the presence of mesenchyme in the infant's middle ear may influence input impedance, as well as forward and backward transmission. The observation that mesenchyme persists in the middle ear for up to 5 months after birth (Spector & Ge, 1981) may explain the changes in tympanometric findings that occur over the same time period (Holte et al., 1991). Mesenchyme may influence middle-ear characteristics by filling spaces that would otherwise contain air and by interfering with the vibration of the ossicular chain and tympanic membrane.

Pneumatization of the temporal bone results from resorption of mesenchyme and leaves air spaces where the mesenchyme had been and by osteoclastic erosion of bone. During fetal development, parts of the bony mastoid are quite dense. The dense bone is eroded (*osteoclasis*) leaving pockets that form the mastoid air cells. In some patients with developmental defects, interruption in the pneumatization process sometimes results in abnormal density of the mastoid. Pneumatization affects middle-ear transmission characteristics because the air enclosed in the middle ear and mastoid influences the vibration of the eardrum. A poorly pneumatized temporal bone contains a smaller volume of air in contact with the eardrum. Because a small volume of air has a high impedance, the poorly pneumatized ear is less efficient in both forward and backward directions.

The eardrum changes in position and structure during the first postnatal year. At birth, the eardrum is nearly horizontal and appears as an extension of the superior ear-canal wall. As the ear develops, it changes to a nearly vertical orientation (Eby & Nadol, 1986). The position of the newborn eardrum makes it difficult to examine with an otoscope (Eavey, 1993), but probably does not affect its function. Like the middle-ear space, the neonate eardrum contains mesenchymal tissue that later is resorbed (Ruah, Schachern, Zelterman, Paprella, & Yoon, 1992). The effect of the structural change on middle-ear transmission characteristics is not known, but it likely influences both forward and backward transmission.

The bony portion of the ear canal is only partially formed at birth (Anson, Bast, & Richany, 1955). The ossification of the canal wall is not well documented, but continues into the postnatal period. The effect of this is evident from pneumatic otoscopy in the newborn period, during which the canal walls move noticeably in response to ear-canal–pressure changes (Holte, Cavanagh, & Margolis, 1990). A number of researchers have suggested that the flaccid nature of the ear-canal wall contributes to tympanometric patterns that occur in newborns (Keefe et al., 1993; Paradise, Smith, & Bluestone, 1976). Holte et al. (1990), however, found no relation between ear-canal–wall movement and tympanometric patterns in full-term newborns. On the other hand, Keefe et al. (1993) was able to account for the impedance characteristics of newborn ears by assuming a flaccid ear-canal wall and a normal middle ear. It has not yet been possible to parcel out the contribution of middle-ear characteristics (e.g., unresolved mesenchyme, incomplete pneumatization) and ear-canal effects in newborn-impedance measurements. It is quite possible, however, that the incomplete development of the ear canal has a substantial influence on OAE measurements in newborns.

OAE characteristics change dramatically during the first few postnatal days. Smurzynski (1994) demonstrated substantial increases in TEOAE and DPOAE amplitudes during the first several weeks of life of preterm infants. Kok, van Zanten, and Brocaar (1992) observed postnatal changes in TEOAE amplitudes that averaged 8 dB over the first few days in full-term babies. The changes were probably due to alterations of the ear canal and middle ear. Chang, Vohr, Norton, and Lekas (1993) demonstrated a substantial effect of cleaning the newborn ear canal on TEOAE amplitudes. Thus, some of the early changes in OAE responses may be due to clearance of vernix and amniotic fluid from the ear canal. Clearance of amniotic fluid and mesenchyme from the middle ear may also contribute to the changes that occur in the first few days.

Case Examples

Case 1: Middle-Ear Pressure

A 7-year old patient has been followed as part of a prospective otitis media study since insertion of his first set of tympanostomy tubes at age 2 years. A second set of tubes was inserted at age 3, and he has had frequent episodes of OM ever since. His audiogram and tympanograms are shown in Figure 7–8. The audiogram indicated a 22-dB air-bone gap on the left (average of 0.25–2.0 kHz). Tympanograms indicated bilateral negative pressure, normal static admittance on the right, high static admittance on the left, and normal tympanometric width bilaterally. The speech recognition threshold on the left was better than the average air-conduction threshold, suggesting that the air-bone gap may not be accurate. Because of the child's atypical behavior, the accuracy of the pure-tone thresholds was questionable. Otoacoustic emission testing was performed to determine if real interaural differences existed. TEOAE recordings were obtained with ambient ear-canal air pressure and with ear-canal pressure set to compensate for the middle-ear pressure. Results for the right ear are shown in Figure 7–9. With ambient ear-canal pressure, no measurable emissions were obtained. When the ear-canal air pressure was adjusted to compensate for the middle-ear pressure, normal emissions were obtained. In the left ear (Figure 7–10), emissions were again absent with ambient pressure. The oscillation that is present at the early part of the recording and the high reproducibility at 4 kHz (84%) is an artifact due to stimulus ringing in the ear canal. Compensating for middle-ear pressure resulted in a small emission, significantly smaller than that obtained from the right ear. A subsequent otomicroscopic examination of the eardrums indicated that the left eardrum was severely retracted and draped over the incus. The robust nature of the OAEs obtained from the right ear with compensating pressure suggests that there was no significant middle-ear transmission problem except for the effect of negative middle-ear pressure. The small emissions obtained from the left ear suggest that a real conductive hearing loss existed in that ear and that the loss could not be fully compensated by ear-canal air pressure.

The poor otoacoustic emissions observed with ambient ear-canal air pressure illustrates the effect of middle-ear pressure on OAE measurement. If this evaluation had been performed for hearing screening purposes, both ears would probably have failed. By compensating for middle-ear pressure, only the abnormal left ear would fail the screening. The case illustrates the potential use of OAE measurement for detecting middle-ear disorders and for evaluating interaural differences.

Case 2: Middle-Ear Fluid

A 60-year old female patient was evaluated for a complex of symptoms including headache, loss of muscle control of the eye, and unilateral hearing loss, all on the right side. She was followed for three years before a magnetic resonance imaging

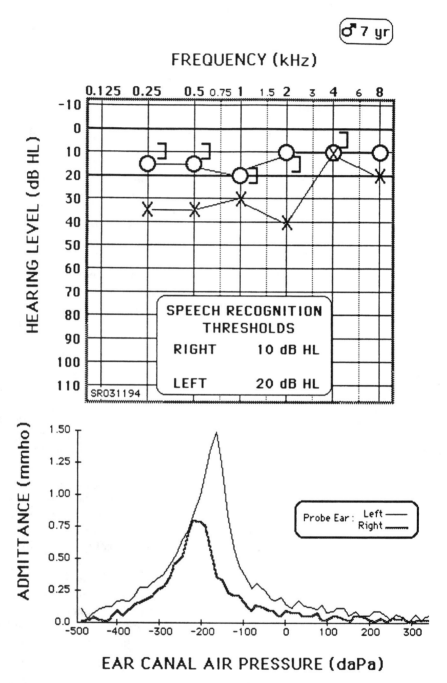

Figure 7–8. Audiogram and tympanograms for a 7-year-old boy. Note that substantial negative pressure indicated on the tympanograms.

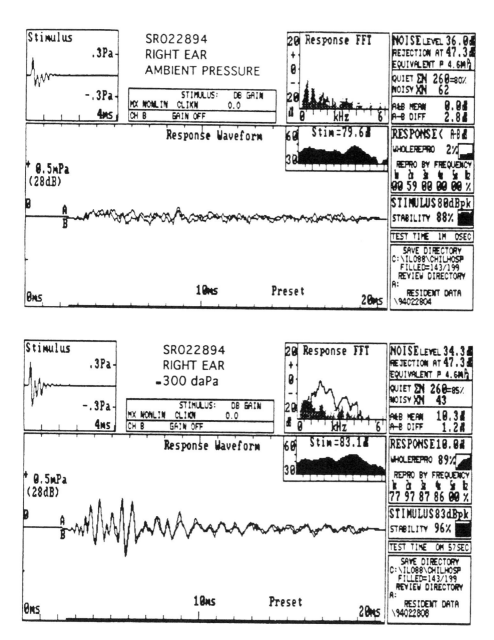

Figure 7–9. TEOAE responses in a 7-year-old boy for the right ear in two pressure conditions. *Top*: With ambient ear-canal pressure there was no response. *Bottom*: When the ear-canal pressure was set to −300 daPa, the emission amplitude increased to 10 dB.

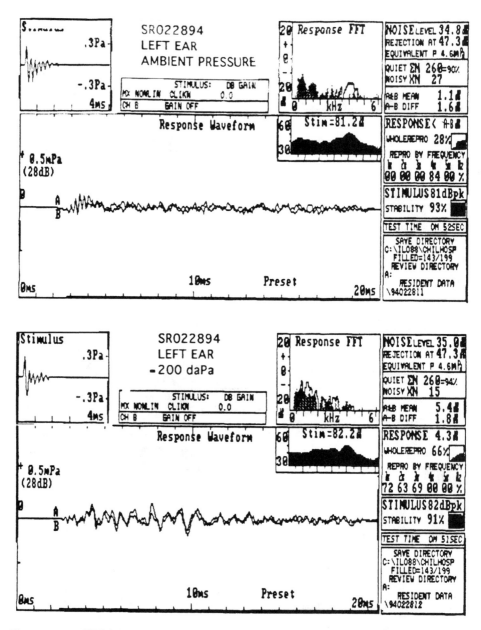

Figure 7–10.   TEOAE responses in a 7-year-old boy for the left ear in two pressure conditions. *Top*: With ambient ear-canal pressure there was no response. *Bottom*: When the ear-canal pressure was set to −300 daPa, the emission amplitude increased to 4.3 dB.

(MRI) scan confirmed the presence of a large (~3 cm) cerebellopontine angle meningioma. Her audiogram indicated a mild sensorineural hearing loss in the right ear with severe speech recognition rollover (Figure 7–11). The tumor was removed and the surgeons were not able to locate the eighth cranial nerve at the conclusion of the resection. Eleven days after surgery, she had a blood-filled middle ear, a flat tympanogram, and no measurable hearing in the right ear. TEOAE recording indicated a normal emission on the left and a small, reproducible emission in the 2 to 3 kHz region on the right; when the patient was seen on a followup visit the response was absent from the operated side (Figure 7–12).

Because of the location of the tumor, the preoperative hearing loss was probably due to compression of the eighth cranial nerve or auditory brainstem and not due to cochlear dysfunction. The postoperative presence of an emission suggests that the intraoperative injury to the auditory system was also retrocochlear. The hemo-tympanum (blood-filled middle ear), not unusual in surgeries of this type, results from exposure of the mastoid air cells and middle ear during the surgery. The middle ear generally clears during the postoperative period through the Eustachian tube. Although middle-ear fluid often eliminates OAEs entirely, an emission can reach the ear canal through a fluid-filled middle ear at sufficient levels to

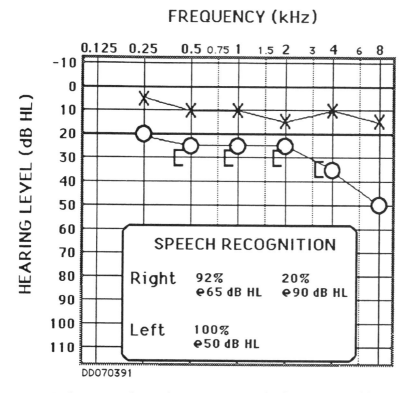

Figure 7–11. Audiogram and speech recognition results for a 60-year-old woman. The patient had a large cerebellopontine angle tumor on the right side.

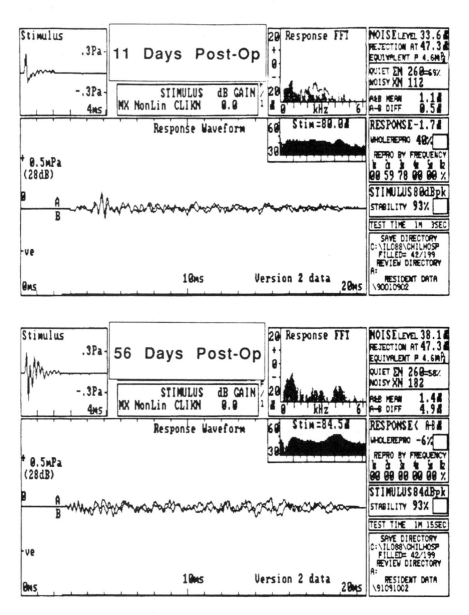

Figure 7–12. TEOAE results for a 60-year-old woman at 11 and 56 days after surgical removal of the large cerebellopontine angle tumor. At 11 days there was a measurable emission in spite of a flat tympanogram and otoscopically evident hemotympanum. At 56 days the emission was absent.

be detected above the noise floor. The absent emission observed on postoperative day 56 probably resulted from cochlear degeneration secondary either to destruction of the eighth nerve or interruption of the cochlear blood supply.

References

Anson, B. J., Bast, T. H., & Richany, S. F. (1955). The fetal and early postnatal development of the tympanic ring and related structures in man. *Annals of Otology, Rhinology, and Laryngology, 64,* 802–823.

Bray, P. J. (1989). Click evoked otoacoustic emissions and the development of a clinical otoacoustic hearing test instrument. London University, Ph.D. Thesis.

Chang, K. W., Vohr, B. R., Norton, S. J., & Lekas, M. D. (1993). External and middle ear status related to evoked otoacoustic emission in neonates. *Archives of Otolaryngology—Head and Neck Surgery, 119,* 276–282.

De Sa, D. J. (1973). Infection and amniotic aspiration of middle ear in stillbirths and neonatal deaths. *Archives of Disorders in Children, 48,* 872–880.

Eavey, R. D. (1993). Abnormalities of the neonatal ear: Otoscopic observations, histologic observations, and a model for contamination of the middle ear by cellular contents of amniotic fluid. *Laryngoscope, 103* (Suppl. 58), 1–31.

Eby, T. L., & Nadol, J. B. (1986). Postnatal growth of the Human temporal bone: Implications for cochlear implants in children. *Annals of Otology, Rhinology, and Laryngology, 95,* 356–364.

Holte, L., Cavanagh, R. M., & Margolis, R. H. (1990). Ear canal wall mobility and tympanometric shape in young infants. *Journal of Pediatrics, 117,* 77–80.

Holte, L., Margolis, R. H., & Cavanagh, R. M. (1991). Developmental changes in multifrequency tympanograms. *Audiology, 30,* 1–24.

Hunter, L. L., Margolis, R. H., & Giebink, G. S. (1994). Identification of hearing loss in children with otitis media. *Annals of Otology, Rhinology, and Laryngology, 103*(Suppl. 163), 59–61.

Keefe, D. H., Bulen, J. C., Arehart, K. H., & Burns, E. M. (1993). Ear-canal impedance and reflection coefficient in human infants and adults. *Journal of the Acoustical Society of America, 94,* 2617–2638.

Kemp, D. T. (1980). Towards a model for the origin of cochlear echoes. *Hearing Research, 2,* 533–548.

Kemp, D. T. (1981). Physiologically active cochlear micromechanics—one source of tinnitus. Ciba Foundation Symposium, *85,* 54–81.

Kemp, D. T., Ryan, S., & Bray, P. (1990). A guide to the effective use of otoacoustic emissions. *Ear and Hearing, 11,* 93–105.

Kok, M. R., van Zanten, G. A., & Brocaar, M. P. (1992). Growth of evoked otoacoustic emissions during the first days postpartum. *Audiology, 31,* 140–149.

Kringlebotn, M. (1988). Network model for the human middle ear. *Scandinavian Audiology, 17,* 75–85.

Margolis, R. H. (1981). Fundamentals of acoustic immittance. In G. R. Popelka (Ed.), *Hearing assessment with the acoustic reflex* (pp. 117–144). New York: Grune and Stratton.

Naeve, S. L., Margolis, R. H., Levine, S. C., & Fournier, E. M. (1992). Effect of ear-canal air pressure on evoked otoacoustic emissions. *Journal of the Acoustical Society of America, 91,* 2091–2095.

Nelson, D. A., & Kimberly, B. P. (1992). Distortion-product emissions and auditory sensitivity in human ears with normal hearing and cochlear hearing loss. *Journal of Speech and Hearing Research, 35,* 1142–1159.

Osterhammel, P. A., Nielsen, L. H., & Rasmussen, A. N. (1993). Distortion product otoacoustic emissions. *Scandinavian Audiology, 22,* 111–116.

Owens, J. J., McCoy, M. J., Lonsbury-Martin, B. L., & Martin, G. K. (1992). Influence of otitis media on evoked otoacoustic emissions in children. *Seminars in Hearing, 13,* 53–64.

Paparella, M. M., Shea, D., Meyerhoff, W. L., & Goycoolea, M. V. (1980). Silent otitis media. *Laryngoscope, 90,* 1089–1098.

Paradise, J. L., Smith, C. G., & Bluestone, C. D. (1976). Tympanometric detection of middle ear effusion in infants and young children. *Pediatrics, 58,* 198–210.

Robinson, P. M., & Haughton, P. M. (1991). Modification of evoked oto-acoustic emissions by changes in pressure in the external ear. *British Journal of Audiology, 25,* 131–133.

Rossi, G., Solero, P., Rolanda, M., & Olina, M. (1989). Are delayed evoked oto-acoustic emissions (DEOE) solely the outcome of an active intracochlear mechanism? *Scandinavian Audiology, 18,* 99–104.

Ruah, C. B., Schachern, P. A., Zelterman, D., Paparella, M. M., & Yoon, T. H. (1992). Age-related morphologic changes in the human tympanic membrane: A light and electron microscopic study. *Archives of Otolaryngology—Head and Neck Surgery, 117,* 627–634.

Schloth, E., & Zwicker, E. (1983). Mechanical and acoustical influences on spontaneous otoacoustic emissions. *Hearing Research, 11,* 285–293.

Smurzynski, J. (1994). Longitudinal measurements of distortion-product and click-evoked otoacoustic emissions of preterm infants. Preliminary results. *Ear and Hearing, 15,* 210–223.

Spector, G. J., & Ge, X. X. (1981). Development of the hypotympanum in the human fetus and neonate. *Annals of Otology, Rhinology, and Laryngology, 88* (Suppl.), 2–20.

Trine, M. B., Hirsch, J. E., & Margolis, R. H. (1993). Effects of middle ear pressure on evoked otoacoustic emissions. *Ear and Hearing, 14,* 401–407.

van Cauwenberge, P. B., Vinck, B., de Vel, E., Dhooge, I. (1995). Tympanometry and click evoked otoacoustic emissions in secretory otitis media: Are C-EOAE really consistently absent in type B tympanograms? Paper presented to the Sixth International Symposium on Otitis Media, Fort Lauderdale, FL.

Veuillet, E., Collet, L., & Morgon, A. (1992). Differential effects of ear-canal pressure and contralateral acoustic stimulation on evoked otoacoustic emissions in humans. *Hearing Research, 61,* 47–55.

Wada, H., Ohyama, K., Kobayashi, T., Sunaga, N., & Koike, T. (1993). Relationship between evoked otoacoustic emissions and middle-ear dynamic characteristics. *Audiology, 32,* 282–292.

Wiederhold, M. L. (1990). Effects of tympanic membrane modification on distortion-product otoacoustic emissions in the cat ear canal. In P. Dallos (Ed.), *The mechanics and biophysics of hearing* (pp. 251–258). Berlin: Springer-Verlag.

Wiederhold, M. L. (1992). Frequency-dependent effect of tympanic membrane loading on reverse middle-ear transmission. In *Abstracts of the fifteenth midwinter research meeting of the Association for Research in Otolaryngology* (Abstract No. 156).

Wilson, J. P., & Sutton, G. J. (1981). Acoustic correlates of tonal tinnitus. *Ciba foundation symposium, 85,* 82–107.

Zwicker, E. (1983). Delayed evoked oto-acoustic emissions and their suppression by Gaussian-shaped pressure impulses. *Hearing Research, 11,* 359–371.

Zwislocki, J. (1962). Analysis of the middle-ear function. Part I: Input impedance. *Journal of the Acoustical Society of America, 34,* 1514–1523.

8

Otoacoustic Emissions and Audiometric Outcomes

Frances P. Harris
Rudolf Probst

Introduction

The early observations made by Kemp in 1978 formed the basis for the association of otoacoustic emissions (OAEs) and auditory functioning in human beings. Kemp documented that otoacoustic emissions were present only when subjective threshold levels were greater (i.e., better) than approximately 30 dB HL. Parallel studies with laboratory animals found that OAEs are highly sensitive to changes in the cochlea that also alter auditory sensitivity. Since these early observations, there have been numerous investigations exploring the relations between OAE parameters and measures of audition in human beings. The results of these investigations are important not only for advancing the status of clinical applications but also for enhancing our understanding of basic cochlear functioning.

The measurement of OAEs for clinical purposes gained prominence after the launch of commercial instrumentation in 1988. In the short time since then, OAEs have already become a preferred method of screening for hearing loss. Additional clinical uses, such as using OAEs for monitoring subtle cochlear changes during administration of ototoxic drugs or from noise continue to be identified.

Three types of OAEs will be included in the chapter: spontaneous OAEs (SOAEs), transient evoked OAEs (TEOAEs) and distortion-product OAEs (DPOAEs). Although stimulus-frequency otoacoustic emissions (SFOAEs) are closely related to cochlear functioning (Avan, Loth, Menguy, & Teyssou, 1991; Brass & Kemp, 1993), they will not be discussed in this chapter because there have been too few investigations of their use for clinical purposes. Tests of OAEs during presentation of a contralateral stimulus are also not included.

The primary emphases of this chapter are (a) results from adults rather than neonates, infants or young children, (b) aspects of individual testing rather than

Steps for Comparing OAEs and Audiometric Outcomes

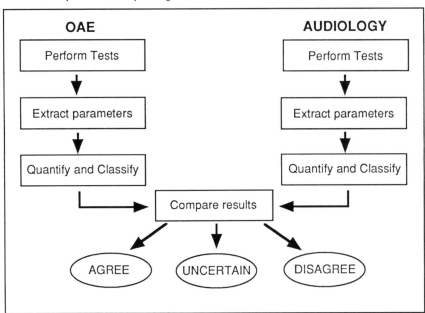

Figure 8–1.   General steps for making comparisons of audiometric outcomes and tests of otoacoustic emissions.

mass screening, (c) cochlear or retrocochlear rather than middle-ear effects. (In this chapter all middle ears function normally unless otherwise specified.)

The basic steps for making comparisons of OAEs and audiometric outcomes are diagrammed in Figure 8–1. Both measurements are made, parameters are extracted from them that are then reported in some meaningful way for comparison; this results finally in a decision about the nature of the correspondence between them. Comparisons have been analyzed and reported both anecdotally and statistically. In the clinical literature on OAEs and audiometric findings, anecdotal evidence for the association of an OAE-test record with the pure-tone audiogram in the form of individual examples has prevailed. Although such examples can be informative, they can also be misleading when used as evidence to support the general case. For making definitive statements about the overall associations of OAE parameters and auditory function, statistical treatment of large samples of data from various groups of subjects with normal and impaired auditory systems is required.

SOAEs

Two types of SOAEs with different audiometric outcomes can be identified: a common "low-level" type that can be recorded in the majority of normally hearing ears and a rare "high-level" type that is clearly related to pathological hearing.

Low-Level SOAEs

The common low-level type of SOAE have been found in up to 78% of subjects with presumed normal hearing, depending on recording methods, age, gender, and race (Burns, Hoberg, Arehart, & Campbell, 1992; Kok, vanZanten, & Brocaar, 1993; Penner, Glotzbach, & Huang, 1993; Talmadge, Long, Murphy, & Tubin, 1993; Whitehead, Kamal, Lonsbury-Martin, & Martin, 1993a). Earlier suggestions that all SOAEs may be a subtle sign of cochlear damage (Clark, Kim, Zurek, & Bohne, 1984; Norton, Mott, & Champlin, 1989; Ruggero, Kramek, & Rich, 1984) are no longer pertinent in view of the high prevalence of SOAEs in both adults and children with normal hearing. Thus, SOAEs can be regarded as a by-product of normal cochlear functioning in most cases. SOAEs are thought to be oscillations generated by an active oscillator within the cochlea (Talmadge, Tubis, Wit, & Long, 1991; van Dijk & Wit, 1990). Indeed, there is evidence that subjects with SOAEs have better hearing sensitivity than those without (McFadden & Mishra, 1993). The difference is about 3 dB and is not likely to be clinically relevant. However, it is tempting to explain such long-established findings as a slightly better hearing sensitivity in women than in men and in Blacks compared to Whites on the basis of differences in cochlear activity that also account for SOAEs (McFadden & Mishra, 1993). Spontaneous otoacoustic emissions are prevalent more in women than in men and more in Blacks than in other racial groups.

Despite the subtle differences within the characterization of SOAEs, the findings point to the fact that SOAEs are related to normal audiometric thresholds in the vast majority of cases. Moulin, Collet, Delli, and Morgon (1991) found a hearing threshold of 10 dB HL or better at 1 kHz and 20 dB HL or better at 0.25, 0.5, and 2 kHz in all ears with sensorineural hearing loss that still had an SOAE. However, the prevalence of SOAEs in such subjects was low (less than 20%). Similar findings were reported by Probst, Lonsbury-Martin, Martin, and Coats (1987) and Bonfils (1989). They reported a low prevalence of SOAEs in ears with sensorineural hearing loss. Pure-tone thresholds for frequencies corresponding to the SOAE (Probst et al., 1987) or subjective click-thresholds (Bonfils, 1989) were always 15 dB HL or better in ears with SOAEs.

The presence of low-level SOAEs always signals hearing better than 20 dB HL in corresponding frequency regions. They are not uncommon in normally hearing ears, and they are rare in ears with sensorineural hearing loss, even if the hearing loss is restricted to certain frequency regions. The presence of SOAEs can exert a strong influence on the amplitude and frequency distribution of other OAE measurements.

High-Level SOAEs

The typical level of SOAEs in adults is around 0 dB SPL and ranges between −10 to 20 dB SPL. OAEs with levels up to 60 dB SPL are rare, but they often attract attention because they may be audible without amplification (Probst, Lonsbury-Martin, & Martin, 1991; Mathis, Probst, De Min, & Hauser, 1991). Generally, the emissions are relatively high in frequency. Case reports of such emissions indicate that as a rule they are present at birth, they may be inherited, and the hearing threshold at the frequency of the emission is pathological. One example of a high-

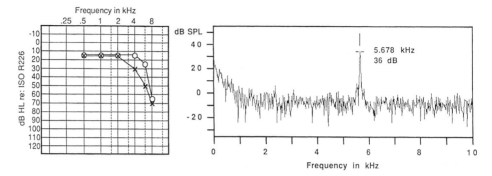

Figure 8–2. Frequency and level of a "high-level" spontaneous otoacoustic emission (SOAE) measured with a B&K 4144 microphone placed at the entrance of the left ear canal of a 2-year-old boy. Subsequent measurement with an ER10A probe sealed in the ear canal identified the SOAE at 5.643 kHz at 55 dB SPL. The SOAE could be heard easily without amplification. The audiogram was obtained when the child was age 3 years. (Adapted from Mathis et al., 1991. Used with permission.)

level SOAE and its associated audiometric outcome was reported by Mathis, Probst, De Min and Hauser (1991) (Figure 8–2). In the report, a child was first identified because his mother heard a clearly audible tonal signal coming from his left ear. Since this case report was published, the child's hearing has remained stable, and he is still not aware of the sound himself. Therefore, a normal audiometric outcome can be expected at the frequency of the vast majority of SOAEs, but some SOAEs may be associated with a pathological state of the cochlea in which case hearing thresholds are generally elevated for the corresponding frequencies.

Except for their unusually high levels and high frequencies, pathological SOAEs cannot be distinguished readily from normal, low-level SOAEs. In addition, it is not known if some low-level SOAEs are also somehow linked to pathological cochlear states. Although most SOAEs are an expression of a particularly sensitive cochlea, the use of SOAE measurements to predict hearing threshold levels is less hindered by knowledge of this caveat than by other factors. These include the idiosyncratic levels and frequencies of SOAEs and the influence of recording methods, which are highly susceptible to background noise.

There are unusual cases of high-level SOAEs in ears with hearing loss. Therefore, some caution must be taken in assuming that hearing is ALWAYS normal when SOAEs are present. Overall, SOAE measurements are not generally necessary for routine audiometric applications.

TEOAES

The main parameters of a TEOAE that have been investigated for their association with audiometric outcomes are illustrated in Figure 8–3. Parameters include (A) overall correlation of two waveforms obtained from time-averaging (*reproducibility*); (B) the overall amplitude of the response in relation to noise in the measure-

Parameters extracted from TEOAE Results

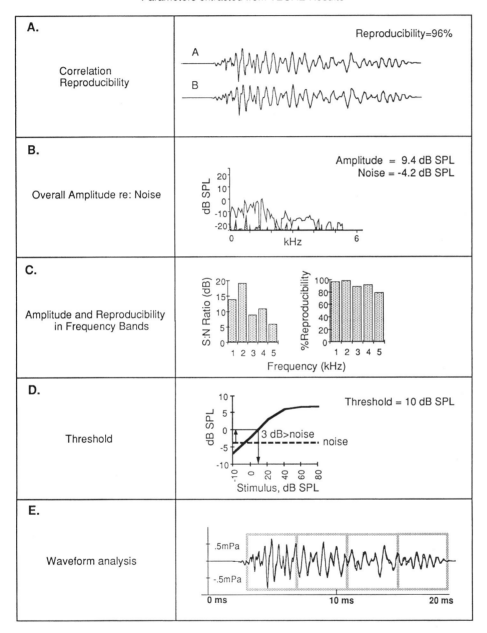

Figure 8–3. Schematic representation of the parameters extracted from measurements of transiently evoked otoacoustic emissions (TEOAEs).

ment; (C) The frequency composition of the response as determined by analysis of the fast Fourier transform (FFT) and the corresponding reproducibility within specific frequency bands; (D) threshold; (E) waveform analysis or other specially derived parameters, such as latency and a response index. After parameters are extracted from the test record, they may be compared with various indices of auditory performance. The relation of TEOAE parameters with hearing thresholds has been of primary clinical interest.

TEOAEs and Pure-Tone Results

The TEOAEs and hearing threshold levels are both derived following stimulation to the cochlea. However, they do not sample the cochlear response in the same way. For measuring TEOAEs, the ear is stimulated by either clicks, tone bursts, or noise bursts that are usually presented at suprathreshold levels. This results in a generalized response from the cochlea that is composed of contributions from sources that are distributed along the cochlear partition (Avan & Bonfils, 1993). The TEOAE has no "true" threshold because its measurement is always constrained by the noise floor of the measuring system. By contrast, a *hearing threshold* is the point where a listener can just detect the presence of a signal at some predefined criterion rate (such as 50% or 75%). A "true" threshold is obtained for the stimulating signal. Despite these methodological differences, TEOAEs and subjective detection thresholds do relate to one another because they share features of a common mechanism. If this mechanism is functioning normally, then the parameters derived from both measures are generally within some grossly normal range. An abnormal mechanism affects both measures.

IDENTIFICATION OF THE OVERALL MAGNITUDE OF HEARING LOSS

Parameters of TEOAEs are influenced strongly by both auditory threshold levels and the frequency distribution of normal versus abnormal hearing in an individual ear. Understanding the nature of these influences is fundamental to the sound interpretation of TEOAEs either for screening or for the prediction of hearing levels by frequency. If the purpose of testing TEOAEs is the identification of hearing loss, parameters for a broad interpretation must be derived. If the purpose is to determine the frequency distribution of a hearing loss, more specific analyses and interpretation of the findings must be made.

The outcomes of the majority of investigations that have been designed to determine the cutoff levels of hearing that can be identified with TEOAEs are summarized in Figure 8–4. There are two distinct situations in which the association of TEOAEs and hearing is straightforward: the case in which overall hearing is better than 20 dB HL (TEOAEs are present in 99% of ears) and the case of sensorineural hearing loss (SNHL) greater than 40 dB HL with no complicating etiological factors (TEOAEs are always absent). This basic dichotomy provides the basis for using TEOAEs in the identification of hearing loss in screening programs. For such purposes, an overall parameter, such as percentage of reproducibility, response level, or a combination of measures, is calculated from the TEOAE and used to determine the presence or absence of hearing loss. When TEOAEs are to be used for general clinical applications, including approximations of hearing levels

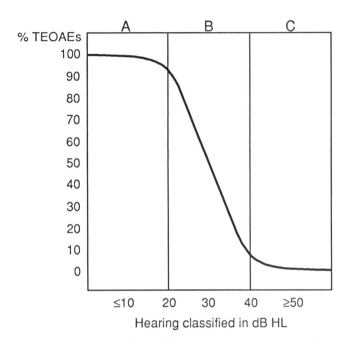

Figure 8–4. Schematic representation of the average pure-tone results associated with percentage of TEOAEs present taken from a compilation of data reported in the literature. *Segment A*: overall hearing is better than 20 dB HL (TEOAEs are present in 99% of ears) (Bonfils, Bertrand, & Uziel, 1988a; Bonfils, Uziel, & Pujol, 1988b; Bonfils, Avan, François, Marie, Trotoux, & Narcy, 1990; Kemp, 1978; Kemp, Bray, Alexander, & Brown, 1986; Probst et al., 1987; Probst et al., 1991; Stevens & Ip, 1988). *Segment C*: SNHL greater than 40 dB HL with no complicating etiological factors: TEOAEs are always absent (Bonfils et al., 1988a; Bonfils et al., 1988b; Bray & Kemp, 1987; Collet, Veuillet, Chanal, & Morgon, 1991; Collet, Levy, Veuillet, Truy, & Morgon, 1993; Collet, Veuillet, Berger-Vachon, & Morgon, 1992; Kemp, 1978; Kemp et al., 1986; Prieve, Gorga, Schmidt, Neely, Peters, Schulte, et al., 1993; Probst et al., 1987; Probst et al., 1991; Robinette, 1992; Stevens & Ip, 1988). The segments A and C can be distinguished clearly from each other. However the value for the cutoff point between sections A and B has varied across studies, depending primarily upon the criteria selected to evaluate both the audiometric outcome and the TEOAE. As a general rule, when average hearing is better than 25 dB HL, TEOAEs are always present. When average hearing is poorer than 45 dB HL, TEOAEs are always absent. Segment B represents a "zone of uncertainty" that extends from approximately 25 to 35 dB HL. In this range, TEOAEs may be present but are generally reduced in amplitude and in frequency content in comparison to findings from ears with thresholds falling within Section A. In the presence of a small amount of hearing loss, a TEOAE may still be measured. It is not certain that a linear relationship exists between decreases in pure-tone threshold and the level and repro-ducibility of TEOAEs. Spectral analyses of TEOAEs can assist in their interpretation because a fragmented response is often associated with partial hearing loss.

by frequency, then the entire function (Figure 8–3) must be taken into account. This includes the "zone of uncertainty," ranging from approximately 25 to 35 dB HL where the interpretation of a TEOAE result is not clear. This uncertainty arises from a combination of factors including methodological differences in deriving both behavioral and TEOAE measures and because the influence of the configuration of the hearing loss is not always accounted for when interpreting the TEOAE. When TEOAEs are evaluated for diagnostic purposes, both broad and more specific interpretations of their association with a range of behavioral values for magnitude and frequency are expected.

When all hearing levels from 0.25 to 8 kHz are better than 20 dB HL, TEOAEs are present in 99% of ears. When all hearing levels from 0.25 to 8 kHz are poorer than 40 dB HL, TEOAEs are absent in 100% of ears with peripheral hearing loss. These guidelines presume that abnormal middle ear function has been ruled out.

An important question when TEOAEs are compared with hearing-test results or used to predict hearing loss is this: Which parameters should be selected from the test results? The choices that are available from most TEOAE results are overall reproducibility, response level and frequency band analyses (Figure 8–3). Audiometrically, pure-tone average (PTA; 0.5, 1, and 2 kHz), threshold at 1 kHz, best threshold and worst threshold have been used. All these possibilities have advantages and disadvantages, and the use of the appropriate parameter can influence the interpretation of the results.

One goal of recent studies by Prieve et al. (1993) and Gorga et al. (1993b) was to determine which TEOAE parameter best predicted hearing levels when worst threshold at 0.5, 1, 2, or 4 kHz was used as the audiometric parameter. They found that the measures of percentage reproducibility, TEOAE level or TEOAE level above noise were highly interrelated, and that they predicted audiometric outcome approximately equally well. The parameter of percentage reproducibility performed slightly better than did the other two. When hearing threshold levels were less (i.e., poorer) than 20 dB HL, TEOAE responses decreased sharply, and there was no direct correspondence between the degree of change in any TEOAE parameter and the magnitude of the hearing loss. Therefore, using any of the TEOAE parameters, a hearing level of 20 dB HL could be used as the cutoff point for predicting the amount of impairment.

Given that percentage reproducibility is a reasonable parameter for differentiating normal from impaired ears, it follows that a criterion level must be selected to make this judgement. In the Prieve et al. (1993) and Gorga et al. (1993b) studies, percentage reproducibility varied from 55 to 70% using their criteria for identification of hearing loss. Whitehead, McCoy, Martin, & Lonsbury-Martin (1993c) reported results from 149 normally hearing ears and 142 ears with high-frequency SNHL with at least a portion of the audiogram better than 25 dB HL. A whole reproducibility score of 50% was able to differentiate ears with hearing loss from those without. Welzl-Müller and Stephan (1994) approached the quantification of TEOAEs in a different way. Results from 525 ears of children from 3 to 11 years of age were classified as present, absent or uncertain by two experienced judges. Numeric values of response level, reproducibility, and of several combination scores devised by the investigators were then calculated. The response level that was found to separate response absent from present was 7.3 dB SPL and for reproducibility it was 56%. As in the Prieve et al. and Gorga et al. results, they also found that the response in relation to the noise was a more sensitive measure than consideration of the response level alone.

The amount of "residual" cochlea contributing to the TEOAE is an important factor in its detection. Robinette (1990) reported results from a group of subjects (n = 226) with high-frequency sensorineural hearing loss (HFSNHL) at various "cut- off" frequencies. He found few TEOAEs present for any band of frequencies from 1 to 4 kHz when the region of HL began above 0.5 kHz; whereas, moving the cut-off frequency progressively upwards increased the number of detectable TEOAEs. This finding was corroborated by Mathis, DeMin and Arnold (1991), who evaluated groups of subjects with hearing loss isolated to either the high, low or mid-frequency range. They determined that the rate of detection of the TEOAE was dependent upon the width of the frequency range of preserved hearing. They also found responses to be highly dependent upon preservation of hearing in the mid frequencies.

The parameter of threshold, which is taken from TEOAE growth functions, has also been used effectively to differentiate normal from abnormal ears (Avan, Bonfils, Loth, Teyssou, & Menguy, 1993; Hauser, Probst, & Löhle, 1991; Stover & Norton, 1993). However, growth functions are time-consuming to obtain, and use of this parameter is not practical for most clinical applications. Because all parameters taken from a TEOAE test record are closely related to each other (Prieve et al., 1993), it is probably not necessary to acquire threshold information for predicting audiometric outcomes. However, when TEOAEs are used for monitoring, such as might be done during the administration of ototoxic drugs, use of a low-level stimulus for gaining information about changes in the cochlea is probably preferable.

For the identification of hearing loss, a percentage-reproducibility score of 50% or better means that a portion of the audiogram has hearing threshold levels better than 25 dB HL. Parameters of percentage reproducibility, response level, and response level above noise are highly interrelated.

IDENTIFICATION OF HEARING LOSS BY FREQUENCY

Examples of the frequency-specific association of the spectral regions of a TEOAE (Figure 8–3) and the configuration of the audiogram in the same ear are pervasive throughout the clinical literature. These examples are conceptually quite convincing of a direct link between the two measures. However, it is not possible to rely on the "shape" of a TEOAE spectrum to predict threshold levels by frequency for several reasons. In addition to methodological differences, factors to consider are (a) the large amount of interindividual variability and the configuration of the spectral distribution of the responses from ears with normal hearing, (b) the contribution of the total amount and configuration of the hearing loss on the transient response and (c) the cause of the hearing loss. When all of these factors are accounted for, reasonable decisions about hearing levels by frequency can be made.

Transient evoked OAEs from ears with normal hearing (NH) are characterized by their individuality across ears. When results are grouped, the frequency components composing the responses are not distributed equally. The percentage of frequency components decreases as frequency increases as described in a study of 265 ears with audiometric thresholds better than 25 dB HL across frequency by

Robinette (1992). He found the distribution of number of responses by frequency to be: 1 kHz, 96%; 2 kHz, 94%; 3 kHz, 89% and 4 kHz, 76%. Moulin et al. (1993) reported similar decreases in 135 ears with normal hearing: 100% occurrence up to about 4 kHz, with occurrence decreasing to around 50% in the 5-kHz region. Examples of the derived spectral distributions from groups of persons with normal hearing are illustrated in Figures 8–5 and 8–14. There is a predominance of energy in the 1 to 2 kHz range and this dominance will occur even in ears with hearing loss.

Investigations of large groups of subjects with varying amounts and configurations of hearing loss have demonstrated that the TEOAEs from ears with hearing loss do depart from results "expected" with normal hearing. These departures are in both the frequency and amplitude domains. A representative example is reproduced as Figure 8–5, which illustrates the results reported by Hauser, Probst and Loehle (1991) for 60 subjects with either normal hearing or sharply falling high-frequency hearing loss above 2 kHz (high-frequency SNHL). Figure 8–5 illustrates several important points. First, results for the two groups are clearly different from each other above approximately 2.5 kHz. Additionally, the low frequency components from the ears with high-frequency SNHL are lower in level than the grouped results from the ears with normal hearing, even though their hearing levels are comparable in this range.

Another question that is often asked about TEOAEs is this: How frequency

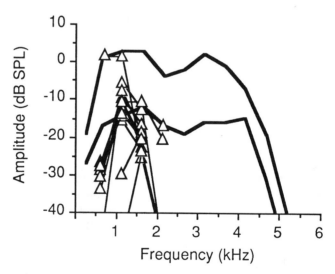

Figure 8–5. Comparison of the 10th and 90th percentiles of the spectra of click-evoked OAEs from 20 ears with normal hearing (*solid lines, no symbols*) and the spectra of 20 ears with hearing loss above 2 kHz (*triangles*). Spectral energy for the ears with hearing loss does not extend above 2.3 kHz. For the majority of ears with high-frequency hearing loss, the response levels are in the lower percentile range when compared with the results for the normally hearing ears. (Adapted from Hauser et al., 1991. Used with permission.)

specific are they? That is, how well can they identify a hearing loss at a specific frequency and can the amount of hearing loss be predicted? Prieve et al. (1993) attempted to answer these questions by determining how well TEOAEs could identify hearing poorer than 20 dB HL at 0.5, 1, 2 or 4 kHz. When data were analyzed into 1000-Hz band segments and then compared with the corresponding frequencies of the audiogram, 2 and 4 kHz could be better differentiated than either 0.5 or 1 kHz using any TEOAE parameter. Avan et al. (Avan, Bonfils, Loth, Narcy, & Trotoux, 1991; Avan, et al., 1993) sought to determine how closely the TEOAE response could be regarded as sensitive to the cochlear state at a particular place in the cochlea. They studied 182 ears from subjects with either normal hearing or hearing loss due to presbycusis or acoustic trauma. Using TEOAE thresholds and amplitudes for their comparisons with pure-tone results, they determined that both parameters are proportional to the total number of "residual active sites" along the organ of Corti. That is, the response is influenced by the entire length of the stimulated part of the cochlea. They also determined that there is a linear relationship between TEOAE threshold and hearing threshold at 2 kHz thus contradicting the notion that TEOAEs could be frequency specific.

The importance of considering the whole audiogram in interpreting a TEOAE result has been illustrated in several studies. Collet et al. (1991) evaluated TEOAE spectra and audiograms from 150 patients and found significant correlations with frequency. However, they noted that the amount of hearing and the configuration of the hearing loss were significant influences on the TEOAE and cautioned against making simple comparisons in a frequency-by-frequency manner. This is an important finding that has been confirmed by other investigators. Harris and Probst (1992) determined from an analysis of click-evoked and 1-kHz tone-burst evoked OAE results from 26 ears affected by Ménière's disease that if any audiometric threshold was better than 30 dB HL at any test frequency from 0.25 to 8 kHz, a TEOAE would be judged as "present." Audiometric threshold at 2 kHz was found to exert a strong influence on the presence of a response, even when the stimulus was a 1-kHz tone burst. They also concluded that one overall score used in isolation, such as percentage reproducibility, was not sufficient to characterize a test outcome for diagnostic purposes. Dominant energy in the low frequencies would inflate the TEOAE level and reproducibility score in relation to the whole time span of analysis (20 ms) and dominant energy in the high frequencies would underestimate the overall response. An individual example illustrating these ideas is displayed in Figure 8–6. Collet et al. (1993), in a report of results from 931 ears, came to a similar conclusion concerning the influence of a "best threshold" on the presence of a TEOAE. When overall hearing loss was greater than 45 dB HL in both ears, TEOAEs could still be detected in some ears, but only if hearing at any frequency from 0.25 to 8 kHz was better than 40 dB HL. The influence of best thresholds was also pointed out by Lind and Randa (1989) in a study of 32 subjects with either high or low- to medium-frequency hearing loss. They found that if hearing was better than 25 to 30 dB HL at 2 kHz, then a response would be present, despite the configuration of the hearing loss.

It has not yet been determined that the most sensitive parameters from TEOAE results for frequency-specific or monitoring applications are being analyzed. Special programs for waveform analyses or other time-domain processing may better

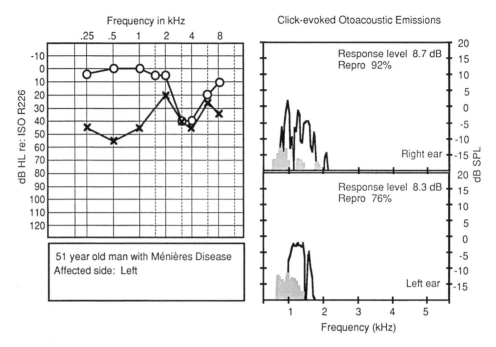

Figure 8–6. Audiogram and TEOAE spectra for both ears of a 51-year old man diagnosed with Ménière's disease. The left ear is the affected ear and symptoms were present for 13 months prior to this evaluation. The example illustrates the influence of "best" threshold on the spectra of the TEOAE and its subsequent interpretation. The best hearing sensitivity for the left ear is at 2 kHz, but the spectra of the TEOAE peaks around 1 kHz. The overall TEOAE response level for the two ears is almost the same despite the differences in audiometric configuration. The example also illustrates that energy in the TEOAE spectra in the 1 to 2 kHz region exerts a strong influence on the overall reproducibility score. For both ears, reproducibility scores were high (+75% in both ears), even though there was no energy in the responses above approximately 2.3 kHz.

serve these purposes (Takeda & Saito, 1991; Wen, Berlin, Hood, Jackson, & Hurley, 1993).

Both the amount and configuration of a hearing loss influence the detection and composition of a TEOAE. When predicting hearing levels by frequency from analysis of a TEOAE spectrum, caution must be exercised.

TEOAEs Stimulated by Tone Bursts

Most clinical tests of TEOAEs have been performed with clicks as stimuli. An important issue is whether another form of stimulation, such as tone bursts, might better sample the frequency-specific cochlear response. Evidence from studies that have used both clicks and tone-burst stimuli for eliciting responses in ears with and without hearing loss have confirmed that there is no significant advantage to using tone bursts as stimuli (Harris & Probst, 1991; Kemp et al., 1986; Norton & Neely,

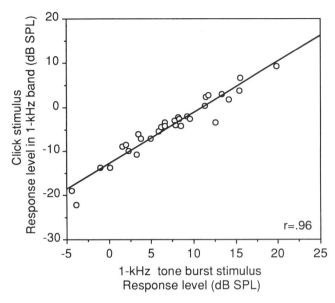

Figure 8–7. Comparison of TEOAE levels at 1 kHz for responses obtained either with 1-kHz tone bursts or clicks. Data are from 31 ears of patients with Ménière's disease. The energy in the 1-kHz spectral band from the click response is compared with the amplitude of the response to the 1-kHz tone burst. The results are highly correlated. (From Harris & Probst, 1991. Used with permission.)

1987; Probst & Harris, 1993a; Probst & Harris, 1993b). If the ear's response to clicks is analyzed into frequency components and the separate components are compared with responses to tone bursts at the same frequencies, the results are almost identical (Hauser, Probst, & Harris, 1991; Probst et al., 1987; Stover & Norton, 1993; Xu, Probst, Harris, & Roede, 1994). An example of this correspondence is illustrated in Figure 8–7.

To emphasize how linearly the ear integrates frequency, responses to individual tone bursts can be used to construct a response that is obtained with a more complex stimulus. For example, in Figure 8–8 results are shown for an ear that has been stimulated with individual tone bursts at 1, 2 and 3 kHz and with a complex tone burst stimulus composed of the same three frequencies. When responses to the individual tone bursts are combined mathematically and compared with the response to the tone burst complex, the results are nearly identical. The only advantage to the tone-burst stimulus is that more energy can be introduced in a specific frequency range than is possible for an equivalent click, which is a more frequency dispersive stimulus. Thus, for example in the high-frequency range where energy in the click begins to fall off, a high-frequency tone burst might be beneficial.

There are no significant advantages to testing transient responses with multiple tone bursts rather than clicks for routine clinical applications.

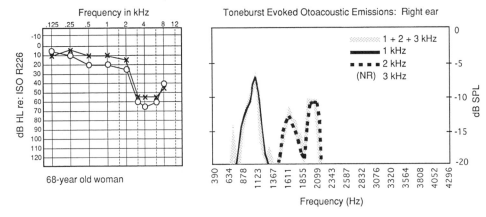

Figure 8–8. Comparison of TEOAEs evoked with single tone bursts at either 1, 2 or 3-kHz and with a multi-tone-burst complex composed of the same three frequencies. The audiometric results for this 68-year old woman reveal a hearing loss above 2 kHz. When the spectra derived from the single tone bursts are compared with the spectra from the multi-tone-burst complex, the results are almost identical. There was no response for stimuli in the 3-kHz region.

Etiology

Because of the link of TEOAEs with cochlear functioning and the strong evidence that outer hair cells probably play a significant role in their generation, it is reasonable to assume that TEOAEs could provide unique information about the etiology of a hearing loss. Apart from some interesting case studies, results from large samples of ears with SNHL to date have not been definitive. In addition, there is a strong influence of the configuration of the audiogram and the best threshold on the interpretation of results, regardless of the cause of the hearing loss. This has not always been taken into account when results have been interpreted from an etiological perspective.

In studies of large numbers of patients with SNHL due to various causes, no characteristic differences in results have been identified that would separate patients etiologically (Avan et al., 1991; Kemp et al., 1986; Probst & Harris, 1993b). There may be differences in results from ears with either sudden hearing loss (SHL) or progressive SNHL. Sakashita, Minowa, Hachikawa, Kubo and Nakai (1991) reported differences in findings for these two patient groups. Results from 42 patients with SHL were compared with results from 46 patients with SNHL of long duration. In roughly one half of the ears from a sample of 42 patients with average SHL worse than 35 dB HL, TEOAEs could be measured. Hearing recovered more often in ears that had OAEs than in those without TEOAEs. In 46 patients with SNHL of long duration, TEOAEs were not detected when average hearing levels exceeded 35 dB HL. Hoth and Bönnhoff (1993) measured TEOAEs serially in 25 patients with SHL. Recovery of TEOAE amplitudes corresponded with improvements in hearing threshold levels. Therefore, there is some evidence that the presence of TEOAEs and their rate of recovery following SHL could be diagnostically significant.

One group of patients that could be expected to have responses in the presence of significant hearing loss are persons with retrocochlear involvement. However, in patients with tumors of the cerebellopontine angle, TEOAEs are rarely present (Bonfils et al., 1988b; Robinette, Bauch, Olsen, Harner, & Beatty, 1992). Bonfils et al. (1988b) reported an incidence of 9% from tests on 28 patients; however, the magnitude of the hearing losses was not reported. In our experience, we have rarely seen a TEOAE when hearing loss at all frequencies from 0.5 to 8 kHz exceeded 30 dB HL. For those rare cases, the location of the tumor was a significant factor. However, it has not yet been established that such findings are diagnostically significant. Another group of patients that could have unexpected TEOAEs are those with central deafness. Bonfils et al. (1988b) measured 24 ears with central deafness, but the criteria for definition of this diagnosis were not provided. Results were the same for this group as for age-matched controls with normal hearing.

Because the putative cause for inner-ear problems experienced by patients with Ménière's disease is believed to involve mechanisms not primarily confined to outer hair cells, it might be expected that TEOAEs would be present despite a moderate to severe hearing loss. This has not been found. In a study of 31 patients with Ménière's disease, Harris and Probst (1992) determined that it was exceptional for an affected ear to have a TEOAE when no auditory thresholds were better than 25 dB HL (Figure 8–6). This investigation was prompted by the report of Bonfils et al. (1988b) that in 5 of 15 patients with MD who had average auditory thresholds greater than 40 dBHL, TEOAEs were present. However, specific information regarding threshold levels by frequency were not provided for these ears. Patients undergoing diagnostic tests with glycerol were also monitored using TEOAEs by Bonfils et al. (1988b). They determined that in 9 of 30 cases, EOAEs were observed after the administration of glycerol when they were not recordable before.

One factor that has been investigated extensively for its influence on TEOAEs is age. There is clearly a difference in TEOAE amplitudes from neonates when compared with adults. Within the adult population, evaluating the influence of age is complicated by the increased presence of hearing loss. Although it has been demonstrated that aging does influence the morphology of TEOAEs, when hearing loss is removed as a covariate, a strong influence of aging on the occurrence of TEOAEs is not present (Collet et al., 1992; Stover & Norton, 1993).

Involvement of the middle ear produces unique changes in the pattern of TEOAEs. Overall, responses decrease in amplitude and become dominated by high-frequency components (Hauser, Probst, & Harris, 1993).

TEOAE characteristics may provide specific information about subtle factors in the cochlea or could be important in differential diagnosis. However, results to date have not shown that tests of TEOAEs can provide specific additional information about the etiology of SNHL. Except in unusual cases, TEOAEs do not provide unique diagnostic information about the specific cochlear factors that have caused a sensorineural hearing loss.

Considerations

Some of the uncertainty in defining the association of TEOAEs and threshold levels arises from differences in the definition of terms. If one ranks only overall amplitude of a click-evoked response with a three-frequency pure-tone average, then a wrong judgment about the presence of residual hearing could be made. The spectrum of the TEOAE in relation to the noise in the measurement or its corresponding reproducibility analyzed into octave bands must be considered. Also, the entire audiometric configuration must be accounted for when comparing TEOAEs and hearing levels. The transient response is composed of components from multiple sources, and these interact in complex ways to provide a final result.

DPOAES

The general properties of distortion generated in the cochlea by bitonal stimulation have been investigated extensively using physiological, psychoacoustic, and acoustic methods in both experimental animals and human subjects. The cumulative results from these studies have provided strong evidence that DPOAE measurements have clinical relevance for the identification of hearing loss by frequency and for monitoring changes in the cochlea during exposure to ototoxic agents. Clinical testing of DPOAEs has developed relatively slowly for several reasons: DPOAEs are small in amplitude in most human ears; they must be measured with high-quality instrumentation and special signal-processing techniques to avoid contamination by artifacts and noise; high-amplitude DPOAEs are generated from a unique combination of stimuli that varies for each individual ear and has hindered the development of standard protocols. However, clinical methods that have overcome many of these limitations are now in use. This has made it possible to conduct large-scaled investigations of the relation of DPOAEs to the magnitude, configuration and etiology of hearing loss.

Stimuli and Parameters

The generation of DPOAEs is dependent on the characteristics of the bitonal stimuli that produce them. Therefore, several basic concepts related to clinical methodology are important: (a) which DPOAEs should be measured, (b) which stimulus frequencies should be selected for comparison with the pure-tone audiogram, (c) the optimal separation of the stimulus frequencies, (d) the selection of stimulus levels, and (e) the general protocols useful for clinical testing.

Although many distortion components arise from bitonal stimulation of the cochlea, the DPOAE at $2f_1 - f_2$ is the highest in amplitude and has been the most frequently measured for clinical purposes. The clinical relevance of other DPOAEs has not yet been determined. The $2f_1 - f_2$ DPOAE is generated in the cochlea where the stimulus tones, F_1 and F_2 interact. Therefore, a frequency corresponding to the cochlear site of this interaction should be used for comparison with audiometric frequencies rather than the DPOAE frequency itself. Reference frequencies for clinical investigations have been either F_2 or the geometric mean ($\sqrt{F_1F_2}$). The two tones must be close enough in frequency to interact within the cochlea, and a ratio of $F_2{:}F_1$ of 1.2:1 will produce high levels of $2f_1 - f_2$ in the majority of human ears.

The levels of the two stimuli must be selected carefully. When stimulus levels exceed 70 to 75 dB SPL, there is a high risk of encountering technical distortion in the instrumentation. This could lead to an invalid interpretation of test results. Additionally, high stimulus levels may be sampling more passive linear mechanisms in the cochlea that are less physiologically vulnerable to injury. Stimulus levels below approximately 60 dB SPL are more likely to be within the physiologically vulnerable range, but may not be of sufficient amplitude to produce distortion in all ears, especially those with peripheral cochlear damage. Reducing L_2 from 6 to 15 dB below an L_1 of 50 to 60 dB SPL is generally adequate to generate DPOAEs that are both detectable and vulnerable (Bonfils & Avan, 1992; Gaskill & Brown, 1990; Sutton, Lonsbury-Martin, Martin, & Whitehead, 1994).

The test protocols that are frequently used for clinical testing of DPOAEs are illustrated, along with the parameters that are extracted from them, in Figure 8–9. In the first protocol, the stimuli remain in a constant level ratio (L_1:L_2) and F_1 and F_2 are varied either separately or together over a range of frequencies. Amplitude of a response by frequency or the best F_2:F_1 for generating high-response levels is acquired from these sweeps. Because a series of discrete frequencies is sampled individually, the results have sometimes been called a "DP-audiogram". However, an audiogram is a behavioral test of a person's ability to detect the presence of a pure tone, and a DPOAE test is not a substitute for this method. Thus, less misleading terms, such as *DP-gram* or *DP-sweep*, are now used. In the second category, F_1 and F_2 are fixed in frequency and L_1 and L_2 are varied either together or separately. From these growth or input/output (I/O) functions, DPOAE amplitude for a specific stimulus level, slope, dynamic range, and threshold have been quantified. This type of protocol may provide more information about the cochlear response when the purpose of testing is diagnostic or monitoring. The clinical significance of latency and phase (Figure 8–9), when used in isolation, has not yet been identified. These protocols and stimulus combinations are typical of those now in use for clinical applications; however, they should not be regarded as standard methods for testing DPOAEs. Test methods are still undergoing considerable development and refinement. There is no standard method for testing DPOAEs. Protocols that are useful for clinical testing are still undergoing development. Because DPOAEs are sampled with discrete frequency stimuli, they have been evaluated primarily for their association with hearing levels by frequency rather than from a composite value that can be used for a general interpretation of the results.

Pure-Tone Results

The association of DPOAEs and pure-tone results has been determined by examining large groups of persons with different pure-tone threshold levels. Results from these investigations are summarized in Figure 8–10. DPOAEs are related in a complex manner to hearing thresholds. This is due to a combination of both methodological and physiological factors. DPOAEs for both high and low levels of stimulation are present across most frequencies at and above 1 kHz in 99 to 100% of ears (Bonfils & Avan, 1992; Gorga, Neely, Bergman, Beauchaine, Kaminski, Peters et al., 1993a; Harris, 1990; Hauser & Probst, 1990; Lonsbury-Martin, Harris, Stagner,

Parameters extracted from DPOAE test protocols

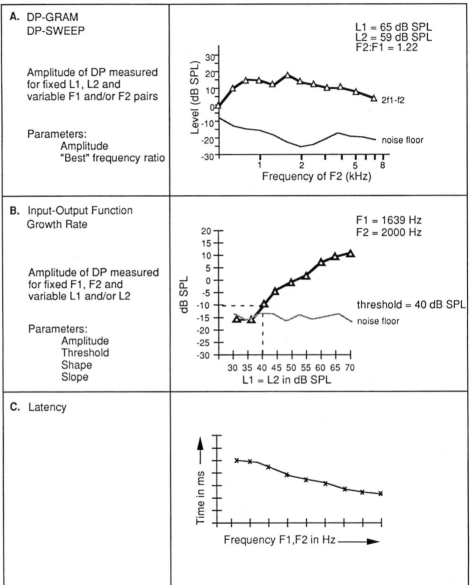

A. DP-GRAM
   DP-SWEEP

   Amplitude of DP measured
   for fixed L1, L2 and
   variable F1 and/or F2 pairs

   Parameters:
      Amplitude
      "Best" frequency ratio

L1 = 65 dB SPL
L2 = 59 dB SPL
F2:F1 = 1.22

Level (dB SPL) / Frequency of F2 (kHz)
2f1-f2
noise floor

B. Input-Output Function
   Growth Rate

   Amplitude of DP measured
   for fixed F1, F2 and
   variable L1 and/or L2

   Parameters:
      Amplitude
      Threshold
      Shape
      Slope

F1 = 1639 Hz
F2 = 2000 Hz

dB SPL / L1 = L2 in dB SPL
threshold = 40 dB SPL
noise floor

C. Latency

Time in ms / Frequency F1,F2 in Hz

Figure 8–9.   Protocols frequently used for clinical testing of DPOAEs and the parameters extracted from them.

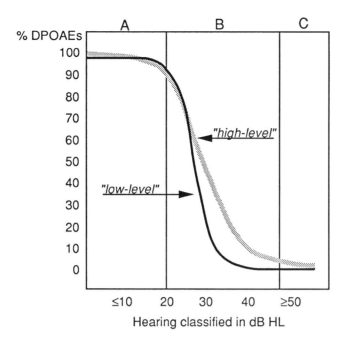

Figure 8–10. Schematic representation of the association of DPOAE presence and average pure-tone threshold levels compiled from reports in the literature. The two curves represent probabilities of obtaining a response for either low-level or high-level stimulation. When hearing is better than 25 dB HL, DPOAEs are routinely present for both high and low-level stimulation for the majority of audiometric frequencies from 1 to 6 kHz, as represented in *Section A*. Depending upon the stimulus parameters, it is possible to generate distortion even when hearing loss exceeds 50 dB HL, represented in the lower portion of the curve (*Section C*). The physiological significance of these DPOAEs in relation to hearing levels is uncertain. When low levels of stimulation are used, DPOAEs are not present above hearing levels of approximately 40 dB HL. The zone of uncertainty represented in *Section B* is wider than that identified for TEOAEs as illustrated in Figure 8–4. This uncertainty can make DPOAE outcomes more difficult to interpret than TEOAEs for purposes of identification of hearing loss.

& Hawkins, 1990; Smurzynski, Leonard, Kim, Lafreniere, & Jung, 1990; Smurzynski & Kim, 1992). For frequencies above 4 kHz, this percentage decreases when stimuli are below 65 dB SPL (Bonfils & Avan, 1992). Between 25 and 50 to 60 dB HL, DPOAE amplitudes are generally reduced or the responses are absent. Detectable DPOAEs may be present for pure-tone threshold levels as high as 50 to 60 dB HL, depending upon the stimulus levels used to produce them (Bonfils & Avan, 1992; Harris, 1990; Probst & Hauser, 1990). Therefore the zone of uncertainty is wider than represented for TEOAEs (Figure 8–4) and can pose problems when DPOAEs are used for screening purposes. Above 50 to 60 dB HL DPOAEs are absent for both high-level and low-level stimulation. Further refinement of these relations and of the frequency-specific correspondence of DPOAE features to hearing thresholds has been a major goal of clinical investigations.

Comparisons of audiometric configurations with DPOAE amplitudes from a DP-sweep paradigm or parameters from I/O functions have shown that there is a general correspondence of the two measures. In ears with SNHL, DPOAEs are generally reduced or eliminated only for the stimulus-frequency regions coincident with the impaired region (Gaskill & Brown, 1990; Harris, 1990; Martin, Ohlms, Franklin, Harris, & Lonsbury-Martin, 1990; Smurzynski et al., 1990). This is illustrated by the scatter plots in Figure 8–11 and Figure 8–12. Both figures are taken from studies of groups of subjects representing a range of pure-tone threshold levels across frequency. In a 1990 study by Harris (Figure 8–11), DPOAE amplitudes at 1 kHz were within the same range for ears in both groups, although all subjects in one group had hearing loss at frequencies above 1 kHz. At 4 kHz, the majority of ears with elevated thresholds had DPOAEs that were below the mean amplitudes − 2 standard deviations for the ears with normal hearing. However, several ears with thresholds of 50 to 60 dB HL had a DPOAE judged present, which illustrates the possibility of an uncertain finding (Figure 8–10). In Figure 8–12, results from a 1990 study by Probst and Hauser of 113 ears with either normal hearing or hearing loss are reproduced. The correlation of DPOAE amplitude and pure-tone threshold level was significant (n = 796, r = 0.52, p <.001). Yet, DPOAEs are still present in some ears when threshold levels exceed 60 dB HL. Therefore, despite the strong negative correlations of DPOAE amplitude and pure-tone threshold by frequency that have been reported by various investigators, DPOAEs cannot be used for precisely predicting hearing threshold levels. To determine if the predictive accu-

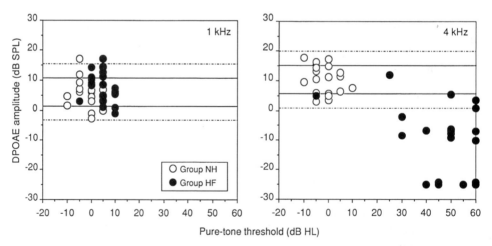

Figure 8–11. Maximum amplitude of DPOAEs generated in the 1 and 4-kHz regions in ears with and without hearing loss (*NH* = normal hearing; *HF* = hearing loss above 1 kHz, N = 20 for each group). The *solid lines* represent the mean ± 1 standard deviation (SD) of the results from Group NH and the broken lines represent ±2 SD. For the 1-kHz stimuli, results from the two groups overlap. At 4 kHz, the two groups differ from each other when thresholds exceed 25 dB HL. However, even with thresholds at 50 and 60 dB HL, DPOAEs falling within the ±2 SD boundaries could be detected. (Adapted with permission from Harris, 1990).

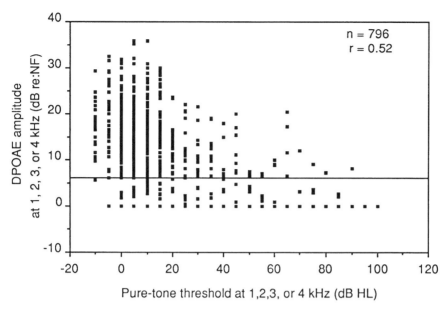

Figure 8–12. Amplitudes of DPOAEs from stimuli at 1, 2, 3, and 4 kHz (re: the geometric mean of F_1 and F_2) as a function of the hearing threshold levels at the same audiometric frequencies. The *horizontal line* indicates the 6-dB criterion that was used to define the presence of a DPOAE. The two parameters of threshold and DPOAE amplitude are correlated, but there are some outlying data points for hearing threshold levels above 60 dB HL. (Adapted from Probst & Hauser, 1990. Used with permission.)

racy of DPOAE measurements could be improved, investigators have explored the use of alternative parameters and analysis methods. These attempts have met with some success.

The threshold and slope of DPOAE growth functions are associated strongly with hearing threshold levels (Harris & Probst, 1991; Kimberley & Nelson, 1989; Martin et al., 1990). Kimberley and Nelson (1989) have suggested that DPOAE thresholds can predict auditory thresholds within 10 dB over a range from 0 to 60 dB SPL. However, threshold values are highly dependent upon the noise present during the measurement series from which they are derived (Whitehead, Lonsbury-Martin, & Martin, 1993b). Whitehead et al. have suggested that defining DPOAE threshold as the lowest stimulus level that elicits a DPOAE greater than a criterion absolute amplitude would be a means of using the threshold parameter without having it unduly influenced by the noise floor. The criterion amplitude would be determined from results of a group of typical subjects. Results from applying this strategy in practice have not been reported.

Bonfils and Avan (1992) developed a method for predicting hearing levels above or below 30 dB HL by analyzing features from a simplified growth series. First, growth functions are stimulated by $L_1 = L_2 = 42, 52, 62,$ and 72 dB SPL. The presence or absence of a response is then judged for stimuli at 52 dB SPL. If a response is present, then hearing is predicted to be better than 35 dB HL. If a response is absent, then the slope of the remaining function is measured. If it is less than or equal to 1, then hearing is judged to be better than 35 dB HL. Using this technique for evaluation of 75 ears representing a range of hearing levels, the sensitivity of the technique was found to be 93 to 100% depending upon the frequency of stimulation. The incidence of false negatives was less than 3% and false positives varied from 0 to 22% yielding good specificity. This is one example of how predictions of elevated hearing levels might be improved by using alternative methods of sampling and analyzing the responses.

Another means of improving the sensitivity and specificity of DPOAE testing is to use an alternative scheme for interpreting the results. For example, Gorga et al. (1993a) applied statistical decision theory to determine which DPOAE measures could best be used to predict hearing loss by frequency. They found in their sample of 180 subjects that hearing levels above and below 20 dB HL could be differentiated on the basis of DPOAE amplitude for specific stimulus frequencies. Best performance was observed for 4 kHz and poorest was for 0.5 kHz. The adverse effects of noise were especially apparent for stimulus frequencies below 2 kHz.

Clinical use of DPOAEs should be enhanced by improved understanding of their specific relation to auditory sensitivity and of the most effective methods of sampling this relation.

In the majority of ears with sensorineural hearing loss, DPOAEs produced by low-level stimuli are reduced in amplitude or are absent when pure-tone threshold levels exceed 25 dB HL. This occurs only for the affected frequency range. Differentiation of normal and impaired hearing using DPOAE amplitudes is better at 4 kHz than at other audiometric frequencies. Noise is a major interfering factor below 2 kHz.

Etiological Influence

Measurements of DPOAEs in persons or small samples of patients with Ménière's disease, SHL, acoustic neuroma, hereditary deafness, drug-induced ototoxicity, and noise-induced hearing loss have been described in the literature, primarily by Lonsbury-Martin and colleagues (Lonsbury-Martin, Whitehead, & Martin, 1991; Lonsbury-Martin, Whitehead, & Martin, 1993; Ohlms, Lonsbury-Martin, & Martin, 1991). The results from these studies are informative because they demonstrate how DPOAE findings can be used to identify processes known to have specific affects on the cochlea. However, definitive categorization of the causes of a hearing loss from DPOAE measurements alone has not been effective. One exception may be in patients affected by Ménière's disease. Ohlms et al. (1991), found that in 14 patients with Ménière's disease, two-thirds had DPOAE configurations that were compatible with their hearing loss and one-third had close to normal results, even in the presence of elevated hearing thresholds. They suggested that such variations could be used to differentiate the cochlear processes underlying progressive phases of the disease. A larger sample of patients in various stages of involvement would be needed to verify this hypothesis. Martin et al. (1990) reported increases in DPOAE amplitudes when patients were given glycerol for diagnostic purposes. This documented that DPOAE measurements may be a sensitive way to monitor changes in the cochlea, but responses must first be present for the method to be effective. This can be a problem when measuring patients with hearing loss.

It is known from studies with experimental animals that the adverse effects of certain ototoxic substances or high levels of noise are largely upon mechanisms in the cochlea that are also responsible for the generation of DPOAEs. Therefore, it is reasonable to expect that DPOAE measurements could be used to monitor changes in the human cochlea from exposure to similar processes. Results of large-scaled studies of persons being monitored with DPOAE measurements during treatment with ototoxic drugs are not yet available. However, case studies confirm that DPOAE amplitudes are affected during the course of such treatment (Ohlms et al., 1991). Results from studies of persons with noise-induced hearing loss are compatible with the general trends that were discussed in the previous section. That is, DPOAEs are affected adversely when hearing loss is present but only for the frequency range restricted to the loss (Harris, Probst, & Matéfi, 1994). Evidence concerning the sensitivity of DPOAEs to the direct effects of noise on the human cochlea is also available from the limited studies of temporary threshold shift (TTS). These results document that the amplitude of DPOAEs (generated by low-level stimuli ($L_1 = 55$ to 60, $L_2 = 30$–35 dB SPL) at frequencies one-half octave above an exposure frequency) decreases after tonal exposure and subsequently recovers after cessation of the exposure (Sutton et al., 1994). These results offer promise that monitoring DPOAEs in persons exposed to noise in the workplace or in the military may be beneficial.

As with TEOAEs, the condition of the middle ear is closely connected with adequate measurement of DPOAEs. Because responses are affected in a fairly predictable way by changes in the middle ear (Hauser et al., 1993), it may also be possible to use tests of DPOAEs as a probe for identifying middle ear problems.

DPOAE measurements may be used to monitor changes in the cochlea during exposure to ototoxic drugs or noise. However, a prerequisite is that responses must be present. This may be a limitation when measuring ears with hearing loss.

Comparison of TEOAEs and DPOAEs

Because TEOAEs and DPOAEs are related to hearing threshold levels, an interrelation of the two emission types would be expected. This has been demonstrated directly by investigations that have compared both DPOAEs and TEOAEs in the same ears (Avan & Bonfils, 1993; Gorga et al., 1993b; Lonsbury-Martin et al., 1991; Moulin et al., 1993; Probst & Harris, 1993a; Probst & Harris, 1993b; Smurzynski & Kim, 1992; Stover & Norton, 1993). In general, when one type of OAE is present, the other will be also. The overall levels of the two responses are correlated. An example of the strength of the correspondence of response amplitudes is illustrated by one study of 166 ears (Figure 8–13). The hearing threshold levels for the ears measured were widely distributed; however, the same high correspondence of response amplitudes also occurs in ears with threshold levels better than 20 dB HL. The presence of SOAEs is a significant contributory factor (Moulin et al., 1993). When selecting an OAE test for clinical purposes, factors such as the relative frequency specificity of TEOAEs and DPOAEs and the frequency range over which they can be tested effectively should be considered.

There is evidence that TEOAEs result from contributions that are distributed over a relatively large portion of the basilar membrane and that their detection and

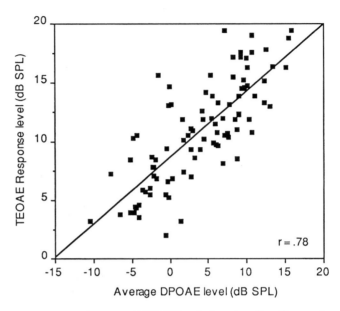

Figure 8–13. Comparison of average DPOAE levels for stimuli at discrete frequencies from 0.75 to 4 kHz with TEOAE response level in 166 ears with a range of hearing levels. A correlation coefficient of 0.78 demonstrated the close correspondence of the two measures. (With permission, Probst & Harris, 1993a).

frequency content are influenced by the status of the whole cochlea (Avan et al., 1991; Probst, Coats, Martin, & Lonsbury-Martin, 1986). By contrast, DPOAEs appear to arise from more localized sources (Avan & Bonfils, 1993). Therefore, when an overall impression of cochlear functioning is desired in a short period of time, such as for screening purposes, acquisition of a click-evoked response may be preferred over a series of DPOAEs. If the goal is to monitor changes in a specific frequency region, then DPOAEs should be considered.

There are differences in the frequency range over which TEOAEs and DPOAEs may be measured effectively. Click-evoked responses are dominated by components in the mid-frequency range, and they are effective in sampling cochlear functioning in that range. DPOAEs can be measured over a broad range of frequencies, but they are present in the high frequencies more often than are TEOAEs. Gorga et al. (1993a, 1993b) have determined that for the identification of hearing loss greater than 20 dB HL, both emissions perform well at 2 kHz, TEOAEs are better than DPOAEs at 1 kHz and DPOAEs are preferable at 4 kHz. Neither emission performs well at 0.5 kHz because the measurements are severely compromised by noise. If one emission type must be selected over another for clinical testing, then the purpose of the test should be considered. For the identification of hearing loss, TEOAEs may be preferable. The test is relatively quick and the zone of uncertainty is smaller than for DPOAEs. For monitoring purposes, DPOAEs may be preferable because they can be measured more easily in the high frequencies where ototoxic or noise-induced changes are more likely to occur.

There is a strong interrelationship between TEOAEs and DPOAEs in the same ear, but there are also differences between them. When only one type of OAE is to be chosen for a clinical evaluation, then the purpose of the testing should be a major factor in determining the selection.

Reporting TEOAE and DPOAE Results

Meaningful formats for reporting OAE test results are an essential part of their use for audiometric purposes. Reporting methods should facilitate interpretation of an individual result and permit comparison of results that have been obtained at different frequencies or with different methods. Several possibilities are available for achieving these aims.

One approach for evaluating an individual result is to compare it with a database composed of results from a representative group of persons with normal hearing (such as neonates or young adults). Statistical treatment of the database can be used to derive standard scores, such as percentiles, against which an individual result can be ranked. An example of how a click-evoked OAE can be evaluated in this way is illustrated in Figure 8–14. Some versions of commercial software now permit the formation of such databases for both TEOAEs and DPOAEs. One example of how an individual DPOAE outcome is ranked within specific percentile categories is illustrated in Figure 8–15. Gorga et al. (1993b) constructed cumulative distributions for DPOAEs at octave intervals from 0.5 to 8 kHz as an additional method for interpretation. From these, one could determine the associated hearing loss for a specified rate of DPOAE identification at any frequency. A primary advantage of converting test outcomes to standard scores is that results for more than one parameter or frequency can be compared directly.

As with many aspects of the clinical applications of OAEs, meaningful formats for reporting results are still being developed. At this time there is no standard method. As the specific relation of OAE parameters to hearing sensitivity is better understood, more effective means of reporting results will be developed.

Summary and Conclusions

SOAEs have limited clinical utility. If they are present, there is a high probability that at corresponding frequencies, hearing thresholds are better than 30 dB HL. However, there are rare instances in which a high-level SOAE can indicate cochlear pathology at the same frequency.

Otoacoustic emissions are linked strongly with normal hearing and are present in close to 100% of healthy ears. Complete absence of OAEs signals a high probability that there are no audiometric thresholds from 0.25 to 8 kHz better than 35 dB HL (TEOAE) or 60 dB HL (DPOAE, stimulated with high levels). Middle ear or retrocochlear factors must be considered in localizing such an outcome. For diagnostic purposes, the prediction of the magnitude of hearing loss by frequency using OAEs is problematic.

The selection of test method depends on the purpose of the test. Current methods of testing TEOAEs provide good information for the classification of hearing in the mid frequencies. Measures of DPOAEs best predict hearing loss at 4 kHz. Within each test, the choice of stimulus parameters is important.

There are similarities and differences in all stimulus-related OAEs from the same

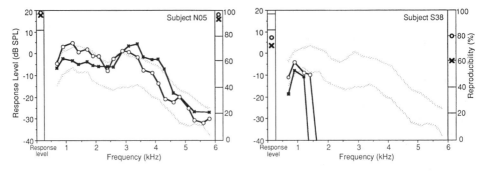

Figure 8–14. Demonstration of how the interpretation of an individual click-evoked response can be facilitated by plotting it against a database of results from ears with normal hearing. The shaded lines in the middle of the graph represent the 10th to 90th percentiles of the spectral distributions for results from 40 ears with normal hearing. The blocked region on the upper portion of the leftmost bar represents the 10th and 90th percentiles for overall response level. The results for Subject N05, who has bilateral hearing sensitivity better than 20 dB HL for all audiometric frequencies, fall well within the normal boundaries. Overall response levels, which are plotted on the leftmost bar are high and reproducibility, which is displayed on the rightmost bar, is above 90% for both ears. This subject has several spontaneous emissions in both ears. On the right graph, results for an individual with a bilateral high-frequency hearing loss above 1 kHz are displayed using the same percentile format. Overall response level is below the 10th percentile for both ears. However, note that reproducibility remains above 50% for both ears. This observation illustrates how reproducibility can be influenced strongly by energy within the mid-frequency range. (Adapted from Harris & Probst, 1991. Used with permission.)

ear. Both TEOAEs and DPOAEs are probably sampling elements of a common mechanism in the cochlea. Both of them will be influenced strongly by the presence of SOAEs, which can either add substantial energy to the responses or interfere with low-level DPOAEs at nearby frequencies. The status of the middle ear may also exert different influences on the reverse transmission of each OAE type.

Results should be analyzed, not only with respect to the overall outcome, but also with respect to specific frequency components. At present, there is no standardized method for reporting results. However, comparison of a test with a database acquired using a fixed set of stimulus parameters and controlled for age of the subjects is useful.

Researchers' understanding of the best methods for using OAEs clinically is still in the developmental stages. However, it is clear that OAE testing can be used effectively as part of a clinical test battery. A significant requirement for advancing the use of OAEs is the improvement of instrumentation. It is expected that in the future test equipment will be simpler to operate, be more portable, and have more stable probes and that calibration methods will be standardized—all of which will facilitate the acquisition of valid test results. Processing of the results will become more automated. Instrumentation that will be capable of combining several OAE tests with other clinical tests, such as immittance is likely to become available.

It is also essential that the direct relationship of OAEs to cochlear functioning be more firmly established for clinical use to develop further. The discussions in this

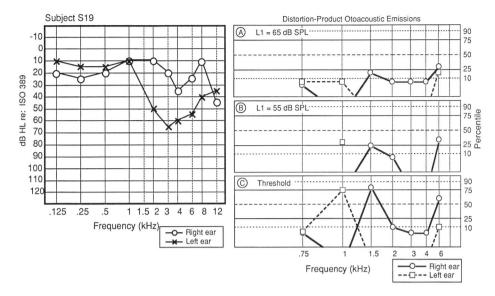

Figure 8–15. Example of a method for plotting DPOAE results against percentile distributions for a group of ears with audiometrically normal hearing. The horizontal solid and dashed lines on each graph represent the percentiles as shown. *Panel A* displays DPOAE results obtained with L1 = 65 dB SPL. Results for the left ear are below the 10th percentile for the lower frequencies and responses could not be measured from 1.5 to 4 kHz. Results in *Panel B* for L1 = 55 dB SPL indicate that a response was present only with stimuli at 1 kHz for the left ear. In *Panel C*, percentiles corresponding to DPOAE threshold are plotted. Results correspond closely with audiometric configuration except at 1 kHz for the right ear. This type of graphic representation not only facilitates interpretation of each individual test, but also permits comparisons across tests acquired using different parameters or analysis methods. (Adapted from Harris & Probst, 1991. Used with permission.)

chapter have been limited almost exclusively to pure-tone results. However, there are many other aspects of auditory function that can be sampled both subjectively and objectively. It may be that OAE results will relate more strongly to measures such as speech understanding ability, tuning, or other psychoacoustic phenomena rather than the detection task used for acquiring pure-tone thresholds in a typical clinical evaluation.

Acknowledgments

This work was supported in part by grant funds from the Swiss National Foundation Project Nr. 32-32348.91.

References

Avan, P., & Bonfils, P. (1993). Frequency specificity of human distortion product otoacoustic emissions. *Audiology, 32,* 12–26.

Avan, P., Bonfils, P., Loth, D., Narcy, P., & Trotoux, J. (1991). Quantitative assessment of human cochlear function by evoked otoacoustic emissions. *Hearing Research, 52,* 99–112.

Avan, P., Bonfils, P., Loth, D., Teyssou, M., & Menguy, C. (1993). Exploration of cochlear function by otoacoustic emissions: Relationship to pure-tone audiometry. In J. H. J. Allum, D. J. Allum-Mecklenburg, F. P. Harris, & R. Probst (Eds.), *Progress in brain research* (Vol. 97, pp. 67–75). Amsterdam: Elsevier Science.

Avan, P., Loth, D., Menguy, C., & Teyssou, M. (1991). Frequency dependence of changes in guinea-pig cochlear emissions after acoustic overstimulation. *Journal of the Acoustical Society of America, 4,* 91–94.

Bonfils, P. (1989). Spontaneous otoacoustic emissions: Clinical interest. *Laryngoscope, 99,* 752–756.

Bonfils, P., & Avan, P. (1992). Distortion-product otoacoustic emissions: Values for clinical use. *Archives of Otolaryngology—Head and Neck Surgery, 118,* 1069–1076.

Bonfils, P., Avan, P., François, M., Marie, P., Trotoux, J., & Narcy, P. (1990). Clinical significance of otoacoustic emissions: A perspective. *Ear and Hearing, 11,* 155–158.

Bonfils, P., Bertrand, Y., & Uziel, A. (1988a). Evoked otoacoustic emissions: Normative data and presbycusis. *Audiology, 27,* 27–35.

Bonfils, P., Uziel, A., & Pujol, R. (1988b). Evoked oto-acoustic emissions from adults and infants: Clinical applications. *Acta Oto-Laryngolica, 105,* 445–449.

Brass, D., & Kemp, D. T. (1993). Suppression of stimulus frequency otoacoustic emissions. *Journal of the Acoustical Society of America, 93,* 920–939.

Bray, P., & Kemp, D. T. (1987). An advanced cochlear echo technique suitable for infant screening. *British Journal of Audiology, 21,* 191–204.

Burns, E., Hoberg Arehart, K., & Campbell, S. L. (1992). Prevalence of spontaneous otoacoustic emissions in neonates. *Journal of the Acoustical Society of America, 91,* 1571–1575.

Clark, W. W., Kim, D. O., Zurek, P. M., & Bohne, B. A. (1984). Spontaneous otoacoustic emissions in chinchilla ear canals: Correlation with histopathology and suppression by external tones. *Hearing Research, 16,* 299–314.

Collet, L., Levy, V., Veuillet, E., Truy, E., & Morgon, A. (1993). Click-evoked otoacoustic emissions and hearing threshold in sensorineural hearing loss. *Ear and Hearing, 14,* 141–143.

Collet, L., Veuillet, E., Berger-Vachon, C., & Morgon, A. (1992). Evoked otoacoustic emissions: Relative importance of age, sex and sensorineural hearing-loss using a mathematical model of the audiogram. *International Journal of Neuroscience, 62,* 113–122.

Collet, L., Veuillet, E., Chanal, J. M., & Morgon, A. (1991). Evoked otoacoustic emissions: Correlates between spectrum analysis and audiogram. *Audiology, 30,* 164–172.

Gaskill, S. A., & Brown, A. M. (1990). The behavior of the acoustic distortion product, $2f_1 - f_2$, from the human ear and its relation to auditory sensitivity. *Journal of the Acoustical Society of America, 88,* 821–839.

Gorga, M. P., Neely, S. T., Bergman, B., Beauchaine, K. L., Kaminski, J. R., Peters, J., & Jesteadt, W. (1993a). Otoacoustic emissions from normal-hearing and hearing-impaired subjects: Distortion product responses. *Journal of the Acoustical Society of America, 93,* 2050–2060.

Gorga, M. P., Neely, S. T., Bergman, B. M., Beauchaine, K. L., Kaminski, J. R., Peters, J., Schulte, L., & Jesteadt, W. (1993b). A comparison of transient-evoked and distortion product emissions in normal-hearing and hearing-impaired subjects. *Journal of the Acoustical Society of America, 94,* 2639–2648.

Harris, F. P. (1990). Distortion-product otoacoustic emissions in humans with high frequency sensorineural hearing loss. *Journal of Speech and Hearing Research, 33,* 594–600.

Harris, F. P., & Probst, R. (1991). Reporting click-evoked and distortion-product otoacoustic emission results with respect to the pure-tone audiogram. *Ear and Hearing, 12,* 399–405.

Harris, F. P., & Probst, R. (1992). Transiently evoked otoacoustic emissions in patients with Meniere's disease. *Acta Oto-Laryngologica, 112,* 36–44.

Harris, F. P., Probst, R., & Matéfi, L. (1994, May). Testing distortion-product otoacoustic emissions in the Swiss Hearing Conservation Program (SUVA). Presented at *Effects of Noise on Hearing Vth International Symposium,* Gothenburg, Sweden.

Hauser, R., & Probst, R. (1990). The influence of systematic primary-tone level variation L2-L1 on the acoustic distortion product emission $2f_1 - f_2$ in normal human ears. *Journal of the Acoustical Society of America, 89,* 280–286.

Hauser, R., Probst, R., & Harris, F. P. (1991). (The clinical use of oto-acoustic emissions of cochlear distortion products) Die klinische Anwendung otoakustischer Emissionen kochleärer Distorsionsprodukte. *Laryngo-Rhino-Otologie, 70,* 123–131.

Hauser, R., Probst, R., & Harris, F. P. (1993). Effects of atmospheric pressure variation on spontaneous, transiently evoked, and distortion product otoacoustic emissions in normal human ears. *Hearing Research, 69,* 133–145.

Hauser, R., Probst, R., & Löhle, E. (1991). Click-and tone-burst-evoked otoacoustic emissions in normally hearing ears and in ears with high-frequency sensorineural hearing loss. *European Archives of Otorhinolaryngology, 248,* 345–352.

Hoth, S., & Bönnhoff, S. (1993). Application of evoked otoacoustic emissions for monitoring inner ear function. *HNO, 41*, 135–45.

Kemp, D. T. (1978). Stimulated acoustic emissions from within the human auditory system. *Journal of the Acoustical Society of America, 64*, 1386–1391.

Kemp, D. T., Bray, P., Alexander, L., & Brown, A. M. (1986). Acoustic emission cochleography-Practical aspects. *Scandinavian Audiology, 25* (Suppl.), 71–96.

Kimberley, B. P., & Nelson, D. A. (1989). Distortion product emissions and sensorineural hearing loss. *Journal of Otolaryngology, 18*, 365–369.

Kok, M. R., vanZanten, G. A., & Brocaar, M. P. (1993). Aspects of spontaneous otoacoustic emissions in healthy newborns. *Hearing Research, 69*, 115–123.

Lind, O., & Randa, J. (1989). Evoked acoustic emissions in high-frequency vs. low/medium-frequency hearing loss. *Scandinavian Audiology, 18*, 21–25.

Lonsbury-Martin, B. L., Harris, F. P., Stagner, B. B., & Hawkins, M. D. (1990). Distortion product emissions in humans. I. Basic properties in normally hearing subjects. *Annals of Otology, Rhinology, and Laryngology, 147* (Suppl.), 3–14.

Lonsbury-Martin, B. L., Whitehead, M. L., & Martin, G. K. (1991). Clinical applications of otoacoustic emissions. *Journal of Speech and Hearing Research, 34*, 964–981.

Lonsbury-Martin, B. L., Whitehead, M. L., & Martin, G. K. (1993). Distortion-product otoacoustic emissions in normal and impaired ears: insight into generation processes. In J. H. J. Allum, D. J. Allum-Mecklenburg, F. P. Harris, & R. Probst (Eds.), *Progress in brain research* (Vol. 97, pp. 77–90). Amsterdam: Elsevier Science.

Martin, G. K., Ohlms, L. A., Franklin, D. J., Harris, F. P., & Lonsbury-Martin, B. L. (1990). Distortion-product emissions in humans. III. Influence of sensorineural hearing loss. *Annals of Otolaryngology, Rhinology and Laryngology, 99*, 30–-42.

Mathis, A., De Min, N., & Arnold, W. (1991). Transient evoked otoacoustic emissions in ears with preserved hearing in high, low or middle frequency ranges. *HNO, 39*, 55–60.

Mathis, A., Probst, R., De Min, N., & Hauser, R. (1991). A child with an unusually high-level spontaneous otoacoustic emission. *Archives of Otolaryngology—Head and Neck Surgery, 117*, 674–676.

McFadden, D., & Mishra, R. (1993). On the relation between hearing sensitivity and otoacoustic emissions. *Hearing Research, 71*, 208–213.

Moulin, A., Collet, L., Delli, D., & Morgon, A. (1991). Spontaneous otoacoustic emissions and sensorineural hearing loss. *Acta Oto-Laryngologica, 111*, 835–841.

Moulin, A., Collet, L., Veuillet, E., & Morgon, A. (1993). Interrelations between transiently evoked otoacoustic emissions, spontaneous otoacoustic emissions and acoustic distortion products in normally hearing subjects. *Hearing Research, 65*, 216–233.

Norton, S. J., Mott, J. B., & Champlin, C. A. (1989). Behavior of spontaneous otoacoustic emissions following intense ipsilateral acoustic stimulation. *Hearing Research, 38*, 243–258.

Norton, S. J., & Neely, S. T. (1987). Tone-burst-evoked otoacoustic emissions from normal-hearing subjects. *Journal of the Acoustical Society of America, 81*, 1860–1872.

Ohlms, L. A., Lonsbury-Martin, B. L., & Martin, G. K. (1991). Acoustic-distortion products: Separation of sensory from neural dysfunction in sensorineural hearing loss in human beings and rabbits. *Otolaryngology—Head and Neck Surgery, 104*, 159–174.

Penner, M. J., Glotzbach, L., & Huang, T. (1993). Spontaneous otoacoustic emissions: Measurement and data. *Hearing Research, 68*, 229–237.

Prieve, B. A., Gorga, M. P., Schmidt, A., Neely, S., Peters, J., Schulte, L., & Jesteadt, W. (1993). Analysis of transient-evoked otoacoustic emissions in normal-hearing and hearing-impaired ears. *Journal of the Acoustical Society of America, 93*, 3308–3319.

Probst, R., Coats, A. C., Martin, G. K., & Lonsbury-Martin, B. L. (1986). Spontaneous, click-, and toneburst-evoked otoacoustic emissions from normal ears. *Journal of the Acoustical Society of America, 21*, 261–276.

Probst, R., & Harris, F. P. (1993a). A comparison of transiently evoked and distortion-product otoacoustic emissions in humans. In J. H. J. Allum, D. J. Allum-Mecklenburg, F. P. Harris, & R. Probst (Eds.), *Progress in brain research* (Vol. 97, pp. 91–99). Amsterdam: Elsevier Science.

Probst, R., & Harris, F. P. (1993b). Transiently evoked and distortion-product otoacoustic emissions. Comparison of results from normally hearing and hearing-impaired human ears. *Archives of Otolaryngology—Head and Neck Surgery, 119*, 858–860.

Probst, R., & Hauser, R. (1990). Distortion product otoacoustic emissions in normal and hearing-impaired ears. *American Journal of Otolaryngology, 11*, 236–243.

Probst, R., Lonsbury-Martin, B. L., & Martin, G. K. (1991). A review of otoacoustic emissions. *Journal of the Acoustical Society of America, 89*, 2027–2067.

Probst, R., Lonsbury-Martin, B. L., Martin, G. K., & Coats, A. C. (1987). Otoacoustic emissions in ears with hearing loss. *American Journal of Otolaryngology, 8*, 73–81.

Robinette, M. S. (November, 1990). Frequency specificity of click evoked otoacoustic emissions for sensorineural hearing loss. Presentation to the American Speech-Language-Hearing Association.

Robinette, M. S. (1992). Clinical observations with transient evoked otoacoustic emissions with adults. *Seminars in Hearing, 13,* 23–36.

Robinette, M. S., Bauch, C. D., Olsen, W. O., Harner, S. G., & Beatty, C. W. (1992). Use of TEOAE, ABR, and Acoustic Reflex measures to assess auditory function patients with acoustic neuroma. *American Journal of Audiology,* 66–72.

Ruggero, M. A., Kramek, B., & Rich, N. C. (1984). Spontaneous otoacoustic emissions in a dog. *Hearing Research, 13,* 293–296.

Sakashita, T., Minowa, Y., Hachikawa, K., Kubo, T., & Nakai, Y. (1991). Evoked otoacoustic emissions from ears with idiopathic sudden deafness. *Acta Oto-Laryngologica, 486* (Suppl.), 66–72.

Smurzynski, J., & Kim, D. O. (1992). Distortion-product and click-evoked otoacoustic emissions of normally-hearing adults. *Hearing Research, 58,* 227–240.

Smurzynski, J., Leonard, G., Kim, D. O., Lafreniere, D. C., & Jung, M. D. (1990). Distortion product otoacoustic emissions in normal and impaired adult ears. *Archives of Otolaryngology—Head and Neck Surgery, 116,* 1309–1316.

Stevens, J. C., & Ip, C. B. (1988). Click-evoked oto-acoustic emissions in normal and hearing-impaired adults. *British Journal of Audiology, 22,* 45–49.

Stover, L., & Norton, S. J. (1993). The effects of aging on otoacoustic emissions. *Journal of the Acoustical Society of America, 94,* 2670–2681.

Sutton, L. A., Lonsbury-Martin, B. L., Martin, G. K., & Whitehead, M. L. (1994). Sensitivity of distortion-product emissions in humans to tonal over-exposure: Effects of L1-L2 differences. *Abstracts of the Association for Research in Otolaryngology* (p. 46). St. Petersburg Beach, FL: ARO.

Takeda, T., & Saito, H. (1991). 100 Hz Narrow-band evoked otoacoustic emissions from ears with sudden deafness. In *Abstracts International Symposium on Otoacoustic Emissions* (pp. 23). Kansas City.

Talmadge, C. L., Long, G. R., Murphy, W. J., & Tubin, A. (1993). New off-line method for detecting spontaneous otoacoustic emissions in humans subjects. *Hearing Research, 71,* 170–182.

Talmadge, C. L., Tubis, A., Wit, H. P., & Long, G. R. (1991). Are spontaneous otoacoustic emissions generated by self-sustained cochlear oscillators? *Journal of the Acoustical Society of America, 89,* 2391–2399.

van Dijk, P., & Wit, H. P. (1990). Amplitude and frequency fluctuations of spontaneous otoacoustic emissions. *Journal of the Acoustical Society of America, 88,* 1779–1793.

Welzl-Müller, K., & Stephan, K. (1994). Confirmation of transiently evoked otoacoustic emissions based on user-independent criteria. *Audiology, 33,* 28–36.

Wen, H., Berlin, C., Hood, L., Jackson, D., & Hurley, A. (1993). A program for quantification and analysis of transient evoked otoacoustic emissions. In *Abstracts of the Association for Research in Otolaryngology,* (p. 102). St. Petersburg Beach, FL: ARO.

Whitehead, M. L., Kamal, N., Lonsbury-Martin, B. L., & Martin, G. K. (1993a). Spontaneous otoacoustic emissions in different racial groups. *Scandinavian Audiology, 22,* 3–10.

Whitehead, M. L., Lonsbury-Martin, B. L., & Martin, G. K. (1993b). The influence of noise on the measured amplitudes of distortion-product otoacoustic emissions. *Journal of Speech and Hearing Research, 36,* 1097–1102.

Whitehead, M. L., McCoy, M. J., Martin, G. K., & Lonsbury-Martin, B. L. (1993c). Click-evoked and distortion-product otoacoustic emissions in adults: Detection of high-frequency sensorineural hearing loss. In *Association of Research in Otolaryngology* (pp. 100).

Xu, L., Probst, R., Harris, F. P., & Roede, J. (1994). Peripheral analysis of frequency in human ears revealed by tone burst evoked otoacoustic emissions. *Hearing Research, 74,* 173–180.

9

Distortion Product Emissions and Sensorineural Hearing Loss

Barry P. Kimberley
David K. Brown
Jont B. Allen

Introduction

Within the realm of the tools now available to the audiologist to assess the peripheral auditory system, evoked otoacoustic emissions (EOAEs) are emerging as being among the fastest and simplest means of detecting cochlear functioning. Attempts to relate otoacoustic emissions (OAEs) and hearing loss were first made with transiently evoked otoacoustic emissions (TEOAEs). Reasonable correlation was found between crude measures of hearing function and TEOAE data (Bonfils, Piron, Uziel, & Pujol, 1988; Kemp, 1978; Probst, Lonsbury-Martin, Martin, & Coats, 1987). More recent reports have indicated that TEOAE measures may also be able to predict frequency-specific hearing ability (Prieve et al., 1993).

The application of distortion product emissions (DPOAEs) to the prediction of hearing status was investigated subsequent to the initial TEOAE work (Allen & Levitt, 1992; Avan & Bonfils 1993; Gaskill & Brown 1993; Gorga et al., 1993; Harris & Glattke, 1988; Kimberley & Nelson, 1989; Martin, Ohlm, Franklin, Harris, & Lonsbury-Martin, 1990; Nelson & Kimberley, 1992). DPOAEs were regarded as particularly attractive because of their inherent frequency specificity. There arose the idea that DPOAEs could be used to predict hearing thresholds for narrow frequency ranges. Early reports found moderately good correlation between DPOAE amplitude and pure-tone threshold in individual cases of cochlear hearing deficit (Lonsbury-Martin & Martin, 1990; Lonsbury-Martin, McCoy, Whitehead & Martin, 1993; Martin, et al., 1990). This paradigm was then extended by combining several DPOAE and demographic features and then comparing this hybrid measure with pure-tone threshold (Kimberley, Hernadi, Lee, & Brown, 1994; Kimberley, Kimberley, & Roth, 1994) for a whole population of both normal and cochlear-impaired ears. For carefully selected cases of cochlear hearing loss, these classification and prediction schemes could achieve approximately 85% correct prediction of normal versus abnormal pure-tone threshold.

One may challenge outright the idea that DPOAEs have a correlation with pure-tone threshold. There is no doubt of the relation between DPOAEs and outer hair-cell physiology. Disrupting the function of the outer hair cells temporarily causes transient changes to the DPOAE; permanent damage translates into irreversible frequency-specific damage. Researchers understand that normal functioning outer hair cells are necessary for normal behavioral thresholds; however there is no physiological evidence that supports the expectation that normal DPOAEs can predict pure-tone thresholds directly. Researchers view the outer hair cells role in sound transduction as one of compressing the large dynamic range of input levels for the limited response range of the inner hair cells. Based on this understanding one could argue that outer hair cell dysfunction and altered DPOAE measures would correlate with recruitment rather than pure-tone threshold (Allen, 1995). Nevertheless, there is enough physiological and empirical data for the pursual of the quantitative relation between DPOAEs and pure-tone thresholds further.

The ability of current DPOAE data to predict pure-tone threshold is not yet robust enough to be clinically useful. Fortunately, it appears that there are various ways in which the DPOAE recording and interpretation can still be improved. At the same time, it is apparent that there are distinct limitations in the DPOAE methodology. For example, it is possible to obtain DPOAE recordings in ears with hearing thresholds as high as 30 dB SPL; the case of isolated neural loss with a normal cochlea (and normal DPOAEs) is a confounding factor in the correlation between DPOAEs and pure-tone thresholds. Additional tests, such as pure-tone audiometry and auditory brain stem responses, can be used to help distinguish neural from sensory losses. Transmission impairments caused by middle ear pathology, such as fluid, can abolish a DPOAE response despite a normally functioning cochlea. Combining middle-ear–impedance measures (reflectance) with DPOAEs may be able to reliably identify emissions weakened by middle-ear problems. Another difficulty in relating pure-tone thresholds and DPOAEs is the existence of ripples in both pure-tone threshold and DPOAE amplitude. This rippling phenomenon, obtained when amplitude or threshold measurements are taken at multiple closely-spaced frequencies, is also known as *auditory microstructure*. To maximize the clinical potential of DPOAEs, current methods need to be improved to better deal with a variety of phenomena such as (a) middle ear transmission problems, (b) isolated neural impairment with a normal cochlea, (c) DPOAE measurement contamination by noise artifact, and (d) confounding DPOAE amplitude microstructure. Ultimately, the noise immunity of a DPOAE measurement algorithm is possibly the most important factor in terms of clinical application.

DPOAE Generation and Normative Data

When using DPOAEs to distinguish individuals with normal hearing from those with hearing losses, one must first define what constitutes a normal emission. Variables that effect the emission, especially in terms of its amplitude, need to be considered in order to make this determination. The absolute amplitude of the emission depends mostly on stimulus recording parameters (Gaskill & Brown, 1990) and hearing threshold (Nelson & Kimberley, 1992). Other investigators (Brown, Sheppard, & Russell, 1994; Lafreniere, Jung, Smurzynski, Leonard, Kim, & Sasek, 1991) have reported that subject age also influenced emission amplitude. It has been common to relate the amplitude of the DPOAE to the mean amplitude ($\pm$ 1 standard deviation [SD]) from a population of normal hearing young adults. Norms should be developed for DPOAE screening in order to determine if the emission is within the range of normal amplitude for that age.

Distortion product emissions are generated by stimulating the cochlea with two tones at frequencies f_1 and f_2 ($f_2 < f_1$); this, in turn, generates the cubic distortion product (DP) at $2f_1 - f_2$ which can be recorded in the ear canal (Figure 9–1). The DPOAE is generated in the frequency region of the basilar membrane (BM) corresponding to the interaction or overlap of the stimulus tones, that is f_1 and f_2 (Furst, Rabinowitz, & Zurek, 1988). The site that makes the most significant contribution to the generation of the DPOAE is controversial, and two possible locations are described in the literature. These are the f_2 place (Brown & Gaskill, 1990; Brown, Gaskill & Williams, 1992; Brown and Kemp, 1984; Fahey and Allen, 1986; Furst et al., 1988; Kimberley, Brown, & Eggermont, 1993; Matthews & Molnar, 1986) and the geometric mean of f_1 and f_2 (Lonsbury-Martin, Whitehead, & Martin, 1991; Martin, Lonsbury-Martin, Probst, Scheinin, & Coats, 1987; Popelka, Karzon, & Arjmand, 1995; Whitehead, Stagner, Lonsbury-Martin, & Martin, 1994). The geometric mean of the primary-tone (or stimulus) frequencies is calculated using $f_1 \times f_2 \times 0.5$. For example, the geometric mean of $f_1 = 1000$ and $f_2 = 1200$ Hz would be 1095.445 Hz and for $f_1 = 10000$ and $f_2 = 12000$ Hz would equal 10954.45 Hz. The difference in frequency between the geometric mean and the f_2 place is 104.555 and 1045.55 Hz,

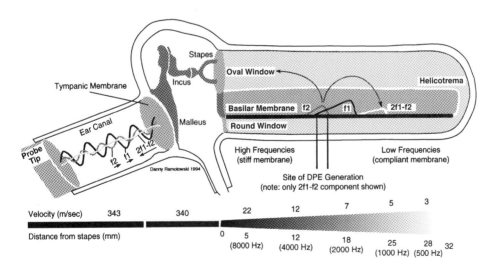

Figure 9–1. The human cochlea "unraveled", showing the generation of a distortion product emission. Lower diagram shows the velocity of sound through the external and middle ear, and the velocity of the traveling wave along the basilar membrane. (From Gould & Sobhy, 1992. Used with permission.)

respectively. This difference is small especially when compared with the audiometric range of frequencies that are typically tested (e.g., 0.25–8 kHz).

The use of f_1, f_2 or the geometric mean of the primaries to compare the frequency of the behavioural threshold is of little consequence when testing an ear with normal hearing. This is because the primaries reach maximum BM displacement over a small frequency range. However, if a loss affects the f_2 frequency and not the f_1 frequency, the behavioural threshold for f_1 will not be affected, but the DPOAE will be affected because of damage in the region of generation (Gaskill & Brown, 1993). DPOAEs are detectable at frequency regions where hearing is normal but are not present for low-level stimuli when behavioural hearing threshold levels are above 15 to 20 dB (Gaskill & Brown, 1993).

Effect of Stimulus Levels on DPOAE Amplitude

Amplitude of the DPOAE is affected by the parameters used to evoke it. The DPOAE is generated by a pair of stimulating tones, f_1 and f_2. The resulting emission is dependent on the intensity, frequency separation or ratio, and level difference between the tones. The level of the primaries influences the amplitude of the emission for normal hearing individuals. In a growth curve, the emission gradually exceeds the noise floor as the intensity of the primary tones increases (Figure 9–2). The stimulus increases from 20 to 60 dB, but emissions at the lowest intensity levels are difficult to distinguish from the noise floor. At high intensity levels, emissions grow to 20 to 30 dB above the noise floor. Figure 9–2 also illustrates

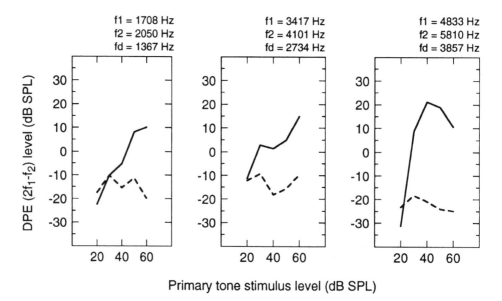

Figure 9–2. DPOAE growth function curves for three different frequencies from a two day old infant. Note that the dip in the growth function curve at $f_2 = 4101$ Hz and the roll-over at $f_2 = 5810$.

some of the different shapes or types of DPOAE growth curves as suggested by Nelson and Kimberley (1992) and Popelka et al. (1995).

A qualitative appreciation for the relation between pure-tone threshold and DPOAE level can be obtained from Figure 9–3.

The intensity of the stimulus used to generate the DPOAE may be low (f < 60–70 dB SPL) or high (<60–70 dB SPL) and result in emissions with categorically

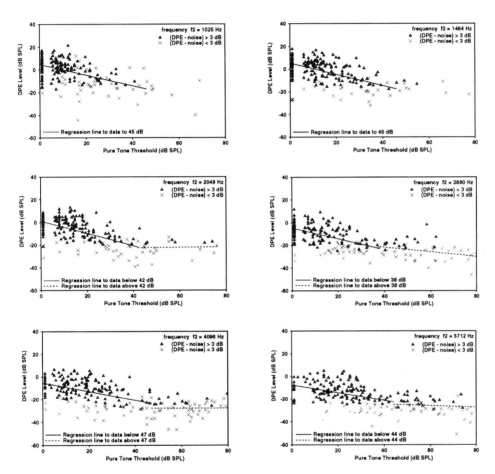

Figure 9–3. Data from 229 ears are presented for six frequencies in scatter plots of DPOAE amplitude versus pure-tone threshold. DPOAE amplitude was measured with L1 = 60 dB SPL and L2 =50 dB SPL. A piece-wise linear regression line was fitted to datapoints both above and below a predetermined pure-tone threshold value. The regression line shows that there is a weak negative correlation between DPOAE amplitude and pure-tone threshold for thresholds less than about 40 dB SPL. The r2 values varied from 0.16 to 0.38, suggesting that DPOAE amplitude alone accounted for only a small amount of the variance associated with changes in pure-tone threshold. For thresholds above 40 dB SPL the mean DPOAE levels become indistinguishable from noise floor levels and are no longer affected by pure-tone threshold.

different features. The DPOAEs elicited from low stimulus levels are dominated by active cochlear mechanical processes, whereas the high stimulus level DPOAEs may be dominated by passive cochlear mechanics (Whitehead, Lonsbury-Martin, & Martin, 1990, 1992a, 1992b). The amplitude of the DPOAEs evoked by low stimulus levels (62 dB SPL) were found to be strongly correlated with the auditory threshold at their geometric mean frequency. Avan and Bonfils (1993) also suggested that the low stimulus level therefore would provide frequency-specific information on the local cochlear state. They also reported that DPOAEs elicited from high stimulus levels (72 dB SPL) are not as sensitive to a decrease in hearing threshold, possibly owing to a broadening of the cochlear tuning.

In addition to the overall level of the primary tone stimuli, the level difference between the two primary tones can affect the DPOAE. The intensity of the two primary tones, L1 and L2, that produced the maximum DPOAE amplitude is dependent on L1, where L1 is the intensity of f_1 and L2 is the intensity of f_2 (Gaskill & Brown, 1990; Whitehead, McCoy, Lonsbury-Martin, & Martin, 1995a, Whitehead, Stagner, McCoy, Lonsbury-Martin, & Martin, 1995b). For high stimulus levels, the maximum DPOAE amplitude was generated when L1 equaled L2 (Rasmussen, Popelka, Osterhammel, & Nelson,1993; Whitehead et al., 1995b;). For low stimulus levels, the optimum level was L1 greater than L2 by 15 dB (Gaskill and Brown, 1990; Whitehead, Lonsbury-Martin, & Martin, 1993). The increase in DPOAE amplitude gained by decreasing the level of L2 was small (i.e., > 3.5 dB at most frequencies) (Whitehead et al., 1995a, 1995b). However, Hauser and Probst (1991) reported that setting L1 greater than L2 could improve the signal-to-noise ratio of the DPOAE and therefore enhance the detectability of the DPOAE.

DPOAE amplitude is also influenced by the ratio (f_2/f_1) of the primary tones. In an early study, Wilson (1980) found maximum DPOAE amplitudes at f_2/f_1 ratios of 1.1 to 1.2. Since then, optimum f_2/f_1 ratios have been studied by others and an f_2/f_1 ratio of approximately 1 to 2 was found (Table 9–1). There is good agreement between these optimum ratios even though they were determined over different frequency ranges and with different methods. Harris, Lonsbury-Martin, Stagner, Coats and Martin (1989) reported that the most effective f_2/f_1 ratio was 1 to 22. However, they also reported an inverse relation between optimal f_2/f_1 ratio and the frequency of the DPOAE. The optimal ratio for low frequency emissions was larger than for high frequency emissions (Figure 9–4). The optimal f_2/f_1 ratio also changes as a function of the intensity of the primary tones. As the intensity of the primary

Table 9–1.   Optimum f_1f_2 Ratios That Generate Maximum DPOAE Amplitudes

Study	Optimum Ratio
Kemp and Brown (1983)	1.25
Harris et al. (1989)	1.22
Gaskill & Brown (1990)	1.225
Bonfils et al. (1991)	1.22
Nielsen et al. (1993)	1.23

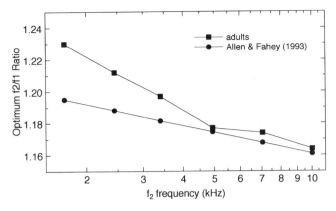

Figure 9–4. f_2/f_1 ratios used to generate maximum DPOAE ($2f_1 - f_2$) amplitudes for different f_2 frequencies. The curve with circle markers is derived from a model by Allen and Fahey (1993).

tones increases, the f_2/f_1 ratio used to elicit maximal DPOAE amplitude also increases (Harris et al., 1989).

Effect of Noise on DPOAE Detection

Another factor that can affect the measurement of an emission is the amplitude of the noise floor. The *noise floor* is defined as the amplitude of background noise that occurs at or near the test frequency at the time of recording. The emission is said to be present if its amplitude is greater than that of the noise floor. The absolute noise floor is governed by noise inherent in the microphone; some microphones, such as the Etymotic Research ER-10C, have a noise floor of -20 dB SPL.

The ease of measuring a DPOAE depends on the noise floor and the sensitivity of the equipment used to measure it (Probst, 1990). One method for estimating the noise floor measures approximately 50, 100, and 150 Hz above and below the $2f_1\text{-}f_2$ frequency. These are averaged together for the duration of testing to yield the noise floor for that DPOAE frequency (Etymotics Research, 1992). Other methods of obtaining noise floor measurements have been reported. These vary from measuring the amplitude of the signal 20 Hz below the DPOAE frequency (Lonsbury-Martin, Harris, Stagner, Hawkins, & Martin, 1990) to estimating the noise floor by averaging eight frequencies below and eight frequencies above the DPOAE frequency (Whitehead et al., 1994). The number of frequencies (or bins from the fast Fourier transform [FFT]) used to estimate the noise floor will affect the variability of the estimate. An increase in the number of frequencies will decrease the variability in the noise floor estimate. The method used to determine the noise floor will influence whether the amplitude of an emission was greater than the noise floor estimate. If the noise floor estimate is too high, a true DPOAE will be obscured by an overestimation of the background noise and thus an emission will not be reported when it was truly present (i.e., a false-negative).

Once the noise floor has been estimated, the next consideration is to determine if a DPOAE is actually present or not. Again, a DPOAE is present if the amplitude of the emission is greater than the estimate of the background noise. The amplitude difference between the noise floor and the emission will determine the false-positive rate (i.e., the reporting of an emission as present when it is not). Differences of as little as 3 dB (Lonsbury-Martin et al., 1990; Smurzynski, 1994) and as much as 11 dB (Popelka et al., 1995) have been suggested. The amplitude difference chosen as the cut-off for an emission to be present is important for the determination of the probability of a false-positive or conversely a false-negative. The number of frequencies chosen to estimate the noise floor will influence the variance and therefore the amplitude difference required to determine if a DPOAE is present. The probability of reporting a false-positive decreases as the amplitude difference between the estimate of the noise floor and the DPOAE increases (Figure 9–5) (Shaw, 1994). If a DPOAE amplitude of 3 dB above the noise floor was used then the probability of saying a DPOAE is present when it is not would be approximately 18%. Increasing the difference between the DPOAE amplitude and the noise floor to 12 dB decreases the probability to approximately zero. Both of these choices have problems: 3 dB allows for too many false-positives, and 12 dB will allow too many false-negatives. Based on the CUBeDIS algorithm (Etymotic Research, 1992), an amplitude of 6 dB above the noise floor will allow for a 5% probability of falsely detecting a emission.

Most adult DPOAE testing occurs in a sound-treated room, where the background noise is minimal and the subjects are cooperative. Testing in such a location yields low noise floor measurements. However, most newborn testing is done in a

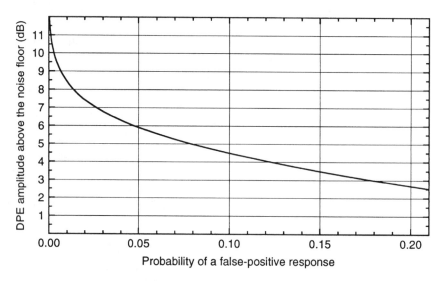

Figure 9–5.   The probability of concluding that a DPOAE is present when it is actually not is determined by the amplitude of the emission above the noise floor. This diagram is based on a six frequency model of noise level calculation with three frequencies above and three frequencies below the $2f_1 - f_2$ frequency.

nursery which will increase the noise floor especially in the low frequencies. Popelka et al. (1995) reported that neonates can add 15 to 30 dB of noise to the noise floor which makes it even more difficult to determine whether or not an emission is present.

Using the DPOAE phase delay is another possible way of determining the presence or absence of a DPOAE at a specific frequency. This approach may prove useful, but has not been extensively pursued to date. Each DPOAE amplitude measurement contains phase information that, given the periodic nature of the DPOAE stimuli and emission, can be used to determine traveling wave delay. This delay is the length of time taken for the stimulus signal to generate the traveling wave that initiates the otoacoustic emission. Thus, phase information can be used to estimate traveling wave delay (TWD) or traveling wave velocity (Figure 9–1) in the cochlea. The delay of the cochlear traveling wave reflects the basic mechanical operation of the organ of Corti. To generate TWD estimates, a number of closely-spaced DPOAE frequencies, related by f_2 frequency, are plotted against the associated DPOAE phase. For normal ears, this relation is linear. This linearity is maintained for some points whose DPOAE amplitude is buried in noise. As long as a few frequencies of the closely-spaced DPOAE measurements are above their noise estimates, the presence or absence of the remaining points may be inferred by the linearity of their phase values to the other points. Phase values which are off this line are likely not present, regardless of the ambient noise.

Traveling wave delay decreases with increasing frequency (Figure 9–6). The linearity of the effect with the logarithm of frequency implies an exponential rela-

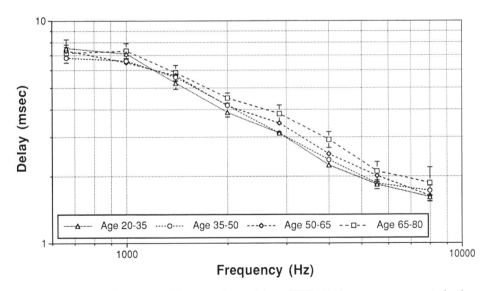

Figure 9–6. Traveling wave delay as estimated from DPOAE phase measurements for four age groups (20–35, $n = 15$; 35–50; $n = 28$; 50–65, $n = 30$, 65–80, $n = 18$). DPOAEs were obtained from ears with pure-tone thresholds ranging from 0 to 40 dB SPL. Error bars are 1 standard error of the mean and are not shown if obscured by their point marker.

tion. There also is a small, but significant effect of age; traveling wave delay apparently increases with age. This suggests an age-dependent change in the mechanics of the basilar membrane, possibly a reduction in the overall stiffness of the membrane.

Effect of Age on DPOAE Amplitude

It has been shown that DPOAE level can distinguish normal and abnormal pure-tone threshold in a large population of adults with varying cochlear losses (Kimberley, Nelson, 1989; Nelson, Kimberley, 1992). However, age likely has a significant effect on DPOAE level (Kimberley, et al., 1994a; Kimberley et al., 1994b; Lonsbury-Martin, Cutler, & Martin, 1991; Nelson & Kimberley, 1992; Stover & Norton, 1994). Specifically, DPOAE levels appear to decrease with age in a manner that is independent of pure-tone threshold. It would thus seem necessary to adjust a prediction scheme based upon DPOAE level according to subject age.

The influence of the aging process on 30 to 60 year olds was investigated by Lonsbury-Martin et al. (1991) who reported that DPOAE amplitude decreased and detection threshold increased with age. Audiometric testing confirmed previous findings in that auditory acuity decreases with age and also with increasing frequency of the test stimuli. Growth curves or input/output functions hold the frequency constant and systematically increase the level of the primaries. The resulting growth curve showed that the oldest ears tended to generate the smallest DPOAEs, especially in the higher frequencies. Differences in absolute amplitude have also been noted when comparing infant data to adult data (Brown et al., 1994; Lafreniere et al., 1991). Whitehead et al. (1994b) have reported that DPOAEs are approximately 3 dB greater in amplitude for infants than for adults. Absolute amplitude of the emission is greater in newborns than in adults (Figure 9–7). The mean absolute amplitudes from adults with normal thresholds indicate that there was a decrease in emission amplitude for the high frequencies with age. However, DPOAEs in the low frequencies were similar across age groups from 18 to 64 years.

The association between DPOAE level and age for ears with normal pure-tone thresholds is illustrated in Figure 9–8, where a weak inverse relation appears to exist over the entire age range. This finding supports the notion that age may be of value in pure-tone threshold prediction and, more generally, that the two are related. One way to deal with the effect of age is to use age-specific normative DPOAE amplitude data to classify DPOAEs. Another method for differentiating between normal and abnormal pure-tone thresholds could be based on a formula that has both DPOAE level and age as weighted variables. Discriminant and neural network analysis are two techniques which can be used to determine optimal weights for dependent variables such as age and DPOAE level.

Empirical Evidence for a Correlation between DPOAES and Pure-Tone Thresholds

Finding a general relation between DPOAEs and pure-tone threshold has proved challenging, especially given the variety of cochlear impairments. DPOAE amplitude and pure-tone threshold are inversely related (Figure 9–3); however, an

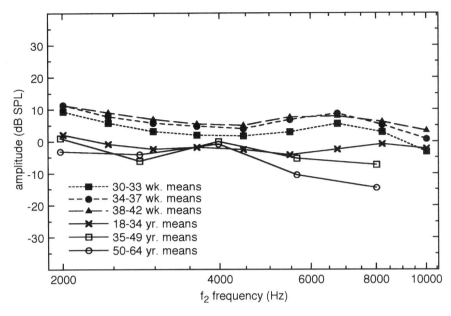

Figure 9–7. DPOAE amplitude as a function of the f_2 frequency for three infants and three adult-age groups.

analytical method to determine normal or elevated pure-tone thresholds could be clinically useful. The difficulties encountered in finding a function that relates these two variables implies that the relation is not straightforward. It would appear that several variables, not just DPOAE level at one frequency, may be used to better predict pure-tone threshold. We have used two analytical techniques to combine variables in a way to optimally characterize normal and abnormal pure-tone threshold: discriminant analysis and a neural network model.

Discriminant analysis is a statistical technique that attempts to define two or more groups on the basis of linear combinations of attributes (*variables*) common to all groups. For example, we were interested in grouping objective attributes, such as DPOAE level and age, into either a normal pure tone group or an abnormal pure tone group. Discriminant functions were used to represent weighted linear combinations of the variables common to both groups. For our study, 45 variables were measured on both the normal and impaired hearing group (Kimberley et al., 1994a). Six discriminant functions, one for each frequency, were computed from our data comprising 115 ears. Table 9–2 indicates that relatively good prediction performance can be achieved with the use of only two variables: DPOAE amplitude associated with stimulus levels of 60 dB SPL and subject age. The results from classifying a number of ears not used in the development of the discriminant model are shown in Figure 9–9.

A neural network approach is another means of finding a generalized relationship between DPOAEs and pure-tone thresholds. Neural networks are computer simulations of arrays of computational elements which individually perform in a

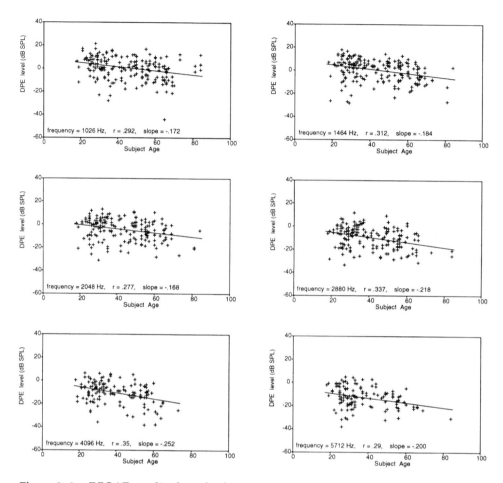

Figure 9–8. DPOAE amplitude and subject age plotted for six f_2 frequencies (n = 181 with normal pure-tone thresholds to 8 kHz).

Table 9–2. Percentages Correctly Classified as Normal or Elevated
Pure Tone Thresholds (PTT) Based on a Discriminant Analysis
with DPOAE Amplitude and Age as Variables

	Normal PTT	Elevated PTT		Normal PTT	Elevated PTT
1025 Hz	90%	70%	2880 Hz	83%	89%
1464 Hz	87%	81%	4096 Hz	88%	57%
2048 Hz	83%	100%	5712 Hz	86%	90%

n = 115 ears

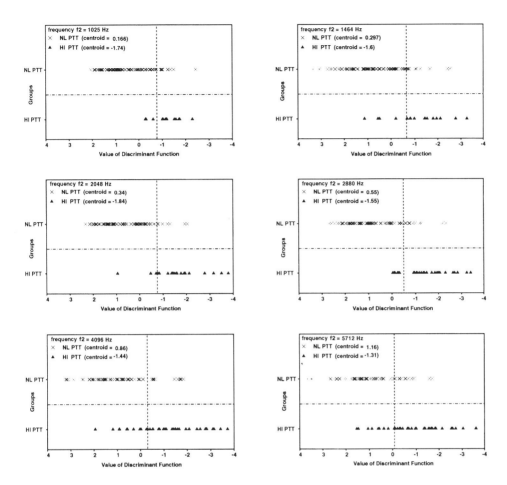

Figure 9–9. Graphical depiction of the prediction accuracy of six frequency-specific functions derived in the discriminant analysis of Kimberley et al. (1994). Of the pure-tone threshold values defined as impaired, the number of ears correctly classified as impaired from DPOAE amplitude, noise floor and age data appear as *triangles* to the right of the vertical pass-fail line (*dashed*). Similarly, the number of *crosses* to the left of the vertical dashed line are the ears with normal pure-tone thresholds that were correctly classified as normal using the DPOAE predictors.

manner similar to elemental neural processes (Mammone & Zeevi, 1991). This relatively new computational approach can deal with nonlinear and noisy data and has little difficulty in classifying outlying data points. We have found this approach to be more accurate than discriminant analysis in the prediction of pure-tone threshold from DPOAE and demographic information (Kimberley et al., 1994b). Figure 9–10 illustrates the schematic of a neural network analysis that could simulate a nonlinear relation between (a) DPOAE and subject data and (b) pure-tone threshold.

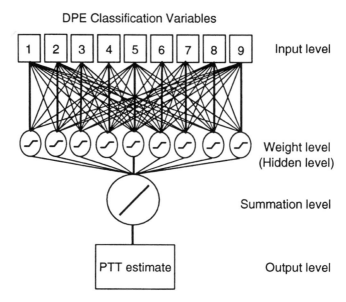

Figure 9–10. Generalized schematic of a neural network as applied to pure-tone threshold prediction. The number of classification variables at the input level are chosen from parameters expected to have an effect at the output. For pure-tone threshold prediction, the classification variables can include DPOAE amplitude (for a variety of stimulus levels), DPOAE phase, and age. Typically, the number of functions in the weight level reflects the complexity of the system being modeled and does not need to equal the number of elements at the input level.

Confounding Phenomena

Age, noise, and stimulus characteristics are not the only factors that can affect how DPOAE level correlates with pure-tone threshold. Harris et al. (1989) observed individual variability in the DPOAE amplitude regardless of the stimulus parameters used. This individuality in DPOAE response may be due to nulls, spontaneous otoacoustic emissions or the microstructure of the individual's cochlea.

Nulls and Dips

Nulls or monotonic dips can be observed in the DPOAE. These may occur in a DP-gram at a single frequency as the DPOAE is measured across a series of frequencies. Gaskill and Brown (1990) suggested that this was due to the f_2/f_1 ratio not having the ideal frequency separation to produce an optimal emission. These nulls are also noticeable in DPOAE growth curves. Some persons may have a sudden decrease in the amplitude of the emission at an individual intensity and then a return to the expected level (Figure 9–2). These dips may be generated by phase cancellation between the acoustic components (Brown, 1987; Schmiedt, 1986) or by the interaction of the two (i.e., low-level and high-level stimuli) generators (Whitehead et al., 1990, 1992a, 1992b). The nulls may occur in a DPOAE recording that may appear as if the emission is not present, when it may be.

Spontaneous Emissions

Spontaneous otoacoustic emissions (SOAEs) can also enhance a DPOAE (Brown et al., 1994; Wit, Langevoort, & Ritsma 1981). A SOAE that occurs within 50 Hz of the frequency of the DPOAE will enlarge the amplitude of the DPOAE (Wier, Pasanen & McFadden, 1988). This can lead to an emission whose amplitude is larger than normal because of the influence by the SOAE. The possibility that a SOAE will be present at the frequency of the emission is small because of the narrow band of the SOAE, but it is possible. If a SOAE is suspected to be present, its influence will be removed by altering the stimulus frequencies and changing the DPOAE frequency slightly.

DPOAE and Pure-tone Threshold Microstructure

When DPOAE amplitude and pure-tone threshold are measured in finer frequency intervals, the smooth curves associated with these features become rougher (Figure 9–11). (This is called microstructure.) If the DPOAE amplitude is measured at a slightly different point than the pure-tone threshold, the troughs and valleys of the DPOAE can affect the final value returned as the DPOAE amplitude. The current popular techniques for measuring pure-tone threshold (audiological and psychophysical techniques) have a precision of up to 5 dB SPL which makes detecting the pure-tone threshold microstructure difficult. Reducing the effect of the DPOAE

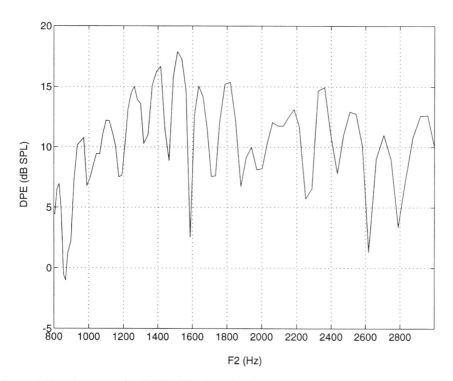

Figure 9–11. An example of DPOAE microstructure.

amplitude microstructure on DPOAE-pure-tone threshold comparisons, therefore, may lead to a better correlation between the two. We have noticed this increased correlation in studies of DPOAE phase and the cochlear traveling-wave delay. The estimation of frequency-specific traveling-wave delay requires multiple DPOAE amplitude measurements to be made at closely-spaced frequency increments very near to each pure-tone threshold frequency tested. Characteristically, there is one DPOAE frequency at which the DPOAE amplitude is a maximum. This is normally at an f_2/f_1 ratio of approximately 1.2, but decreases slightly for higher frequencies (Figure 9–4). Comparing this optimal ratio DPOAE amplitude value against pure-tone threshold increases the correlation between the two measures by a factor of two over that of a simple DPOAE amplitude measurement.

Using DPOAE measurements taken at multiple f_2/f_1 ratios has been suggested by Smurzynski et al. as one way to avoid being mislead by DPOAE or pure-tone threshold microstructure (Smurzynski & Kim, 1992; Smurzynski, Leonard, & Kim, 1990). For persons with normal hearing, there is a linear decrease of DPOAE maximum amplitude with pure-tone threshold; frequency does not appear to affect the slope of this trend (Figure 9–12). The value of the y-intercepts for Figure 9–12 change with frequency and may reflect the sensitivity of the normal cochlea to that frequency (i.e., bearing some relation to an iso-loudness curve). Figure 9–13 suggests that DPOAE maximum amplitude falls as age increases, again showing little frequency effect between the age groups. Further study in the use of the DPOAE maximum may lead to the development of better techniques for correlating DPOAE and demographic features with normal or mildly impaired pure-tone threshold.

Figure 9–14 shows a narrow band of hearing data for a single subject and

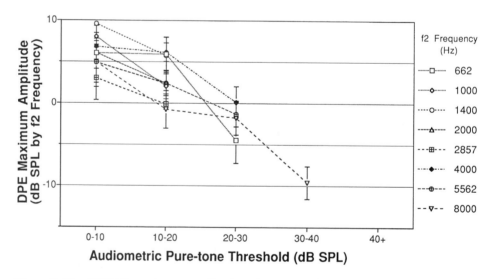

Figure 9–12. DPOAE maximum amplitude as it varies with audiometric pure-tone threshold over ages 20–65 (n = 37). Error bars are 1 standard error of the mean.

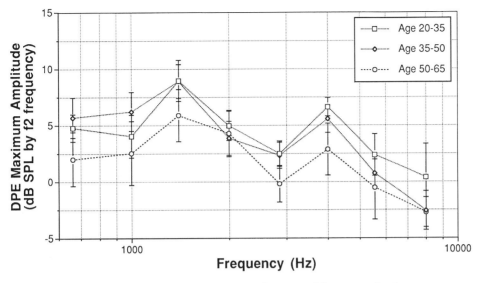

Figure 9–13.   DPOAE maximum amplitude as a function of frequency for three age groups (20–35 $n = 12$, 35–50 $n = 16$, 50–65 $n = 8$), plotted on a semilog scale. Error bars are 1 standard error of the mean.

incorporates pure-tone threshold, DPOAE, and magnitude reflectance data. The DPOAE magnitude is plotted against the frequency of the emission—that is, not against the frequency of either of the stimulating tones. Reflectance is simply the complex ratio of output pressure to input pressure upon stimulation of the ear with a single tone. This is another way of looking at single frequency otoacoustic emission information.

There is a frequency correspondence between the locations of the rippling behaviours of the three phenomena. The dip in pure-tone threshold data nearly matches the rather sharp dip in reflectance data. A low point in reflectance corresponds to a high point in absorbed sound energy. Thus, for this example, the ear apparently hears better in the frequency region where the most sound energy is absorbed. The DPOAE data also shows a rippling behaviour that is slightly offset from the other two measures (Voss & Allen, 1994).

Signal Processing Considerations

Some of the difficulties encountered in measuring DPOAEs are related to auditory physiology. Other problems exist in trying to isolate the low amplitude emission from background noise. There are two basic methods of signal processing and artifact rejection that are useful in f_2 estimation: filtering and time averaging. These two signal processing schemes are linear techniques that combine the different portions of a time signal and reduce them to a number that represents the f_2 magnitude (i.e., pressure).

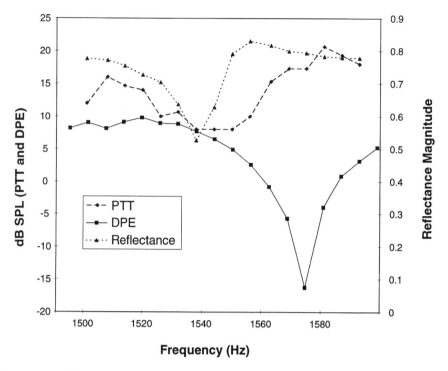

Figure 9–14. Relation between DPOAE, pure-tone threshold, and reflectance micro-structures.

Filtering

Filtering a signal is a linear process that emphasizes certain frequency components in the signal and deemphasizes others. If a narrow band filter having a 1 Hz pass band was designed, it would be possible to selectively look at the energy at a f_2 frequency, while excluding the energy at the stimulus frequencies. Such a filter would need to have very high precision arithmetic for two reasons. First, the filter would need a high rejection ratio for the high level stimuli at f_1 and f_2. Second, it would need a very narrow bandwidth to remove noise near the f_2 frequency. High precision arithmetic (*digital*) or very stable components (*analogue*) are needed to meet these two requirements. Because of these sensitive issues, filtering is not usually considered to be a reasonable solution for extracting f_2s. Analogue systems that use this method are likely to be unstable, while digital filtering systems can be noisy.

Time Averaging

While it is possible to use filtering to isolate a f_2, alternative solutions use time averaging and the Fourier transform (FT) to extract the spectral information. Both averaging and the FT are linear processes, like filtering. Time averaging schemes however do not have sensitive coefficients, nor do they depend on differences between two nearly identical numbers. These methods include power spectral estimation, windowed time-synchronous averaging (WTSA), and transient suppressed time-synchronous averaging (TS-TSA).

WINDOWED METHODS

Spectral estimation and the short-time Fourier transform (STFT) are the most common form of windowed signal averaging. Power spectral estimation is based on asynchronous averaging of the magnitude of the FT of the windowed signal. A signal, $s(t)$, is time shifted by time T, and multiplied by a time symmetric window, $w(t)$, forming the signal, $w(t)s(t - T)$. The window function is a high quality low-pass filter; the FT of $w(t)$, which we designate $W(f)$ is small in magnitude at high frequencies. The FT of the windowed signal is a complex spectrum—simply meaning that each point in the spectrum has magnitude and phase components. The magnitudes of many of these spectra are averaged together to form an estimate of the spectrum of $s(t)$. The variance of the estimate of the spectrum depends on the number of signals averaged together as well as the signal to noise ratio within the pass-band of $W(f - fd)$, where fd is the frequency of the f_2 (e.g., $fd = 2f_1 - f_2$). The bandwidth of the window depends critically on its length. Every window may be characterized by a parameter called its time-bandwidth product (TB). This is defined as the time duration of the window multiplied by its bandwidth. The time-bandwidth product is typically a number like 3 or 4. If we know the TB product and we know the bandwidth, B, one needs to attain a certain signal to noise ratio specification in order to calculate the time duration of the window, T. For example, a 1 Hz bandwidth with a window like a Hamming window, which has TB of 4, requires a duration of 4 seconds. This Hamming window will attenuate by about 42 dB all signals which are more than 0.5 Hz away from the frequency of the DPOAE that one is trying to detect.

Windows were developed to reduce the effects of the transients which accompany an abruptly turned on signal. Signal transients accompany the onset of the primary signals as well as the resulting f_2s. The window tapers the signal, bringing it gradually to full magnitude. However, this taper also reduces the magnitude of the signal and removes what might be important signal information where the effects of the window are greatest. One solution for this problem is to overlap many windows (typically 2–4 times overlap) so that each data sample is processed between 2 to 4 times, but at different places in the window. This reduces the loss of signal information at the cost of reduced processing efficiency. Another problem with windowing is that a window smears the signal energy by an amount that is equal to the bandwidth of the window. This makes it difficult to estimate the noise near a signal component because the signal "leaks" into the channel where the noise is being estimated (i.e., the channels are no longer independent). The solution to the leakage problem is to use a window with the smallest possible TB value. Another solution is to not use any window, in which case the transient is likely to dominate the response.

Because they average the magnitude of the FT of the windowed signal, window methods cannot take advantage of the phase of the periodic stimulus signal. As a result, windowed methods are inferior to time synchronous averaging methods that do not require a window.

TIME-SYNCHRONOUS AVERAGING

When time averaging in a synchronous manner, window can be used if the signal transient can not be avoided. However, if this transient is suppressed, the window is unnecessary. This form of artifact rejection is called *transient suppressed time-synchronous averaging* (TS-TSA). TS-TSA relies on the fact that one can have precise control over the stimulus signal. This knowledge can give a large signal processing advantage because one can make certain assumptions about the behaviour of the signal. The only requirement is that the length of the FFT be greater than the memory in the system—namely the length of the anti-aliasing filter and the settling time of the f_2s after the primary signals are turned on. As long as this condition is true, TS-TSA processing allows the window and all of its problems to be avoided. It follows that each frequency bin in the FFT is independent, and that the window leakage is zero. This type of processing is used by CUBeDIS (Mimosa Acoustics) and SYSid (Ariel). CUBeDIS makes the assumption that the noise is smooth across frequency and uses a neighboring frequency 48 Hz away to get the noise estimate.

A unique parameter that CUBeDIS uses is the pressure measured in the ear canal, normalized by the pressure measured in a DB-100 (i.e., a Zwislocki coupler). Below about 3 or 4 kHz, this measure is related to the relative impedance of the ear. It can be very useful in determining whether or not a good seal has been established by the foam eartip in the ear canal because a reliable seal is critical to good measurements.

A mathematical consequence of TS-TSA is that the measurement bandwidth is inversely proportional to the duration of the time average. Because there is no leakage, the FFT frequency bins on either side of the tone stimulus are at the level of the noise floor. The noise floor level, which is determined by the bandwidth, is given by the reciprocal of the averaging time. The level of the noise floor can be varied by simply changing the averaging time.

Assuming that the noise is similar for frequencies in the neighborhood of the f_2 frequency and given that there is no leakage, one can estimate the noise at the measurement frequency. Typically one FFT bin is 24 or 49 Hz wide. For example, if the sampling rate is 50 kHz, and the FFT is 1024 points long, the FFT bins are spaced by 50,000/1024, or approximately 48.83 Hz. If the FFT is 2048 points long, the spacing is 24.4 Hz. To reduce the variance of the noise estimate, a few FFT bins on either side of the DPOAE frequency are least squares averaged, yielding a very robust noise estimate. If three bands are averaged on either side of the $2f_1$-f_2 f_2 frequency, the variance reduction would be about a factor of 2.4 (i.e., 1/60.5), assuming an FFT length of 1024 and uniform noise over a frequency range of 3 × 49 Hz.

An important advantage of this noise estimation method is that it is made for the same period that the DP signal estimate is made. This can be important if noise levels vary with time, as in the case of breathing, coughing, crying, and other transient type noise.

A more common type of noise rejection is to interleave the measurements, for example into even and odd presentations (i.e., one FFTs' worth of signal apiece). Two separate averages are maintained for each of the even and odd samples. The two sets of averaged signals are then windowed, and added in one term and subtracted in another. The addition term is twice the signal. For the subtraction term, the signal part is assumed to cancel, giving an estimate of the random noise. A problem with this scheme is that the results are typically windowed. More important, it is assumed that the noise and the signal are stationary. Even slight variations in either the signal or the noise show up as errors in the noise estimate. This is a very subtle type of error that would be difficult to identify. Causes of this type of error include movement of the transducer in the ear canal during the measurement and a pop or transient noise that occurs during the even presentation but not during the odd. This type of error can be avoided if the noise is estimated from the neighboring FFT bins within 150 Hz of the f_2 frequency.

There is, however, a problem with the neighboring FFT bin estimation procedure. At low frequencies (i.e., <1 kHz) the noise from a DPOAE microphone, such as the ER-10C, increases and can become the dominate system noise. This noise increases as the measurement frequency decreases. As an example, let the upper stimulus frequency f_2 be 500 Hz and assume that $f_2/f_1 = 1.2$ and that the FFT bins are spaced every 48 Hz. If three FFT bins below fd = f_2 (2/1.2 − 1) = 333.3 Hz are used to estimate the noise, then the lowest frequency used is about 333 − (3 × 49) = 186 Hz. Therefore, the noise floor displayed at 500 Hz would contain a component of noise at 186 Hz, where microphone noise is high. A large slope on low frequency microphone noise can therefore bias the estimate of the noise at 333 Hz, so the measurement will appear to have excessive noise for low frequencies.

The low frequency noise problem may be avoided by using fewer number of frequency bins in the noise estimate, or by choosing a larger FFT length. The first solution has the disadvantage of raising the variance of the noise estimate, while the second increases the time to compute an FFT. On fast computers or digital signal processors the latter is less important. The FFT calculation time may be overlapped with the time taken for signal averaging; thus, the FFT processing time will not be the limiting time in the data collection process.

Summary and Conclusions

This chapter focused on important details concerning the distortion product otoacoustic emission and how it is affected by pure-tone threshold, noise, age, and individual factors. It should be clear that in spite of the technical advancements made in detecting these low level responses, the relation between the DPOAEs and sensorineural hearing loss is not fully understood. There is no physiological basis for assuming that DPOAE measures ought to perfectly correlate with pure-tone threshold, even in the case of a purely cochlear hearing loss. For example, DPOAEs alone will not help with the distinction between a neural transmission loss and normal hearing. Currently available empirical evidence, however, suggests that the general relationships between pure-tone threshold and DPOAE will serve as an important tool for the audiologist. DPOAEs have attracted special interest because of their ease of use and inherent frequency specificity. The implementation of advanced DPOAE recording and noise estimation methods maximizes the opportunity to observe a good DPOAE–pure-tone–threshold correlation. In addition, techniques based on the interaction of multiple variables, such as neural network analysis and discriminant analysis, can be used to enhance the prediction of hearing thresholds from DPOAE and demographic data. Eventually, DPOAE measurements will be incorporated into a larger objective testing regime involving the simultaneous recording of DPOAEs, middle ear reflectance, and auditory brain stem response.

References

Allen, J. B. (1995, June) DeRecruitment by multi-band compression in hearing aids. Paper presented at the Boystown Conference on the Modeling of Cochlear Hearing Loss, Omaha, NE.

Allen, J. B., & Fahey, P. F. (1993) A second cochlear-frequency map that correlates distortion product and neural tuning measurements. *Journal of the Acoustical Society of America, 94*, 809–816.

Allen, J. B., & Levitt, H. (1992) A comparison of pure tone and distortion product audiometric thresholds. *Unpublished manuscript.*

Avan, P., & Bonfils, P. (1993) Frequency specificity of human distortion product otoacoustic emissions. *Audiology, 32*, 12–26.

Bonfils, P., Avan, P., Londero, A., Trotoux, J., & Narcy, P. (1991) Objective low-frequency audiometry by distortion-product acoustic emissions. *Archives of Otolaryngology—Head and Neck Surgery, 117*, 1167–1171.

Bonfils, P., Piron, J. P., Uziel, A., & Pujol, R. (1988). A correlative study of otoacoustic emission properties and audiometric thresholds. *Archives of Otorhinolaryngology, 245*, 53–56.

Brown, A. M. (1987). Acoustic distortion from rodent ear: A comparison of responses from rats, guinea pigs and gerbils. *Hearing Research, 31*, 25–38.

Brown, A. M., & Gaskill, S. A. (1990). Can basilar membrane tuning be inferred from distortion measurement? In P. Dallos, C. D. Geisler, J. W. Matthews, M. A. Ruggero, & C. R. Steele (eds.): *Mechanics and biophysics of hearing* (pp. 164–169). New York: Springer-Verlag.

Brown, A. M., Gaskill, S. A., & Williams, D. M. (1992). Mechanical filtering of sound in the inner ear. *Proceedings of the Royal Society of London. Series B: Biological Sciences, 250*, 29–34.

Brown, A. M., & Kemp, D. T. (1984). Supressibility of the $2f_1 - f_2$ stimulated acoustic emissions in gerbil and man. *Hearing Research, 13*, 29–37.

Brown, A. M., Sheppard, S. L., & Russell, P. T. (1994). Acoustic distortion products (ADP) from the ears of term infants and young adults using low stimulus levels. *British Journal of Audiology, 28*, 273–280.

Etymotic Research. (1992). User manual for the CUBeDIS distortion product measurement system. Version 2.40. Elk Grove Village, IL.

Fahey, P., & Allen, J. (1986). Characterization of cubic intermodulation distortion products in the cat external auditory meatus. In J. Allen, J. L. Hall, A. Hubbard, S. T. Neely, & A. Tubis (eds): *Peripheral auditory mechanisms* (pp. 314–321). New York: Springer-Verlag.

Furst, M., Rabinowitz, W. M., & Zurek, P. M. (1988). Ear canal acoustic distortion at $2f_1 - f_2$ from human ears: Relation to other emissions and perceived combination tones. *Journal of the Acoustical Society of America, 84*, 215–221.

Gaskill, S. A., & Brown, A. M. (1990). The behavior of the acoustic distortion product, $2f_1 - f_2$, from the human ear and its relation to auditory sensitivity. *Journal of the Acoustical Society of America, 88*, 821–839.

Gaskill, S. A., & Brown, A. M. (1993). Comparing the level of the acoustic distortion product $2f_1 - f_2$ with behavioural threshold audiograms from normal-hearing and hearing impaired ears. *British Journal of Audiology, 27*, 397–407.

Gorga, M. P., Neely, S. T., Bergman, B., Beauchaine, K. L., Kaminski, J. K., Peters, J., & Jestead, W. (1993). Otoacoustic emissions from normal-hearing and hearing-impaired subjects: Distortion product responses. *Journal of the Acoustical Society of America, 93*, 2050–2060.

Gould, H. J., & Sobhy, O. A. (1992). Using the derived auditory brain stem response to estimate traveling wave velocity. *Ear and Hearing, 13*, 96–101.

Harris, F., & Glattke, T. (1988). Distortion product emissions in humans with high-frequency sensorineural hearing loss. *Journal of the Acoustical Society of America, 84*, s74.

Harris, F. P., Lonsbury-Martin, B. L., Stagner, B. E., Coats, A. C., & Martin, G. K. (1989). Acoustic distortion product in humans: Systemic changes in amplitude as a function of f_2/f_1 ratio. *Journal of the Acoustical Society of America, 85*, 220–229.

Hauser, R., Probst, R. (1991). The influence of systematic primary-tone level variation $L2 - L1$ on the acoustic distortion product emission $2f_1 - f_2$ in normal human ears. *Journal of the Acoustical Society of America, 89*, 280–286.

Kemp, D. T. (1978). Stimulated acoustic emissions from the human auditory system. *Journal of the Acoustical Society of America, 64*, 1386–1391.

Kimberley, B. P., Brown, D. K., & Eggermont, J. J. (1993). Measuring human cochlear traveling wave delay using distortion product emission phase responses. *Journal of the Acoustical Society of America, 94*, 1343–1350.

Kimberley, B. P., Hernadi, I., Lee, A. M., & Brown, D. K. (1994). Predicting pure-tone thresholds in normal and hearing-impaired ears with distortion product emission and age. *Ear and Hearing, 15*, 199–209.

Kimberley, B. P., Kimberley, B. M., & Roth, L. (1994). A neural network approach to the prediction of pure-tone thresholds with distortion product emissions. *ENT Journal, 73*, PAGES–PAGES.

Kimberley, B. P, & Nelson, D. A. (1989). Distortion product emissions and sensorineural hearing loss. *Journal of Otolaryngology, 18*, 365–369.

Lafreniere, D., Jung, M. D., Smurzynski, J., Leonard, G., Kim, D. O., & Sasek, J. (1991). Distortion-product and click-evoked otoacoustic emissions in healthy newborns. *Archives of Otolaryngology—Head and Neck Surgery, 117*, 1382–1389.

Lonsbury-Martin, B. L., Cutler, W. M., & Martin, G. K. (1991). Evidence for the influence of aging on distortion-product otoacoustic emissions in humans. *Journal of the Acoustical Society of America, 89*, 1749–1759.

Lonsbury-Martin, B. L., Harris, F. P., Stagner, B. B., Hawkins, M. D., & Martin, G. K. (1990). Distortion product emissions in humans I. Basic properties in normally hearing subjects. *Annuals of Otology, Rhinology, and Laryngology, 147*, 3–14.

Lonsbury-Martin, B. L., & Martin, G. K. (1990). The clinical utility of distortion-product otoacoustic emissions. *Ear and Hearing, 11*, 144–154.

Lonsbury-Martin, B. L., McCoy, M. J., Whitehead, M. L., & Martin, G. K. (1993). Clinical testing of distortion product emissions. *Ear and Hearing, 1*, 11–22.

Lonsbury-Martin, B. L., Whitehead, M. L., & Martin, G. K. (1991). Clinical applications of otoacoustic emissions. *Journal of Speech and Hearing Research, 34*, 964–981.

Mammone, R., & Zeevi, Y. (1991). *Neural networks—Theory and application*. New York: Academic Press.

Martin, G. K., Lonsbury-Martin, B.L., Probst, R., Scheinin, S. A., & Coats, A. C. (1987). Acoustic distortion products in rabbit ear canal. II. Sites of origin revealed by suppression contours and pure-tone exposures. *Hearing Research, 28*, 191–208.

Martin, G. K., Ohlms, L. A., Franklin, D. J., Harris, F. P., & Lonsbury-Martin, B. L. (1990). Distortion product emissions in humans III. Influence of sensorineural hearing loss. *Annals of Otology, Rhinology, and Laryngology, 99*, 30–42.

Matthews, J. W., & Molnar, C. E. (1986). Modeling intracochlear and ear canal distortion products. In J. Allen, J. L. Hall, A. Hubbard, S. T. Neely, & A. Tubis (eds.): *Peripheral auditory mechanisms* (pp. 258–265). New York: Springer-Verlag.

Nelson, D. A., & Kimberley, B. P. (1992). Distortion-product emissions and auditory sensitivity in human ears with normal hearing and cochlear hearing loss. *Journal of Speech and Hearing Research, 135*, 1142–1159.

Nielsen, L. H., Popelka, G. R., Rasmussen, A. N., & Osterhammel, P. A. (1993). Clinical significance of probe-tone frequency ratio on distortion product otoacoustic emissions. *Scandinavian Audiology, 122*, 159–164.

Popelka, G. R., Karzon, R. K., Arjmand, E. M. (1995). Growth of the $2f_1 - f_2$ distortion product otoacoustic emission for low-level stimuli in human neonates. *Ear and Hearing, 16*, 159–165.

Prieve, B. A., Gorga, M. P., Schmidt, A., Neely, S., Peters, J., Schultes, L., & Jesteadt, W. (1993). Analysis of transient-evoked otoacoustic emissions in normal-hearing and hearing-impaired ears. *Journal of the Acoustical Society of America, 93*, 3308–3320.

Probst, R. (1990). Otoacoustic emissions: An overview. *Advances in Oto-Rhino-Laryngology, 44*, 1–91.

Probst, R., Lonsbury-Martin, B. L., Martin, G. K., & Coats, A. (1987). Otoacoustic emissions in ears with hearing loss. *American Journal of Otolaryngology, 8*, 73–81.

Rasmussen, A. N., Popelka, G. R., Osterhammel, P. A., & Nielsen, L. H. (1993). Clinical significance of relative probe-tone levels on distortion product otoacoustic emissions. *Scandinavian Audiology, 22*, 223–229.

Schmiedt, R. A. (1986). Harmonic acoustic emissions in the ear canal generated by single tones: Experiments and a model. In J. B. Allen, J. L. Hall, A. Hubbard, S. T. Neely, & A. Tubis (eds): *Peripheral auditory mechanisms* (pp. 330–337). New York: Springer-Verlag.

Shaw, G. (1994) On the setting of a threshold level in DPE testing. Unpublished data.

Smurzynski, J. (1994). Longitudinal measurements of distortion-product and click-evoked otoacoustic emissions of preterm infants: Preliminary results. *Ear and Hearing, 15*, 210–223.

Smurzynski, J., & Kim, D. O. (1992). Distortion-product and click evoked otoacoustic emissions of normally-hearing adults. *Hearing Research, 58*, 227–240.

Smurzynski, J., Leonard, G., Kim, D. O., Lafreniere, D., & Jung, M. (1990). Distortion product otoacoustic emissions in normal and impaired adult ears. *Archives Otolaryngology—Head and Neck Surgery, 116,* 1309–1316.

Stover, L., & Norton, S. J. (1993). The effects of aging on otoacoustic emissions. *Journal of the Acoustical Society of America, 94,* 2670–2681.

Whitehead, M. L., Lonsbury-Martin, B. L., & Martin, G. K. (1990). Actively and passively generated acoustic distortion at 2f1 − f2 in rabbits. In P. Dallos, C. D. Geisler, J. W. Matthews, M. A. Ruggero, & C. R. Steele (eds.): *Mechanics and biophysics,* VOL, PAGE–PAGE.

Whitehead, M. L., Lonsbury-Martin, B. L., & Martin, G. K. (1992a). Evidence for two discrete sources of $2f_1 − f_2$ distortion-product otoacoustic emission in rabbit. I. Differential dependence on stimulus parameters. *Journal of the Acoustical Society of America, 91,* 1587–1607.

Whitehead, M. L., Lonsbury-Martin, B. L., & Martin, G. K. (1992b). Evidence for two discrete sources of $2f_1 − f_2$ distortion-product otoacoustic emission in rabbit. II. Differential physiological vulnerability. *Journal of the Acoustical Society of America, 92,* 2662–2682.

Whitehead, M. L., Lonsbury-Martin, B. L., & Martin, G.K. (193). The influence of noise on the measured amplitudes of distortion-product otoacoustic emissions. *Journal of Speech and Hearing Research, 36,* 1097–1102.

Whitehead, M. L., McCoy M. J., Lonsbury-Martin, B. L., & Martin G. K. (1995a). Dependence of distortion-product otoacoustic emissions on primary levels in normal and impaired ears. I. Effects of decreasing L2 below L1. *Journal of the Acoustical Society of America, 97,* 2346–2358.

Whitehead, M. L., Stagner, B. B., Lonsbury-Martin, B. L., & Martin, G.K. (1994). Measurement of otoacoustic emissions for hearing assessment. *IEEE Engineering in Medicine and Biology, Apr/May,* 210–226.

Whitehead, M. L., Stagner, B. B., McCoy, M. J., Lonsbury-Martin, B. L., & Martin, G. K. (1995b). Dependence of distortion-product otoacoustic emissions on primary levels in normal and impaired ears. II. Asymmetry in L1,L2 space. *Journal of the Acoustical Society of America, 97,* 2359–2377.

Wier, C. C., Pasanen, E. G., & McFadden, D. (1988). Partial dissociation of spontaneous otoacoustic emissions and distortion product during aspirin consumption in humans. *Journal of the Acoustical Society of America, 84,* 230–237.

Wilson, J. P. (1980). The combination tone $2f_1 − f_2$, in psychophysics and ear-canal recording. In G. van den Brink & F. A. Bilsen (eds.): *Psychophysical, physiological and behavioural studies in hearing* (pp. 43–52). Delft, The Netherlands: Delft University Press.

Wit, H. P., Langevoort, J. C., & Ritsma, R. J. (1981). Frequency spectra of cochlear acoustic emissions ("Kemp-echoes"). *Journal of the Acoustical Society of America, 70,* 437–445.

Voss, S. E., & Allen, J. B. (1994) Measurement of acoustic impedance and reflectance in the human ear canal. *Journal of the Acoustical Society of America, 95,* 372–384.

10

Contributions of Evoked Otoacoustic Emissions in Differential Diagnosis of Retrocochlear Disorders

Martin S. Robinette
John D. Durrant

Introduction

Evoked otoacoustic emissions (EOAEs) are believed to be generated by electro-motile activity of the outer hair cells of the cochlea, and without question, they represent a preneural phenomenon (although they are subject to some influence by the descending auditory pathway). The clinical implications of having a noninvasive direct "window" into the cochlea are exciting. Early, objective methods in the clinical evaluation of auditory function failed to provide direct measures of cochlear hydromechanical function, let alone the functional state of the outer hair cells. OAEs are believed to provide a direct functional view of outer hair cells (Kemp, 1978, 1988; Probst, 1990). The outer hair cells are implicated in the fine-tuning of cochlear micromechanics and the underlying nonlinear processes (Geisler, 1985; Neely & Kim, 1986). Consequently, the outer hair cells are of interest by virtue of their putative contribution to the sensitivity and frequency selectivity of the hearing organ.

This chapter focuses on the applications of EOAE measures intended to discriminate between cochlear and neural functioning and, thereby, assist in differential diagnosis of auditory disorders. First, the preneural characteristics of EOAEs are described based upon observations in both animals and humans. Second, the diagnostic value of EOAEs in patients found to have eighth cranial nerve tumors is examined, as well as their value in monitoring the subsequent effects of eighth-nerve–tumor surgery on cochlear and neural functioning. In this endeavor, EOAE measures will be compared with the results of auditory brainstem response (ABR) testing. Third, case examples are presented to demonstrate the diagnostic value of EOAE measures in the evaluation of other retrocochlear auditory disorders of the eighth cranial nerve and more central structures.

Preneural Origin of EOAEs

Many reports have suggested that EOAEs may be produced and measured independent of the neural integrity of the auditory system. Kim (1980) demonstrated that afferent neurons are not necessary to generate distortion product otoacoustic emissions (DPOAEs). He perfused a chinchilla's scala tympani with cyanide, which resulted in the permanent elimination of the whole-nerve neural-action potential. Yet, the magnitude of the DPOAEs, as well as the cochlear microphonic, showed complete recovery within 4 min. Similarly, using tetrodotoxin (TTX)—a sodium channel blocker that inhibits all synaptic transmission—Arts, Norton, and Rubel (1990) found the DPOAE to be unaltered in gerbils. On the other hand, click-evoked ABR's were essentially eliminated. The findings provide strong evidence that EOAE generation does not require afferent neural activation.

Other evidence of the preneural nature of EOAEs includes the observations that DPOAEs were unaltered following surgical sectioning of the auditory portion of the eighth cranial nerve in rabbits (Ohlms, Lonsbury-Martin, Martin, 1991). Furthermore, Robinette (1992a.) observed transient evoked otoacoustic emissions (TEOAEs) in a patient whose eighth cranial nerve was sacrificed during surgery to remove a vestibular schwannoma. Even though EOAEs may be altered by efferent stimulation (Collet, Veuillet, Bene & Morgan, 1992; Rossi, Actis, Solero, Rolando & Pejrone, 1993) an intact efferent system is not necessary for their generation per se (Durrant, Kamerer, & Chen, 1993). Norton (1992, p. 9) wrote, "It is important to remember when applying OAEs to clinical populations that their generation is preneural and independent of both afferent and efferent innervation. That is, if a lesion is central to outer hair cells, OAEs could be present and behavioral and neural responses depressed."

EOAEs in Patients with Eighth-Nerve Tumors

The applications of EOAEs in the evaluation of patients with eighth cranial-nerve tumors are for (a) the differential diagnosis, (b) the monitoring of cochlear function before, during and after surgery to remove the tumor, and (c) the prediction of residual hearing following eighth-nerve surgery.

Diagnosis

Review of the literature suggests that the presence of TEOAEs indicates peripheral hearing sensitivity of 25 to 30 dB HL or better at emission frequencies from 1000 through 4000 Hz (Probst, Lonsbury-Martin, & Martin, 1991). Consequently, the observation of TEOAEs in ears with severe to profound sensorineural hearing loss has been found helpful in the diagnosis of retrocochlear disorders (Lutman, Mason, Sheppard, & Gibbon, 1989; Robinette, 1992a, 1992b; & Robinette and Facer, 1991). The case studies of these reports demonstrated TEOAEs, despite profound hearing losses measured behaviorally. The observations have indicated satisfactory cochlear functioning, with retrocochlear dysfunction determined to be responsible for the hearing losses. Therefore, TEOAE assessment offers the possibility to distinguish sensory hearing loss from neural hearing loss.

Even so, routine use of TEOAEs in the diagnostic workup to differentiate between cochlear and eighth-nerve disorders has been disappointing (Bonfils & Uziel, 1988; Cane, Lutman, & O'Donoghue, 1994; Prasher, Tun, Brooks, & Luxon, 1995; Robinette & Bauch, 1991). Table 10–1 provides a summary of the reports, including a recent sample from the Mayo Clinic. As shown, TEOAEs were present in 112 (47%) of the tumor ears. Hearing sensitivity was within normal limits for 69 of the 112 ears and therefore the presence of TEOAEs was expected for those ears. For the remaining 43 ears (18% of the total sample) there was significant hearing loss, yet TEOAEs were present confirming cochlear integrity. For these 43 patients, the TEOAE indication of good cochlear reserve suggests that the hearing loss was due primarily to the retrocochlear pathology.

Reports on DPOAE measures for 80 patients (collectively) with eighth-nerve tumors have shown similar results (Durrant, 1992; Telischi, Roth, Stagner, Lonsbury-Martin & Balkany, 1995a). Durrant reported that of 36 patients with surgically confirmed eighth nerve tumors, DPOAEs for 8 (22%) supported the diagnosis of retrocochlear hearing loss. Similarly, Telischi, et al. found 13 of 44 patients (30%) with acoustic neuromas had DPOAEs despite significant hearing loss. Thus, in only about one quarter of patients with eighth-nerve tumors are EOAE measures expected to support the diagnosis of retrocochlear hearing loss.

The implication of these studies is that EOAE measurement (TEOAE or DPOAE) has limited diagnostic potential in the identification of eighth-nerve tumors (providing a hit rate of 20–30%). This lack of diagnostic precision is attributable to the cochlear hearing losses that frequently accompany eighth-nerve tumors. The associated cochlear hearing losses in these patients is thought to be due to the restriction of the blood supply to the cochlea provided by the internal auditory artery

Table 10–1. TEOAE and Diagnosis of VIIIth Nerve Tumors

	Tumors (No.)	Present No.	%	TEOAEs Present Normal Audiogram (No.)	TEOAEs Present H-loss Audiogram (No.)	Important in Diagnosis No.	%
Bonfils & Uziel, 1988	28	9	31	4	5	5/28	18
Robinette & Bauch, 1991	65	34	52	22	12	12/65	18
Robinette (1992–1995)	72	41	57	28	13	13/72	18
Cane et al., 1994	45	21	47	9	12	12/45	27
Prasher et al., 1995	26	7	27	6	1	1/26	4
Total	236	112	47	69	43	43/236	18

(Levine, Ojeman, Montgomery, & McGaffigan, 1984). Expansion of the tumor in the internal auditory meatus probably limits the blood supply and the oxygen and nutrients required by the cochlea. Clearly, other auditory tests, such as acoustic reflex measures and ABR, are more sensitive in the identification of eighth-nerve lesions (Turner, Shepard, & Frazer, 1984).

On the other hand, EOAE testing of patients who may not be candidates for electrophysiological measures and are suspected to have eighth-nerve disorders may provide diagnostic information in ears with moderate to profound hearing losses. For example, Cane et al. (1994) reported that just under half of their 45 patients with eighth-nerve tumors had a best two-frequency average (500–4000 Hz) less than 70 dB HL, which is near the upper limit of hearing sensitivity for obtaining diagnostic information from either ABR or electrocochleography (ECochG) (Durrant & Wolf, 1991; Jacobson, Jacobson, Ramadan & Hyde, 1994). Therefore, findings of EOAEs in an ear with a moderate or greater sensorineural hearing impairment are highly specific. They provide strong evidence of good outer hair-cell function and indicate a retrocochlear lesion, as long as nonorganic hearing loss (i.e., pseudohypacusis) has been ruled out.

Monitor Cochlear Function

Another application of EOAE testing is to monitor cochlear function during and following surgery to remove eighth-nerve tumors (Cane, O'Donoghue, & Lutman; Telischi, Widick, Lonsbury-Martin, & McCoy, 1995b). The feasibility of intraoperative monitoring via TEOAEs was first reported by Cane et al. (1992). They found that TEOAEs could be measured and remained stable during breaks in the drilling of the petrous bone and other surgical procedures prior to the manipulation of the brainstem. When the tumor was dissected from the eighth cranial nerve, the TEOAE gradually decreased and was lost over a 30 minute period. Hearing thresholds measured post-operatively revealed a total loss of hearing. It was assumed that cochlear function was compromised by reduced blood supply during the removal of the tumor. The high level of noise in the operating room was the only material problem encountered, and this was not sufficient to prevent recording identifiable TEOAE waveforms. Noise levels varied from 50 dBA when only vital equipment was running to 90 dBA during drilling.

Telischi, Widick, Lonsbury-Martin, and McCoy (1995b) also reported successful intraoperative measurements of cochlear and neural function during eighth-nerve tumor surgery. DPOAEs were measured from 2000 to 4000 Hz with primary tone levels of 75 dB SPL for f_1 and f_2. The same transducer was used for alternating tests of ABR and DPOAE. In addition, direct recordings from the eighth cranial nerve were monitored. They noted that in two cases the EOAEs were stable through the drilling process, but were extinguished during tumor removal; changes in the EOAE occurred about 90 seconds before the noted changes in ABR-wave morphology.

These case studies support the hypothesis of Cane et al. (1992) that cochlear damage is not related to acoustic trauma from drilling, but most likely associated with the interruption of the cochlear blood supply during tumor removal. From these observations it appears that EOAEs, as well as ABR and ECochG testing, can provide information about the mechanisms of injury from the removal of eighth-nerve tumors.

Preoperative and postoperative tests of cochlear and neural function for patients with eighth-nerve tumors have shown that cochlear function often decreases, but that neural function is maintained or improved postoperatively. Postoperative results for 11 Mayo Clinic patients with eighth-nerve tumors who had measurable TEOAEs preoperatively and measurable ABRs both preoperatively and post-operatively is displayed in Table 10–2. Tumors were removed by a suboccipital surgical approach which resulted in saving the eighth nerve anatomically. None of the patients showed post-operative improvement in general auditory function as measured by pure-tone sensitivity (represented by the three-frequency pure-tone average [PTA]), by speech reception thresholds (SRT) or by word recognition scores (measured at 26 or 40 dB SL). Threshold sensitivity based on PTAs or SRTs was equally divided between "no change" and "worse". Word recognition scores were less affected: nine showed "no change" and two showed "worse" (as determined by the Raffin & Thornton [1980] criteria for critical differences).

While measures of pure-tone sensitivity and word recognition do not differentiate changes between cochlear and neural function, assessment of the postoperative ABR measures (absolute wave V latency and the I-V interpeak interval) and acoustic reflex measures [acoustic reflex (AR) threshold and reflex decay (RD)], can provide indications of changes in neural function after tumor removal. The majority of ears showed improved neural function according to ABR measures: 7 of the 11 ears (64%) had wave V latencies more than 0.2 msec earlier, and 6 of them (54%) had I-V interpeak intervals shortened by more than 0.2 ms. Changes from abnormal to normal acoustic reflex thresholds and/or elimination of reflex decay (Silman & Gelfand, 1991) also occurred for 5 (45%) of the 11 ears postsurgically. On the other hand, TEOAEs, which were present for all 11 patients pre-operatively, were decreased or absent for 8 ears (73%) postoperatively. For the 11 patients, the postoperative measures of cochlear and neural function showed that most patients suffered outer hair-cell damage, but experienced improved neural function, pre-

Table 10–2.   11 VIII Nerve Tumor Ears with Measurable OAEs Preoperatively and Measurable ABRs Pre- and Postoperatively

Auditory Measure	Improved	No Change	Worse	Absent
≥10 dB PTA	0	6	5	0
≥10 dB SRT	0	5	6	0
Word recognition*	0	9	2	0
≥0.2 ms ABR V	7	2	2	0
≥0.2 ms ABR I–V	6	2	3	0
AR/RD	5	2	4	0
≥4 dB TEOAE	0	3	4	4
Tumor size	Small	≤1.0 cm	5	
	Medium	1.1–2.0 cm	4	
	Large	>2.0 cm	2	

*Raffin & Thornton, 1980.

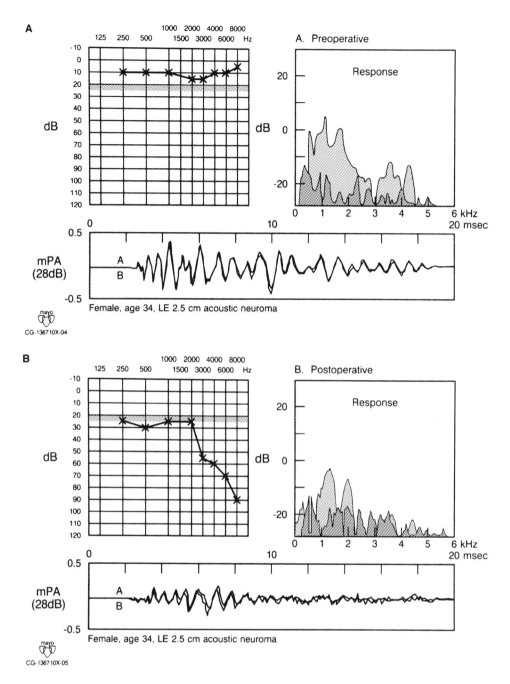

Figure 10–1. Illustrative example of the pre-operative (*1a*) and post-operative (*1b*) Audiologic evaluation of a patient with an eighth nerve tumor. The top left box of each picture shows the audiogram. The top right box labeled "Response" shows the frequency spectrum of the TEOAE as the light shaded area under the curve; the noise spectrum is indicated by the darkly shaded area. The lower box shows the two overlapped emission waveforms in the time domain from 2.5 ms to 20 ms. Test data show that postoperatively hearing sensitivity and TEOAE amplitude and frequency spectrum decreased. On the other hand, acoustic reflex thresholds and decay went from abnormal to normal and ABR results went from only a Wave I to showing Waves I, III, and V. (Adapted from Robinette, Bauch, Olsen, Harner, & Beatty [1992]. Used with permission.)

sumably from the release of pressure on the eighth nerve due to surgical removal of the tumor.

An example of improved neural function and reduced cochlear function following eighth-nerve tumor removal is illustrated in Figure 10–1.

Prediction of Residual Hearing

Because tumor removal generally results in a significant decrease in cochlear function, it is tempting to speculate that patients with an acoustic neuroma and hearing loss may have a better chance of residual hearing post-operatively if they have normal cochlear function preoperatively (i.e., the more cochlear reserve before the operation, the better the chance of some cochlear reserve after). Indeed, Kileny (1995) reported a case having a 2.5 cm meningoma, with an extension into the internal auditory canal. A profound hearing loss and normal cochlear function were revealed with the measurement of pure-tone threshold and EOAEs. Because of the cochlear reserve, a suboccipital surgical approach was used in an attempt to preserve the eighth cranial nerve. The reported results were dramatic. Not only was hearing preserved, but fell within the normal hearing range after the operation.

Cases as dramatic as this are rare. Nonetheless, the importance of EOAE testing for this patient is clear. We looked at 104 patients with surgically confirmed vestibular schwannomas in an attempt to assess pre-operative nonsurgical factors predictive of hearing preservation (Robinette, Bauch, Olsen, Harner, & Beatty, 1996). However, for these patients, cochlear reserve as measured by EOAEs was not found to be a significant protective factor.

Differential Diagnosis

The validation of the clinical importance of EOAE measures as part of an audiological evaluation occurs when EOAE results (a) contribute to the diagnosis, or (b) produce changes in medical or audiological management of the patient. Thus, while the benefit of EOAE testing seems limited in the detection of acoustic tumors, this does not diminish the importance of EOAE testing in differential diagnostic testing per se.

Some patients with idiopathic sudden hearing (ISHL) loss have EOAEs, despite sensorineural hearing loss. Sakashita, Minowa, Hachikawa, Kubo, and Nakai (1991) presented data on a control group of 46 patients (50 ears) with long-standing sensorineural hearing loss of unknown causes and an experimental group of 42 patients (43 ears) who suffered from ISHL within 14 days preceding the hearing evaluation. Seven of the 50 ears with long standing hearing loss and 20 of the 43 ears with ISHL had moderate to severe hearing loss >35 dB HL for the frequencies of 0.5 through 4 K Hz. None of the seven ears with long term hearing loss demonstrated EOAES, but 11 (55%) of the ISHL ears had EOAEs. In fact, three ears with EOAEs had hearing losses greater than 80 dB HL for the frequencies of 0.5 through 4 K Hz. Because retrocochlear lesions were ruled out in all patients by measurements such as ABR and computed tomography (CT) scans, Sakashita and coworkers concluded that in patients with ISHL greater than 35 dB HL and with EOAEs, the inner-ear injury was not to the outer hair cells, but to other structures.

Of course, sudden hearing loss may also involve the eighth nerve or central auditory tracts. In the following case examples, EOAEs helped confirm cochlear origin in *Case 1* and *Case 2*, and helped confirm retrocochlear origins in *Case 3* and *Case 4*. In the other cases examples, EOAE findings often altered audiological and medical management.

Case 1

A 60-year-old female suffered a sudden left-ear hearing loss in the 24-hours before the audiological evaluation. As shown in Figure 10–2 (a), hearing sensitivity was within normal limits for the frequencies of 250 through 1000 Hz followed by a precipitous drop to 55 dB HL at 1500 Hz, gradually returning to 25 dB at 8000 Hz. EOAEs were only detected from about 800 to 1300 Hz. Acoustic reflex, reflex decay, and ABR test results were normal. In a follow-up evaluation conducted 1 month, pure-tone thresholds for all tested frequencies were normal. EOAEs also showed a much wider frequency spectrum extending from about 800 to 3000 Hz. The loss of EOAEs corresponding to frequencies of hearing loss and the subsequent return of EOAEs with the recovery of hearing sensitivity supported the conclusion the sudden hearing loss was of cochlear origin.

Case 2

A 36-year-old male was awaken in the middle of the night by an intense ringing tinnitus in his left ear, and he subsequently experienced a sense of hearing loss in that year. He went to the audiology center in the morning. Pure-tone audiometry corroborated his complaint of an acute loss of hearing (albeit mild), which appeared as a notch around 2 kHz (Figure 10–3). From the patient's history and the results of follow-up ABR testing (which were negative [Figure 10–4A]), the loss was concluded to be of cochlear origin. The DPOAE results, which showed a corresponding frequency "island" of depression (Figure 10–4B), confirmed the diagnosis and suggested that the outer hair cells were the specific site of the lesion. Within a week, the patient experienced complete recovery of hearing, as confirmed by the retest audiogram. The DPOAE amplitude at this juncture also had nearly completely recovered. This case demonstrates the sensitivity of EOAE tests to cochlear lesions.

Case 3

A self-referred 30-year-old male was seen in the Otolaryngology Department, reporting sudden left-ear hearing loss, vertigo, and constant, intolerable left-ear tinnitus. The onset had occurred the previous month. He was in a wheelchair and reported that he had multiple sclerosis. The results of a physical examination of the ears, nose, and throat was negative. Clinical fistula-test results were difficult to interpret, but were judged to be negative. An audiological evaluation (Figure 10–5) revealed a profound hearing loss for the left ear (95–115 dB HL from 250–2000 Hz; speech awareness occurred at 80 dB HL). The right ear showed normal hearing through 4000 Hz, a 6000 Hz notch, and normal hearing at 8000 Hz. Tympanometry was normal bilaterally; no acoustic reflexes were obtained when the left ear was stimulated. The pure-tone Stenger test results were negative. Results from a CT

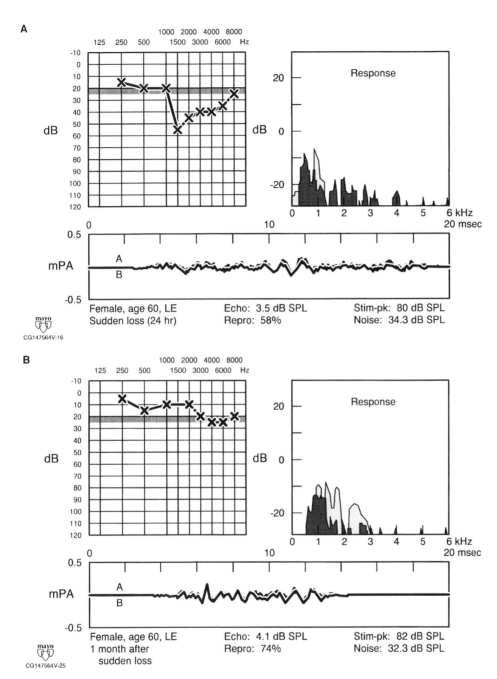

Figure 10-2. (Case 1) Audiometric and TEOAE findings for a 60-year-old woman with a sudden left ear hearing loss. *A*: The box labeled *Response* shows the frequency spectrum of the TEOAE as the light shaded area under the curve; the noise spectrum is indicated by the dark area. Below the *Response* box is the replicated echo shown in the time domain from 2.5 ms to 20 ms following each stimulus pulse. *B*: Results of a 1-month follow-up evaluation. (Adapted from Robinette, 1992a. Used with permission.)

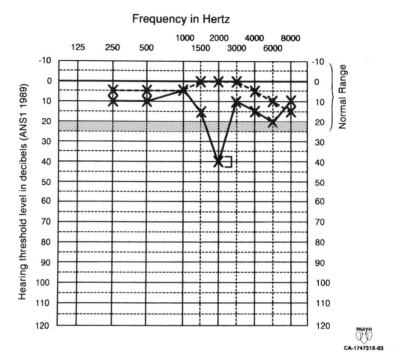

Figure 10–3. (Case 2) Pure-tone audiometry results for a 36-year-old man with a mild left ear hearing loss of sudden onset. Solid line shows sudden loss audiogram. Dashed line shows follow-up audiogram one week later.

scan of the head, with high-resolution views of the petrous bone, were negative. Review of a magnetic resonance imaging (MRI) study that he brought with him showed widespread increased T_2 signal, consistent with the previously diagnosed multiple sclerosis.

In light of the negative CT results, the initial clinical impression of the left-ear hearing loss was that is was profound, sudden sensorineural hearing loss either due to multiple sclerosis or possibly cochlear dysfunction, such as a perilymph fistula. However, sudden, profound unilateral hearing loss is not normally associated with multiple sclerosis (Drulovic, Ribaric-Jankes, Kostic, & Sternic, 1994); therefore, a perilymph fistula was suspected.

TEOAEs were measured for both ears (Figure 10–6). The elicited emission amplitudes were nearly identical for the two ears at 11.7 dB for the right ear and 12.0 for the left ear. The TEOAE spectrum was also similar extending from 0.49 to 3.76 K Hz in the right ear and 0.54 to 3.08 K Hz in the left. The TEOAEs were interpreted as being within normal limits for both ears.

The findings of normal TEOAEs in an ear with a profound hearing loss ruled out a perilymph fistula or other cochlear causes, so retrocochlear dysfunction or pseudohypacusis were suspected. But the negative findings for the Stenger test ruled out pseudohypoacusis, and the CT results ruled out a space-occupying

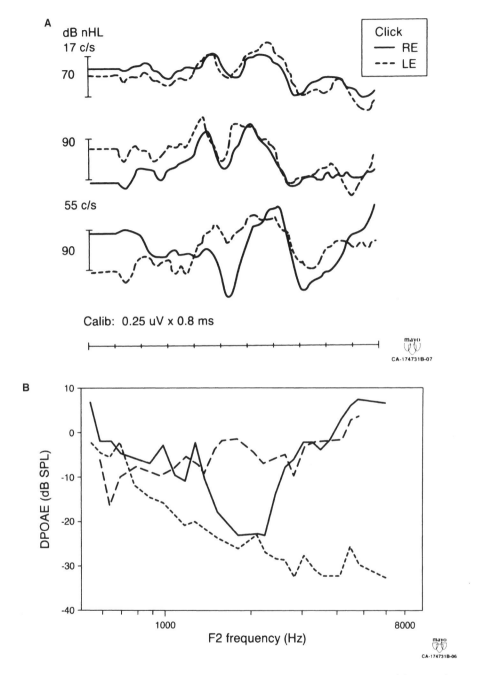

Figure 10–4.   (Case 2) *A*: ABR test results for a 36-year-old man at the time of the initial visit. The ABRs were recorded using a montage of forehead-hairline to ipsilateral mastoid (30–3,000 Hz, −12 dB/OCT, N = 2048). Clicks were presented at 70 and 90 dB nHL at 17.1 per second and 55 per second (90 dB only). *B*: DPOAEs for left ear only. Solid line shows initial visit, and dotted line the noise floor from the initial test.

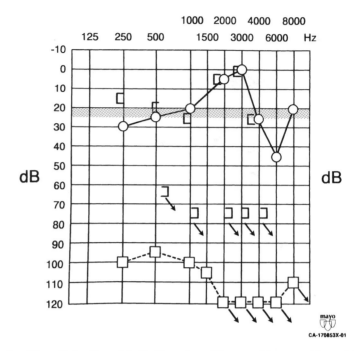

Figure 10–5. (Case 3) Audiometric findings for a 30-year-old man with multiple sclerosis and sudden left-ear hearing loss with roaring tinnitus. (Adapted from Robinette & Facer, 1991. Used with permission.)

lesion. In the final analysis, the hearing loss was concluded to be due to an exacerbation of the multiple sclerosis. Furman, Durrant, and Hirsch (1989) reported a case of multiple sclerosis and root entry involvement of the eight cranial nerve, in which the patient presented with a reversible, profound high-frequency sensorineural-hearing loss. The lesion in that case was vivid in the MRIs.

This patient was treated with a short course of steroids, and 2 weeks later experienced complete recovery of hearing in his left ear. (Adapted from Robinette & Facer, 1991.)

Case 4

A 33-year-old male with a complaint of sudden hearing loss in his left ear that occurred 4 weeks previously was seen for a medical and audiological evaluation. He reported no previous ear problems and had no complaint of vertigo or tinnitus. The results of pure-tone audiometry revealed a mild- to moderate-sensorineural-hearing loss in the left ear. The audiometric configuration for the right ear showed a slight, low frequency loss at 500 Hz and a mild, high frequency hearing loss above 3000 Hz (Figure 10–7). His word recognition score (W-22 lists) was 80% for the left ear and 100% for the right ear at a sensation level of 40 dB SL. Tympanometry indicated normal, bilateral middle-ear functioning. Ipsilateral and contralateral acoustic reflexes were absent for pure-tone stimuli to the left ear.

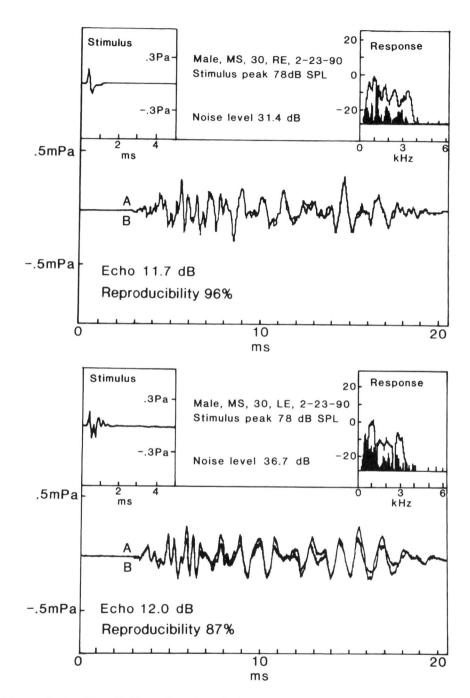

Figure 10–6. (Case 3) Normal TEOAE findings for both ears of a man with multiple sclerosis and profound left-ear sensorineural hearing loss. The box labeled *Response* shows the frequency spectrum of the TEOAE as the unshaded area. (Adapted from Robinette & Facer, 1991. Used with permission.)

TEOAE amplitude for the right ear was 3.6 dB above the noise floor, and the emission-frequency spectrum extended from 1200 through 2300 Hz (Figure 10–7). Left-ear TEOAE amplitude was 4.8 dB above the noise floor, and the emission frequency spectrum extended from 600 through 1200 Hz. DPOAEs were also measured. Primary tones F_1 and F_2 were presented at 70 dB SPL at an F_1/F_2 ratio of 1.2. The evoked distortion product measured at $2F_1 - F_2$ was displayed graphically at the F_2 place (Figure 10–7). In the right ear, DPOAEs were elicited from about 1200 through 1800 Hz and again from 2500 through 4000 Hz. DPOAEs in the left ear were elicited from about 800 through 6000 Hz, with the possible exception of the quarter octave between 3000 and 4000 Hz, where the response was obscured by noise artifact. The combination of the otoacoustic emission measures was interpreted as showing normal to near-normal cochlear functioning for the majority of the frequency range from 1000 through 4000 Hz in each ear, despite the marked difference in pure-tone thresholds between ears.

The ABR results in Figure 10–8 show normal absolute and interpeak wave latencies for the right ear and an abnormal wave I absolute latency of 2.16 ms (normal being <1.88 ms) for the left ear. No other repeatable waveform peaks could be identified for the left ear. An MRI scan showed no lesions in the area of the internal auditory canals, but did show several small- to moderate-size T_2 signal abnormalities in the periventricular white matter of both cerebral hemispheres consistent with the diagnosis of multiple sclerosis.

The prevalence of hearing loss as one of the initial symptoms in persons with multiple sclerosis is estimated to be 1% (Kahana, Leibowitz, & Alter, 1973), and reports of sudden hearing loss as the only initial symptom are particularly rare (Durlovic et al., 1994). For this patient, the evidence suggests that sudden, unilateral hearing loss was the first clinically recognized sign of multiple sclerosis. The disorder is associated with multiple focal demyelinating plaques throughout the white matter of the central nervous system. In order for one or more of the plaques to produce unilateral loss (as occurred in this case and *Case 3*), it has been hypothesized that the lesion must lie distal to the cochlear nucleus complex and central to the neurilemmal-neuroglial junction on the auditory nerve, i.e., the root-entry zone (Antonelli et al., 1986; Furman et al.,1989; Hallpike, 1967; Robinette & Facer).

Case 5 (Deaf Child)

A male infant who initially failed ABR screening bilaterally as a newborn was seen at age 4 months. The audiological evaluation supported the diagnosis of profound hearing loss. No behavioral responses to noisemakers were observed. Tympanometry was normal bilaterally. An ABR evaluation given to the infant while under sedation revealed a questionable response at 95 dB nHL for the right ear and no response for the left ear. Management at this time included a binaural fitting of behind-the-ear (BTE) hearing aids and enrollment in an early-language stimulation program.

On a 10-month follow up, the mother said that she observed a startle response to loud sounds and that he participated in imitative vocal play both with and without his hearing aids. Behavioral audiometry revealed some localization response to

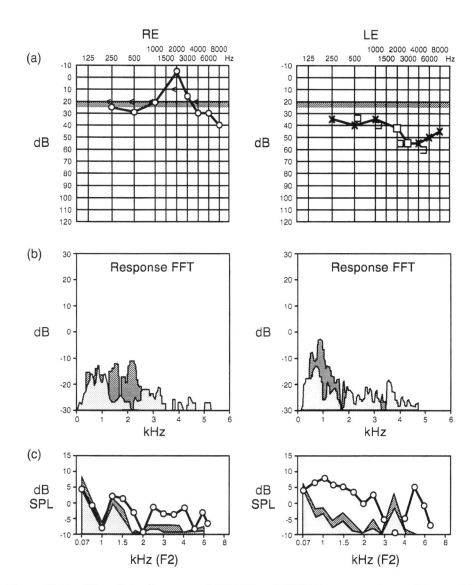

Figure 10–7.   (Case 4) Audiogram and TEOAE and DPOAE measures from a 33-year-old man with sudden left ear hearing loss. *A*: puretone audiogram. *B*: TEOAE frequency spectrum (lightly shaded shows the noise floor; dark area shows emission); *C*: DPOAE (open circles are the cubic distortion product; light and dark areas represent 1 and 2 standard deviations, respectively, above the mean level of the noise). (Adapted from Cevette, Robinette, Carter, & Knops, 1995. Used with permission.)

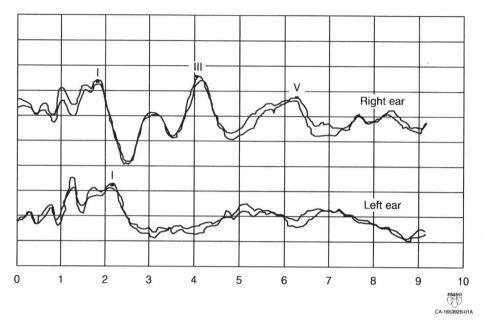

Figure 10–8. (Case 4) ABR tracings for a 33-year-old man with sudden left-ear hearing loss. The top tracings are replicated right ear normal waveforms. The bottom tracings are the replicated abnormal left ear waveforms. Stimuli were rarefaction clicks at a level of 85 dB nHL at a rate of 11.1 per sec. (Adapted from Cevette, Robinette, Carter, & Knops, 1995. Used with permission.)

noise makers (maraca 70 dB SPL). Still, he did not condition for visual reinforcement audiometry (VRA) testing. Another ABR under sedation yielded, again, no response bilaterally. However, ipsilateral acoustic reflexes were elicited bilaterally at 85 to 100 dB HL for 500, 1000, and 2000 Hz tones. Contralateral acoustic reflexes were obtained bilaterally for 2000 Hz at 105 dB HL, but no responses were observed for 500 or 1000 Hz stimulation at 110 dB HL. The acoustic reflex responses were unexpected because of the lack of ABR response. TEOAE testing proved particularly valuable. As shown in Figure 10–9, TEOAEs were present bilaterally. The right-ear emission spectrum covered the range of 1500 through 3500 Hz with an emission amplitude of 11.9 dB SPL. The left-ear emission spectrum covered the range of 1500 through 5000 Hz, with an amplitude of 11.2 dB SPL. For both ears the emission amplitude was more than 3 dB above the uncorrelated noise floor.

The presence of otoacoustic emissions indicated that the severe to profound hearing loss was primarily retrocochlear. One possible explanation of the ABR and acoustic reflex data was that as a consequence of the delayed neurological development eighth-nerve firing to acoustic stimuli occurred with sufficient amplitude to elicit an ipsilateral acoustic reflex, but insufficient synchrony to obtain an ABR. The ability to obtain ipsilateral, but not contralateral, acoustic reflexes in brainstem lesions has been reported (Jerger & Jerger, 1977). The hearing aid use was discontinued.

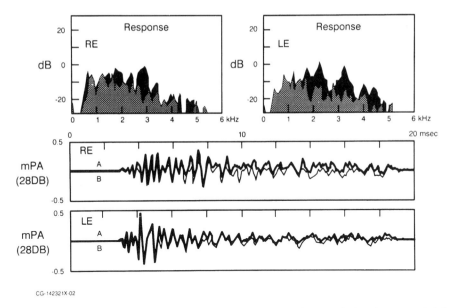

CG-142321X-02

Figure 10–9. (Case 5) TEOAE findings for a 10-month-old boy with developmental delay, seizure disorder, and profound bilateral sensorineural-hearing loss. No response was obtained from ABR testing; however ipsilateral acoustic reflexes were present. The box labeled *Response* shows the frequency spectrum of the TEOAE as the dark area under the curve; the noise spectrum is indicated by the shaded area. Below the *Response* box is the replicated echo shown in the time domain from 2.5 ms to 20 ms following each stimulus pulse. (Adapted from Robinette, 1992b. Used with permission.)

Case 6 (Delayed Speech Development)

The parents of a 15-month-old girl brought their daughter for examination because delayed speech development. They reported a normal birth, postnatal development, and medical evaluations. They also reported that she did not respond consistently to sound and that one needed to tap her shoulder to obtain her attention. Pure-tone Visual Response Audiometry (VRA) testing showed a profound sensorineural-hearing loss (Figure 10–10). Tympanometry was within normal limits, and acoustic reflexes could not be elicited. Four-channel ABR recordings to an 85-dB-nHL rarefaction clicks (Figure 10–11) were also abnormal, with only a reproducible wave I for the right ear. The usual management for a profound hearing loss with absent or questionably absent ABR waveforms is to fit binaural hearing aids, refer the patient for genetic counseling, initiate a language-stimulation program, and consideration a cochlear implant. The measurement of robust normal EOAEs (Figure 10–12), however, altered clinical management considerations. Recommendations included referral for a genetic work-up, a temporal-bone imaging, a vibrotactile type aid to present sound stimuli to the skin, and language stimulation. While not an isolated case (Norton, 1995), this is a rather uncommon case of measured EOAEs for a child with a severe- to profound-hearing loss because their were no indications of any developmental dysfunction, except for the

Female Age 15 Months

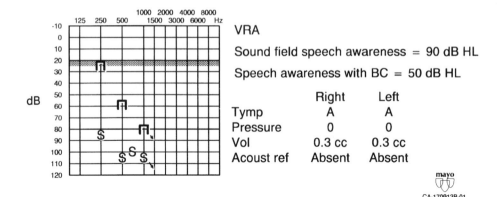

VRA

Sound field speech awareness = 90 dB HL

Speech awareness with BC = 50 dB HL

	Right	Left
Tymp	A	A
Pressure	0	0
Vol	0.3 cc	0.3 cc
Acoust ref	Absent	Absent

CA-170913B-01

Figure 10–10. (Case 6) Visual response audiometry (VRA) and acoustic immittance findings for a 15-month-old girl with delayed speech development.

Female Age 15 Months

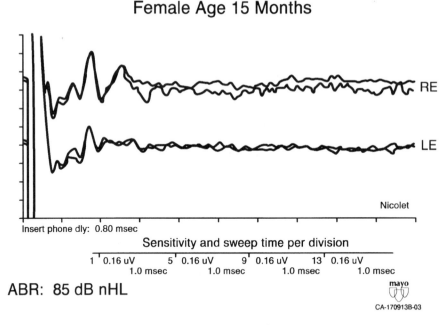

RE

LE

Nicolet

Insert phone dly: 0.80 msec

Sensitivity and sweep time per division

1 0.16 uV	5 0.16 uV	9 0.16 uV	13 0.16 uV
1.0 msec	1.0 msec	1.0 msec	1.0 msec

ABR: 85 dB nHL

CA-170913B-03

Figure 10–11. (Case 6) ABR tracings for a 15-month-old girl with delayed speech development. The top tracings are replicated right-ear waveforms and the bottom are replicated left -ear waveforms. Stimuli were rarefaction clicks at a level of 85 dB nHL at a rate of 11.1 per second. Only wave I for her right ear was judged to be present. The large positive deflection preceding wave I appears to be wave I prime or conceivably the summating potential (Moore, Semela, Rakerd, Robb, & Ananthanarayan, 1992; Schwartz, Morris, & Jacobson, 1994).

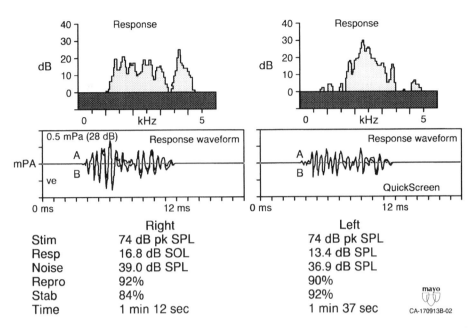

Female Age 15 Months

	Right	Left
Stim	74 dB pk SPL	74 dB pk SPL
Resp	16.8 dB SOL	13.4 dB SPL
Noise	39.0 dB SPL	36.9 dB SPL
Repro	92%	90%
Stab	84%	92%
Time	1 min 12 sec	1 min 37 sec

Figure 10–12. (Case 6) TEOAE findings for a 15-month-old girl with delayed speech development. The box labeled *Response* shows the spectrum of the TEOAE above the subtracted noise floor. Below is the replicated echo shown in the time domain from 2.5 ms to 12.5 ms following each stimulus pulse.

retrocochlear hearing loss. In addition, the child's 5-month-old brother also was evaluated and had similar results (i.e., normal EOAEs and absent ABR and acoustic reflexes). EOAE screening alone would have passed these children, thereby missing the retrocochlear disorder; this case, as well as *Case 6*, are poignant reminders that EOAE measurements reflect responses of the peripheral auditory system through outer hair-cell function.

Case 7 (Congenital "Mixed" Sensory-Neural Hearing Loss)

A 9-year-old boy had been followed audiologically from a young age for a well-documented bilateral, congenital sensorineural-hearing loss. He had suffered repeated ear infections, speech and language delays, and seizures. Over the years, audiometric results became reasonably stable and showed a mild-to-severe high-frequency loss with an intricate configuration on the right (Figure 10–13). ABR tests performed at other facilities had yielded variable results, but were interpreted to suggest retrocochlear involvement (later supported by results of a central auditory processing battery). Speech recognition ability was also quite variable (76–92% on the right and 44–72% on the left). The referring audiologist sought to further clarify the results by defining the cochlear component of the hearing loss (if any)

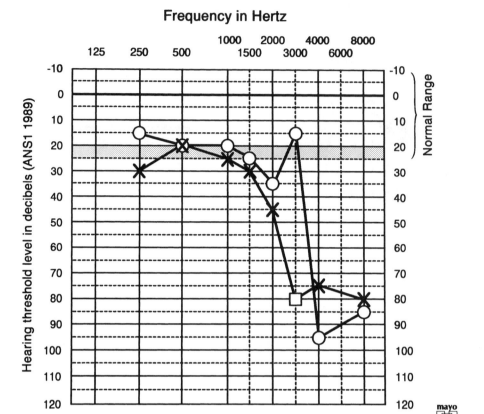

Figure 10–13. (Case 7) Audiogram of a 9-year-old boy having a congenital hearing loss with a central auditory processing disorder.

for which DPOAE testing was proposed. Additional ABR testing at the Center for Audiology failed to demonstrate the presence of any reproducible components in the click-evoked response (Figure 10–14). A 1-kHz tone pip evoked a small response, but its latency was delayed. The DPOAE results (Figure 10–15) suggested some probable end-organ involvement, but, the DPOAEs (above 3 kHz) were not depressed to the extent expected from the audiogram. The results were interrupted to reflect a mixed sensory-neural hearing loss.

Naturally, a considerable concern of the audiologist was the appropriateness of hearing aids in this case. The DPOAE findings helped to validate the decision to use hearing aids.

The patient was reexamined several years later at the Medical Center. The hearing loss was essentially symmetrical: The hearing in the right ear had decreased, and the left hear had changed little. DPOAEs were barely detectable only above 4 kHz in the right ear and not detectable in the left ear. The results were taken to indicate that the progression hearing loss was cochlear and further justifying the use of hearing aids.

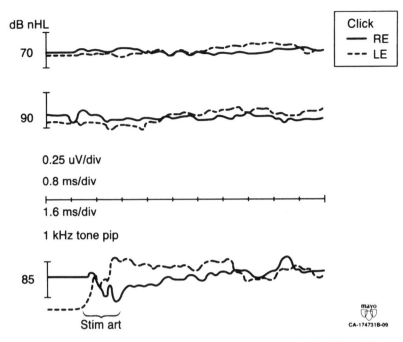

Figure 10–14. (Case 7) ABR test results using clicks at 70 and 90 dBn HL at 17.1 per second and the tone pips of 1 kHz at 85 dB. These results were interpreted to reflect no significant response by click stimulation and questionable with tone pips.

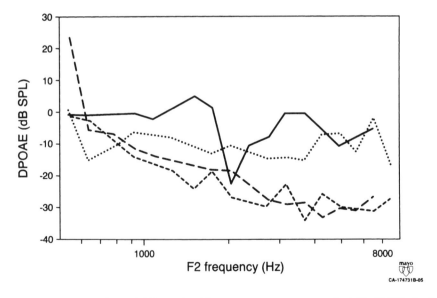

Figure 10–15. (Case 7) DPOAE results. Test tones were presented at 65 dB SPL for both primarlis with $F_2/F_1 = 1.2$. Solid line represents right ear DPOAE amplitude, and the dotted line left ear amplitude. The long and short dashed lines represent the noise floor for the right and left ears respectively.

Case 8: (Cochlear Implant Candidate)

A 28-year-old female woman with a profound bilateral sensorineural-hearing loss was brought by her parents to the Clinic to seek advice about cochlear implants. The patient suffered the hearing loss three years previously because of an automobile accident. She was a quadriplegic with some upper-left and lower-extremity motion. Results of a physical examination of the ears, nose, and throat were negative. Binaural BTEs had been tried and were reported not to help. A behavioral audiological evaluation suggested a bilateral profound hearing loss (Figure 10–16). The patient was nonverbal; responses were head nods to pure-tone stimuli. Tympanometry was normal bilaterally, and acoustic reflex thresholds suggested that her hearing sensitivity was better than found during audiometric testing. Specifically, contralateral–acoustic reflex thresholds to right ear stimulation were 95, 95, 95, and 110 dB HL for the frequencies of 500, 1000, 2000, and 4000 Hz, respectively. For the left ear, acoustic reflexes were observed for 105, 110 dB HL for tones at 500 and 1000 Hz, respectively. No acoustic reflex responses were obtained at 110 dB HL for 2000 or 4000 Hz. ABR testing was attempted both without and with sedation. However, excessive myogenic activity made ABR interpretation impos-

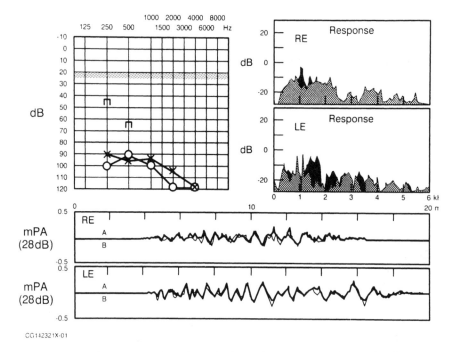

CG142321X-01

Figure 10–16. Audiometric and TEOAE findings for a 28-year-old quadriplegic woman, under review as a cochlear implant candidate. The box labeled *Response* shows the frequency spectrum of the TEOAE as the dark area under the curve; the noise spectrum is indicated by the shaded area. Below the *Response* box is the replicated echo shown in the time domain from 2.5 ms to 20 ms following each stimulus pulse. (Adapted from Robinette, 1992b. Used with permission.)

sible. TEOAEs were observed bilaterally. The left ear emission spectrum covered the range of 1000 through 3500 Hz, with an emission amplitude of 9.7 dB SPL. A smaller TEOAE was recorded from the right ear, with an emission spectrum of only 1000 through 1500 Hz, and an amplitude of 5.8 dB SPL. For both ears, the emission amplitude was more than 3 dB above the uncorrelated noise floor. The results were interpreted as showing normal cochlear functioning for the left ear and some cochlear functioning for the right ear. The presence of EOAEs indicated that the profound hearing loss was primarily retrocochlear. Therefore, the TEOAE test results clearly demonstrated that a cochlear implant was not warranted. The surgery not only would have destroyed a satisfactorily functioning cochlea, but the cochlear implant would have failed because of the retrocochlear dysfunction.

Case 9 (Adult With Viral Neuritis Due to Human Immunodeficiency Virus Infection)

A 35-year-old male with the complaint of nasal and left-aural fullness was seen for an audiological evaluation. He already had been diagnosed as with human immunodeficiency virus (HIV) infection. Several days later, he developed a hearing loss in his left ear and dizziness (Figure 10–17). His speech-recognition ability was within normal limits.

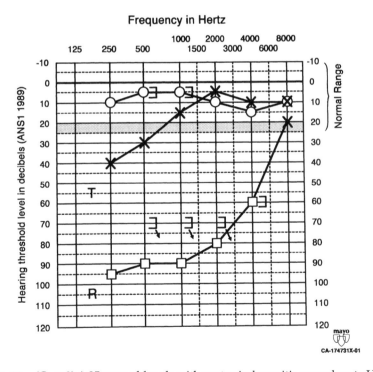

Figure 10–17.   (Case 9) A 35-year-old male with acute viral neuritis secondary to HIV+. The initial test (T) audiogram and the retest (R) four days later following complaint of worsening symptoms.

ABR testing demonstrated normal responses on the right, but little reproducible response after wave I (Figure 10–18). Electrocochleography demonstrated robust compound-action potentials bilaterally; the DPOAE results demonstrated symmetrical distortion product (DP)–grams in contrast to the considerable audiometric asymmetry (Figure 10–19). About 1 month later, an audiogram showed that the hearing loss in the left ear had profoundly deteriorated, but the DPOAE output was unchanged. The results were taken to suggest this case to be an eighth-nerve–lesion or "disconnect" syndrome. Indeed, MRI demonstrated an enhancement in the cerebellopontine angle. (Adapted from Hirsch, Durrant, Yetiser, Kamerer, and Martin, 1996.)

Case 10 (Nonverbal Adult)

A 46-year-old female patient was referred to a clinic for EOAE testing only. She was previously diagnosed with mild-to-moderate mental retardation, essentially nonverbal, and hearing-impaired. Specifically, ABR testing 8 years previously suggested severe-to-profound bilateral hearing loss. Recently, however, behavioral audiometry yielded the impression of a "less than profound hearing loss." Hearing aids had been tried, but were not tolerated by the patient. Interestingly, the staff that provided her care indicated that she often responded to her name when

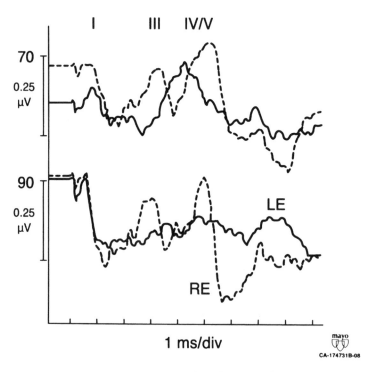

Figure 10–18. (Case 9) ABR testing obtained at the time of the "retest" (R) audiogram (Figure 10–17). Click stimuli were at 70 and 90 dBn HL and a rate of 17.1 per second.

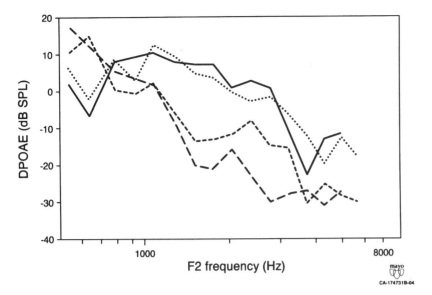

Figure 10–19. (Case 9) DPOAE results from a HIV-infected man at the time of the "retest" (R) audiogram (Figure 10–17). Primary tones were presented at 65 dB SPL with $f_1/f_2 = 1.2$. Solid line represents right ear DPOAE amplitude, and dotted line left ear amplitude. The long and short dashed lines represent the noise floor for the right and left ears, respectively.

spoken at normal conversational levels and that on rare occasions she had spoken with essentially normal articulation and voice quality. Another auditory assessment had been performed just before this referral (Figure 10–20). Play audiometry revealed a mild to moderate sensorineural hearing loss. Tympanograms were normal, but acoustic reflexes were absent. In addition, to the previous auditory assessment, TEOAE and DPOAE analysis was conducted (Figure 10–20). The EOAEs were robust and suggested normal to near-normal cochlear functioning. This information was valuable to the referring audiologist and led to a revision of diagnosis and to the discontinuation of recommendations for amplification.

Summary and Conclusions

The clinical value of EOAEs is the opportunity (under conditions of normal external and middle ear function) to separately assess sensory function and, specifically, to document normal to near-normal cochlear function. An additional value is that the clinical measurement is objective, efficient, and noninvasive. The disadvantage, however, is that the absence of EOAEs does not reflect the actual magnitude of the sensory component of the hearing loss (i.e., mild, moderate, severe, or profound).

Even with this limitation, in the 10 case examples presented in this chapter, the employment of EOAEs as part of the diagnostic test battery helped confirm the cochlear, retrocochlear, or mixed origin of the disorders. Researchers have much to learn about the usefulness of this new clinical tool. The data presented here from

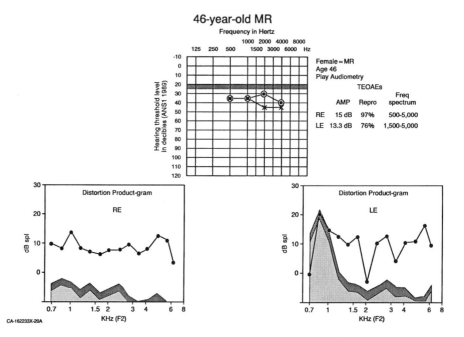

Figure 10–20. (Case 10) Play audiometry and TEOAE and DPOAE findings for a 46-year-old woman, reported as non-verbal, hearing impaired, and mentally retarded. On the distortion product–gram, circles represent the cubic distortion product, light and dark shaded areas represent 1 and 2 standard deviations, respectively, above the mean level of the noise.

patients with surgically removed acoustic neuromas and patients with other retro-cochlear hearing loss provides clear evidence of the increasing value of EOAE measures in audiological evaluations.

References

Antonelli, A. R., Bellotto, R., Bertazzoli, M., Busnelli, G. P., Nunez Castro, M., Felisali, G., & Romagnoli, M. (1986). Auditory brainstem response test battery for multiple sclerosis patients: evaluation of test findings and assessment of diagnostic criteria. *Audiology, 25,* 227–238.

Arts, H. A., Norton, S. J., & Rubel, E. W. (1990). Influence of perilymphatic tetrodotoxin and calcium concentration on hair cell function. *Abstracts of the thirteenth midwinter meeting: Association for Research in Otolaryngology 13th ARO mid-winter meeting.*

Bonfils, P., & Uziel, A. (1988). Evoked otoacoustic emissions in patients with acoustic tumors. *American Journal of Otology, 9,* 412–417.

Cane, M. A. Lutman, M. E., & O'Donoghue, G. M. (1994). Transiently evoked otoacoustic emissions in patients with cerebellopontine angle tumors. *The American Journal of Otology, 15,* 207–216.

Cane, M. A., O'Donoghue, G. M., & Lutman, M. E. (1992). The feasibility of using evoked oto-acoustic emissions to monitor cochlear function during acoustic neuroma surgery. *Scandinavian Audiology, 21,* 173–176.

Cevette, M. J., Robinette, M. S., Carter, J., & Knops, J. L. (1995). Otoacoustic emissions in sudden unilateral hearing loss associated with multiple sclerosis. *Journal of the American Academy of Audiology, 6,* 197–202.

Collet, L., Veuillet, E., Bene, J., & Morgon, A. (1992). Effects of contralateral white noise on click-evoked emissions in normal and sensorineural ears: towards an exploration of the medial olivocochlear system. *Audiology, 31*, 1–7.

Durrant, J. D. (1992) Distortion-product OAE analysis: is it ready for broad clinical use? *The Hearing Journal, 45*, 42–45.

Durrant, J. D., Kamerer, D. B., & Chen, D. (1993). Combined OAE and ABR studies in acoustic tumor patients. In D. Hoehmann (ed.), *ECoG, OAE and intraoperative monitoring* (pp. 231–239). Amsterdam: Kugler.

Durrant, J. D., & Wolf, K. E. (1991). Auditory evoked potentials: Basic aspects. In W. F. Rintlemann (ed.), *Hearing assessment* (2nd ed., pp. 321–381). Austin: Pro-Ed.

Durlovic, B., Ribaric-Jankes, K., Kostic, V., & Sternic, N. (1994). Multiple sclerosis as the cause of sudden "pontine" deafness. *Audiology, 33*, 195–201.

Furman, J. F. R., Durrant, J. D., & Hirsch, W. L. (1989) Eighth nerve signs in a case of multiple sclerosis. *American Journal of Otolaryngology, 10*, 376–381.

Geisler, C. D. (1985). A model of the effect of outer hair cell motility on cochlear vibrations. *Hearing Research, 6*, 35–39.

Jacobson, G. P., Jacobson, J. T., Ramadan, N., & Hyde, M. (1994). Auditory brainstem response measures in acoustic nerve and brainstem disease. In J. T. Jacobson (ed.), *Principles and applications in auditory evoked potentials* (pp. 387–486). Boston: Allen & Bacon.

Jerger, S., & Jerger, J. F. (1977). Diagnostic value of crossed vs. uncrossed acoustic reflexes. *Archives of Otolaryngology, 103*, 445–453.

Hallpike, C. S. (1967). The loudness recruitment phenomenon: A clinical contribution to the neurology of hearing. In A. B. Graham (ed.), *Sensorineural hearing processes and disorders* (pp. 488–99). Boston: Little, Brown.

Hirsch, B. E., Durrant, J. D., Yetiser, S., Kamerer, D. B., & Martin, W. H. (1996). Localizing retrocochlear hearing loss. *American Journal of Otology*, in press.

Kahana, E., Leibowitz , U., & Alter, M. (1973). Brainstem and cranial nerve involvement in multiple sclerosis. *Acta Neurology Scandinavian, 49*, 269–279.

Kemp, D. E. (1978). Stimulated acoustic emissions from within the human auditory system. *Journal of the Acoustical Society of America, 64*, 1386–1391.

Kemp, D. E. (1988). Developments in cochlear mechanics and techniques in noninvasive evaluation. *Advances in Audiology, 5*, 27–45.

Kileny, P. (1995, April). Recent trends in clinical auditory neurodiagnostic measures. Presented at American Academy of Audiology Seventh Annual Convention, Dallas, TX.

Kim, D. O. (1980). Cochlear Mechanics: Implications of electrophysiological and acoustical observations. *Hearing Research, 2*, 297–317.

Levine, R. A., Ojemann, R. G., Montgomery, W. W., & McGaffigan, P. M. (1984). Monitoring auditory evoked potentials during acoustic neuroma surgery: Insights into the mechanism of the hearing loss. *Annals of Otology, Rhinology and Laryngology, 93*, 116–123.

Lutman, M. E., Mason, S. M., Sheppard, S., & Gibbin, K. P. (1989). Differential diagnostic potential of otoacoustic emissions: A case study. *Audiology, 28*, 205–210.

Moore, E. J., Semela, J. J. M., Rakerd, B., Robb, R. C., & Anathanarayan, A. K. (1992). The I' potential of the brain-stem auditory-evoked potential. *Scandinavian Audiology, 21*, 153–156.

Neely, S. T., & Kim, D. O. (1986). A model for active elements in cochlear biomechanics. *Journal of the Acoustical Society of America, 79*, 1472–1480.

Norton, S. J. (1992). Cochlear function and otoacoustic emissions. *Seminars in Hearing, 13*, 1–14.

Norton, S. J. (1995). Personal communication.

Ohlms, L. A., Lonsbury-Martin, B. L., & Martin, G. K. (1991). Acoustic distortion products: Separation of sensory from neural dysfunction in sensorineural hearing loss in humans and rabbits. *Otolaryngology—Head and Neck Surgery, 104*, 159–174.

Prasher, D. K., Tun, T., Brookes, G. B., & Luxon, L. M. (1995). Mechanisms of hearing loss in acoustic neuroma: An otoacoustic emission study, *Acta Oto-Laryngologica, 115*, 375–381.

Probst, R. (1990). Otoacoustic emissions: An overview. *Advances in Oto-Rhino-Laryngology, 44*, 1–91.

Probst, R., Lonsbury-Martin, B. L., & Martin, G. K. (1991). A review of otoacoustic emissions. *Journal of the Acoustical Society of America, 89*, 2027–2067.

Raffin, M. J. M., & Thornton, A. R. (1980). Confidence levels for differences between speech-discrimination scores: A research note. *Journal of Speech and Hearing Research, 23*, 5–18.

Robinette, M. S. (1992a). Clinical observations with transient evoked otoacoustic emissions with adults. *Seminars in Hearing, 13*, 23–26.

Robinette, M. S. (1992b). Otoacoustic emissions in cochlear vs. retrocochlear auditory dysfunction. *The Hearing Journal, 45*, 32–34.

Robinette, M. S., & Bauch, C. B. (1991, April). Pre- and postoperative EOAE and ABR results on selected patients with eighth nerve tumors. Poster presented at Third Annual Convention of the American Academy of Audiology, Denver, CO.

Robinette, M. S., Bauch, C. B., Olsen, W. O., Harner, S. G., & Beatty, C. W. (1992). Use of TEOAE, ABR, and acoustic reflex measures to assess auditory function in patients with acoustic neuroma. *American Journal of Audiology, 1*, 66–72.

Robinette, M. S., Bauch, C. B., Olsen, W. O., Harner, S. G., & Beatty, C. W. (1996, May 4). Non-surgical factors predictive of postoperative hearing for vestibular schwannoma patients. *American Neutrology Society* Scientific Program, Orlando, FL.

Robinette, M. S., & Facer, G. W. (1991). Evoked otoacoustic emissions in differential diagnosis: A case report. *Otolaryngology—Head & Neck Surgery, 105*, 120–123.

Rossi, R., Actis, P., Solero, M., Rolando, M. D., & Pejrone, M. D. (1993). Cochlear interdependence and micromechanics in man and their relations with the activity of the medial olivocochlear efferent system (MOES). *The Journal of Laryngology and Otology, 107*, 883–891.

Sakashita T., Minowa, Y., Hachikawa, K., Kubo, T., & Nakai, Y. (1991). Evoked otoacoustic emissions from ears with idiopathic sudden deafness. *Acta Oto-Laryngologica, 486* (Suppl.), 66–72.

Schwartz, D. M., Morris, M. D., & Jacobson, J. T. (1994). The normal auditory brainstem response and its variants. In J. T. Jacobson (Ed.), *Principles and applications in auditory evoked potentials* (p. 144). Boston: Allyn & Bacon.

Silman, S., & Gelfand, S. A. (1981). The relationship between magnitude of hearing loss and acoustic reflex threshold levels. *Journal of Speech and Hearing Disorders, 46*, 312–316.

Telischi, F. F., Roth, J., Stagner, B. B., Lonsbury-Martin, B. L., & Balkany, T. J. (1995). Patterns of evoked otoacoustic emissions associated with acoustic neuromas. *Laryngoscope, 105*, 675–682.

Telischi, F. F., Widick, M. P., Lonsbury-Martin, B., and McCoy, M. J. (1995). Monitoring cochlear function intraoperatively using distortion product otoacoustic emissions. *American Journal of Otology, 16*, 597–608.

Turner, R. G., Shepard, F. T., and Frazer, C. J. (1984). Clinical performance of audiological and related diagnostic tests. *Ear and Hearing, 5*, 187–194.

11

Neonatal Screening via Evoked Otoacoustic Emissions

N. Brandt Culpepper

Introduction

One widespread clinical application of evoked otoacoustic emissions (EOAEs) is the detection of peripheral auditory dysfunction in neonatal-hearing screening programs. Numerous investigations and clinical experiences in hospital-based programs have demonstrated that EOAEs have many favorable attributes for use with neonates, particularly transient evoked otoacoustic emissions (TEOAEs). The use of distortion product otoacoustic emissions (DPOAEs) has also been suggested for newborn-hearing screening and has been attempted to a limited degree. This chapter focuses on some of the clinical, practical, and logistical issues surrounding the use of EOAEs with neonates and summarizes the issues of establishing an EOAE-based neonatal hearing screening program.

Early Identification and Intervention

Although early identification has been advocated in the United States since 1947 (Ewing & Ewing, 1947), recent estimates suggest that less than 3% of all newborns are screened for hearing loss (Bess, 1993). The unsatisfactory situation has not improved substantially over the past fifty years. Programs have traditionally targeted only neonates and infants at risk for hearing loss (American Speech-Language-Hearing Association [ASHA], 1989, 1991), despite the fact that using a high-risk based approach has a maximum potential of identifying only 50% of infants with hearing loss (Elssmann, Matkin, & Sabo, 1987; Mauk, White, Mortensen, & Behrens, 1991). Unfortunately, many parents and caretakers do not bring their infants in for the necessary follow-up visits. For example, in Utah's High-Risk Hearing Screening program, which is known for its longevity (it was founded in 1978) and its relative success, only about a quarter of the infants who are invited to come back for audiological testing actually do so, despite extensive follow-up efforts. Based on prevalence data that assumes that 3 to 4 per 1000 infants will have hearing loss, (Culpepper, 1995), however, the program identifies only 10% of the infants who have congenital hearing impairments (Mahoney, 1993).

In the United States, the average age at which children with significant hearing impairment are identified is estimated as being between 18 and 30 months of age (U.S. Department of Health and Human Services, Public Health Service, 1990; Strong, Clark, Johnson, Watkins, Barringer, & Walden, 1994. Until recently, universal detection of hearing loss in all live-births was not considered feasible due to the validity, practicality, and cost efficiency of existing techniques. Although some professionals disagree that universal neonatal hearing screening is justified (Bess & Paradise, 1994), many professionals from across disciplines are advocating screening for all neonates (Goldberg, 1993; Meister, 1993; Northern & Hayes, 1994; Robinette, 1994; Robins, 1990, 1991; White & Behrens, 1993; White & Maxon, 1995). EOAEs may finally provide the health care system in the United States the impetus necessary to reduce the average age of identification of hearing loss to 12 months of age, in accordance with goal 17.16 in *Healthy People 2000* (U.S. Department of Health and Human Services, Public Health Service, 1990). As the former Surgeon General of the United States Koop stated in 1993:

"The power and convenience of TEOAE as a newborn screening tool solves many of the most persistent problems that have prevented us from identifying children with hearing impairments before their first birthdays. With this new tool and our continued efforts, the goal we set in 1989, which many thought was unattainable, can become a reality by the year 2000."

Neonatal Otoacoustic Emissions

Otoacoustic emissions (OAEs) measurable in healthy adult ears are also measurable in healthy neonatal ears, including spontaneous OAEs (SOAEs) and the EOAEs, which include TEOAEs, DPOAEs, and stimulus frequency otoacoustic emissions (SFOAEs). Several consistent differences may be noted, however, between neonatal OAEs and adult OAEs. Owing in part to anatomical differences, emission response amplitudes from neonates are greater by 10 dB or more and typically have a higher resonant frequency for both the stimulus and the response spectra than EOAEs observed for adults (Figure 11–1). In addition, adult responses often have notches while neonates typically have smooth, flat response spectra (Burns, Arehart, & Campbell, 1991; Kemp, Ryan, & Bray, 1990; Norton & Widen, 1990; Prieve, 1992).

Although the presence of SOAEs is good indicator of a normal, healthy cochlea (Bonfils, 1989) and middle-ear system, they have limited value for use for neonatal hearing detection because current measuring techniques do not detect SOAEs in all ears with normal hearing. Therefore, the use of SOAEs in screening programs would result in excess referrals. Similarly, SFOAEs are not likely to be widely used for neonatal hearing screening because they provide similar information to that provided by TEOAEs, but require more time to record and more complex calculations to separate stimulus from response. The two remaining forms of EOAEs— TEOAEs and DPOAEs—remain to be considered for neonatal hearing screening.

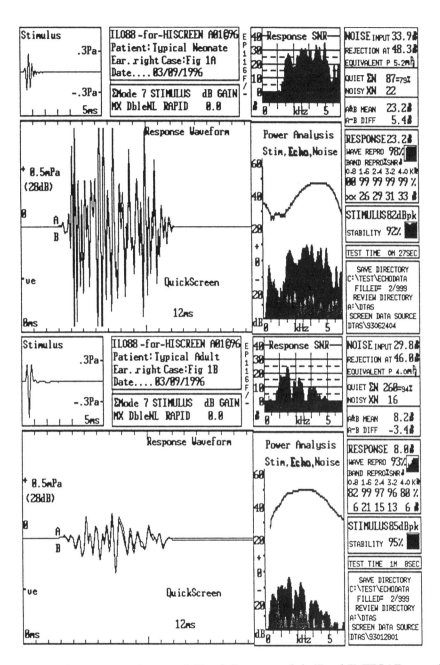

Figure 11–1. Comparison of neonatal (*Panel A*) versus adult (*Panel B*) TEOAEs recorded using *Quickscreen*. Notice the neonatal response has higher frequency stimulus and response spectral maximums. The neonatal response is also more robust than the adult TEOAE.

Although several reports have appeared regarding the use of DPOAEs with neonates (Brass & Kemp, 1994; Lafreniere, Jung, Smurzynski, Leonard, Kim, & Sasek, 1991; Lasky, Perlman, & Hecox, 1992; Popelka, Karzon, & Arjmand, 1995; Smurzynski, 1994; Smurzynski et al., 1993), TEOAEs are the most thoroughly investigated OAE regarding the screening of peripheral auditory functioning of neonates (Bonfils, Uziel, & Pujol, 1988; Johnsen, Bagi, Parbo, & Eberling, 1983; Norton, 1994; Stevens, Webb, Hutchison, Connell, Smith, & Buffin, 1989, 1990; White & Behrens, 1993; White, Vohr, Maxon, Behrens, McPherson, & Mauk, 1994). Because of the overwhelming abundance of literature and clinical experience regarding the successful use of TEOAEs in neonatal hearing screening programs, this chapter will primarily focus on TEOAEs. There are still relatively few published studies regarding the use of DPOAEs for neonatal screening, no large clinical trials have been completed, and few reports of studies including follow-up behavioral auditory assessments of the infants. Even so, many of the basic-screening concepts and program elements discussed in this chapter will be similar for using DPOAEs for neonatal screening and some will also be relevant for screening programs using auditory brainstem response (ABR) or automated ABR measures.

The only commercially available equipment clinically available for recording TEOAEs in the United States is the ILO88 Otodynamic Analyzer. DPOAE systems are commercially available from Grason-Stadler, Virtual, Biologic, Etymotic Research, and Madsen, in addition to Otodynamics. It is also important to recognize that the measurement of EOAEs is still being refined. Advances in the knowledge base and improvements in technology, instrumentation, and software are inevitable. For instance, recent investigations in adults have demonstrated that EOAEs may be recorded at more rapid stimulus rates using clicks presented according to maximum length sequences (Picton, Kellett, Vezsenyi, & Rabinovitch, 1993). Additionally, new software that integrates the screening software with a database tracking system for data management has already been distributed. Although it may seem at times impossible to keep up with continuous advances, persons who develop an understanding of the concepts fundamental to EOAEs and to audition should make transitions with relative ease. Indeed, the majority of the software modifications stem from requests and feedback obtained from personnel using the system. Although computer hardware which provides expanded capabilities consistently is being developed, changes in the hardware needed to measure EOAEs are not anticipated. Therefore, programs that have purchased systems may need to upgrade software on occasion, but it is unlikely that existing hardware will need to be replaced.

Establishing a Universal Neonatal Hearing Screening Program

There are several steps or phases that must be completed in the establishment of universal neonatal-hearing screening programs. The phases may or may not follow an anticipated time line, and phases assumed to be completed may have to be reentered repeatedly. The steps in developing a program are: (a) financing, (b) preparation, (c) organization and training, (d) implementation, and (e) quality assurance.

Financing

Third party reimbursement for performing EOAEs is not firmly established in the United States. However, in December 1993, Rhode Island was successful in passing legislation requiring that all health insurers cover newborn hearing screening as a reimbursable benefit. States that can include a similar provision will have a financial foundation that will allow their neonatal hearing screening programs to become largely self-sustaining (Johnson, Mauk, Takekawa, Simon, Sia, & Blackwell, 1993). One event that assisted the use of EOAEs for neonatal hearing screening was the publication of Common Procedural Terminology (CPT) codes for otoacoustic emissions (limited and comprehensive) in the 1995 CPT manual (Table 11–1) (ASHA, 1994). The availability of CPT and other classifications (e.g., the ninth revision of International Classification of Diseases and Related Health Problems [ICD-9]) is an important development for obtaining reimbursement for services provided from governmental health-care providers and insurance carriers.

One important issue about the financial aspects of a massive screening program using EOAEs is the cost of performing the procedure for each child. Although several estimates have been reported in the literature, the individuality of each program requires a cautious approach when estimating the procedural expense for each program. As stated in the 1994 Position Statement by the Joint Committee on Infant Hearing (JCIH):

"Cost/benefit analysis of infant hearing programs should include consideration of direct cost assessment, identification, and intervention. In addition, it may be valuable to determine the cost savings that accompany early detection and the subsequent management of the child with hearing loss. Each infant hearing program should develop the cost/benefit analysis associated with its specific protocol. The results of cost/benefit analysis vary widely because of differences in protocol, location, geographic and economic considerations, and other factors." (p. 153)

The Rhode Island Hearing Assessment Program (described in White, Vohr, & Behrens, 1993), uses TEOAE for first-stage screening, TEOAE rescreening for those who are referred, followed by ABR for those who again fail. Their estimated total costs for completing the screening was $26.05 per infant screened (Maxon, White, Behrens, & Vohr, 1995). These estimates include equipment amortization, screening supplies, hospital overhead, and all requisite personnel (Table 11–2). Another estimate, which used the same pass-refer statistics as those in Rhode Island and a protocol including the fees of the diagnostic audiological and medical evaluation in a different setting (the Mayo Clinic), calculated a screening cost of $36 per infant (Robinette, 1994). A third estimate from the Hearing Health Institute in Fort Worth,

Table 11–1.   CPT Codes for Otoacoustic Emissions*

92587	Evoked otoacoustic emissions; limited (single stimulus level, either transient or distortion product).
92588	comprehensive or diagnostic evaluation (comparison of transient and/or distortion product otoacoustic emissions at multiple levels and frequencies).

1996 nosology

Table 11–2. Actual Costs of Operating
a Universal Newborn-Hearing Screening Program*

	Cost**
Personnel: screening technicians (avg. 103 hrs./week), clerical (avg. 60 hrs./week), audiologist (avg. 18 hrs./week), coordinator (avg. 20 hrs./week),	$ 60,654
Fringe benefits (28% of salaries)	16,983
Supplies, telephone, postage	12,006
Equipment	6,575
Hospital overhead (24% of salaries)	14,557
Total cost	**$110,775**

*Costs incurred at Women and Infants Hospital of Rhode Island from July 1, 1993 to December 31, 1993.

**Cost Per Infant Screened = $26.05.

Texas, included the costs of the initial screening, but not costs of clerical time for data management, equipment, or supervision. That estimate was given as $13.65 per neonate (Albright, Allen, Carlock, Wolters, & Finitzo, 1995).

Another way of preparing estimates of program finances is to consider screening costs according to category (White, 1995). Figure 11–2 illustrates the percentage of costs allocated to each category for Women and Infants' Hospital of Rhode Island. From the data, it is apparent that the majority of the costs associated with a screening program accrue to salary expense. If a program plans to utilize existing personnel to conduct the hearing screening program rather than hiring more staff, it may also be useful to estimate of staff time necessary for operating a successful TEOAE-neonatal hearing screening program. For every 1000 babies born annually in a hospital, it is estimated that a 0.25 Full Time Equivalent (FTE) is needed for TEOAE screening, a 0.15 FTE is needed for clerical assistance, and audiologist or coordinator support would require a 0.10 FTE (White, 1995).

Although information from other programs may be reviewed to determine what financial issues needed to be considered, it must be remembered that each program is unique. In many hospitals it is often difficult to determine which services are and which services are not being reimbursed during the neonatal period. As such, it is not advisable to wait until all questions are answered before beginning programs, because the universal hearing screening programs may be delayed indefinitely. There are, however, three financial aspects of the program that need exploration prior to program initiation. The first is patient demographics, related to population enrollment in different types of insurance programs, such as diagnostically related groups (DRGs), health maintenance organizations (HMOs), Medicaid, and other insurance carriers. Second, what are the reimbursement policies and schedules of the various local agencies and insurance carriers for neonatal hearing screening? Third, do hospital accounting procedures itemize services and allocate reimbursement to specific programs? Programs may find it advantageous to have a standing order stating that hearing screenings will be performed as a standard of care for all neonates before discharge from the hospital nursery.

Cost of Universal Newborn Hearing Screening According to Category

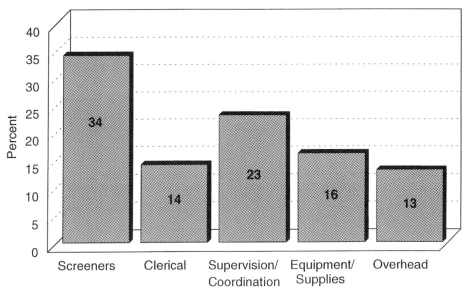

Figure 11–2. Percentage of cost by category for universal newborn hearing screening in the Rhode Island Hearing Assessment Program.

Preparation

When preparing to initiate a neonatal hearing screening program, there are numerous factors that must be considered. While it is not necessary to develop a program entirely from scratch, there is no single "packet" or "module" that can be plugged into an existing system. Each site has unique characteristics, protocols, written and unwritten rules, and structures—all of which should be considered in the planning phase. Human factors play a huge role in the ultimate success of the program. In the preparation phase, several distinct activities are important: documenting the need, generating support from people with influence on the hospital's programs (e.g., administrators, professionals, parents); meeting with key administrators and personnel; and addressing equipment, instrumentation, and clinical issues.

Documenting Need

Documenting the need for establishing a program is fairly straightforward and may be accomplished through the use of literature, national and local demographic data, and nursery statistics (e.g., number of births per a given time period, average age of neonates at discharge, and estimate of the ratio of well-baby to special-care births). In addition, it may be helpful to determine the number of children being identified by the existing program, if any, and compare that to the reported incidence and prevalence of hearing loss for similar neonatal populations. Although the prevalence estimate of 1 per 1000 child having a severe to profound bilateral sensorineural hearing loss is still accepted, several existing universal screening programs have shown that when infants with milder degrees of hearing loss and unilateral hearing losses are included, the prevalence figures rise considerably. Table 11–3 presents prevalence data based on infants with confirmed hearing loss for several universal neonatal hearing screening programs. On average, it appears that a typical program may anticipate identifying 3 to 4 neonates with hearing loss for every thousand screened. In general, the prevalence of hearing loss will also be higher for special-care neonates when compared to full-term, healthy neonates. Owing to the relatively low occurrence of congenital hearing loss, the prevalence figures will fluctuate over time and among programs. For instance, the prevalence rate for confirmed congenital hearing loss in the initial Rhode Island Hearing Assessment Program cohort at Women and Infants' Hospital of Rhode Island was 5.95 per thousand (White et al., 1993). Because the hospital has a higher percentage of special-care babies than a typical hospital, the prevalence rate for the first cohort was a slightly lower 4.6 per thousand when adjusted to reflect the typical newborn population and has ranged from 1.5 to 7.5 per thousand for different cohorts (Table 11–4).

Many professionals may be located in areas that provide few or seemingly inadequate early intervention services. Some may argue that neonates with hearing loss need not be identified if appropriate referral sources are not in place. However, much of today's health care becomes available on a supply and demand basis. If neonates, infants, and young children with hearing loss are not being identified, appropriate early interventions services will not become available.

Table 11–3. Sample Size and Prevalence of Hearing Loss per Thousand for Six Universal Screening Programs

Location	Dates	Sample Size	Prevalence per 1000
Women and Infants' Hospital of Rhode Island	3/91 to 6/94	31,948	3.4*
Colorado**	5/92 to 2/95	20,700	4.58
Logan Regional Hospital	7/93 to 12/94	1,900	4.20
Hawaii	1/94 to 9/94	7,031	3.27
Walter Reed Army Medical Center	3/94 to 1/95	745	4.03
Texas**	7/94 to 1/95	3,722	1.61

*Adjusted for percentage of babies in special care nurseries so that reported prevalence represents a typical neonatal population. Women and Infants' Hospital of Rhode Island has a higher percentage of neonates born into special care nurseries than the general population. Since a higher prevalence of hearing loss is found in special care nurseries as opposed to well-baby nurseries, prevalence rates for each nursery were determined. The percentage of special care nursery neonates was reduced to reflect that found in a typical hospital, and prevalence rates were adjusted proportionally.

**Based on programs using primarily automated auditory brainstem response measures. Audiologists confirmed hearing loss for these programs by pediatric audiometric assessments consisting of a combination of behavioral and electrophysiologic tests, such as immittance, auditory brainstem response (ABR), and Behavioral Observation Audiometry (BOA), Distraction Audiometry or Visual Reinforcement Audiometry (VRA).

Table 11–4. Sample Size and Prevalence of Confirmed Hearing
Loss at Women and Infants' Hospital of Rhode Island

Dates of Cohort	No. in Cohort	Adjusted Prevalence Per 1000*
8/15/90 to 2/28/91	1,850	4.6
3/1/91 to 12/22/91	4,492	3.2
12/23/91 to 5/31/92	2,285	7.5
6/1/92 to 3/21/93	6,946	1.3
3/22/93 to 12/31/93	9,200	2.4
1/1/94 to 6/3/94	7,175	1.5

*Adjusted for percentage of babies in special care nurseries so that reported prevalence
represents typical population.

Therefore, arguments against initiating neonatal hearing screening programs
based the unavailability of adequate services may be short-sighted.

Compelling support for neonatal hearing screening is found in the conclusions
reached at the National Institutes of Health (NIH)–sponsored Consensus Development Conference on Early Identification of Hearing Impairment in Infants and
Young Children (1993). The abstract of the resulting Consensus Statement states:
"… the panel concluded that (1) all infants admitted to the neonatal intensive
care unit be screened for hearing loss prior to discharge; (2) universal screening be
implemented for all infants within the first 3 months of life; (3) the preferred model
for screening should begin with an evoked otoacoustic emissions test and should
be followed by an auditory brainstem response test for all infants who fail the
evoked otoacoustic emissions test; (4) comprehensive intervention and management programs must be an integral part of a universal hearing screening program;
(5) universal neonatal screening should not be a replacement for ongoing surveil-
lance throughout infancy and early childhood; and (6) education of primary caregivers and primary health care providers on the early signs of hearing impairment
is essential."

Similarly, the Joint Committee on Infant Hearing 1994 Position Statement "…
endorses the goal of universal detection of infants with hearing loss as early as
possible. All infants with hearing loss should be identified before 3 months of age,
and receive intervention by 6 months of age" (p. 152). In addition, there are
numerous articles on the use of EOAEs for newborn hearing screening conducted
at different facilities around the world (Bonfils et al., 1988; Bonfils, Dumont, Marie,
Francois, & Narcy, 1990; Johnsen et al., 1983; Kennedy et al., 1991; Plinkert, Sesterhenn, Arold, & Zenner, 1990; Stevens et al., 1989, 1990; Uziel & Piron, 1991; White
& Behrens, 1993; White et al., 1994). The most prominent study that has provided
the largest clinical trial is the Rhode Island Hearing Assessment Program. Many of
the clinical and practical issues surrounding the use of TEOAEs for universal
neonatal-hearing screening were explored at Women and Infants' Hospital of
Rhode Island. The findings of the project were widely disseminated in the February 1993 issue of Seminars in Hearing entitled *The Rhode Island Hearing Assessment
Project: Implications for Universal Newborn Hearing Screening*. The publication pro-

vides a valuable resource for professionals involved in EOAE hearing screening programs.

Generating Support

After documenting the need for the program, it is necessary to generate support both from people who are influential in making decisions regarding the hearing screening program and from the persons who will be involved in the program. This typically includes personnel from several different departments (e.g., nursing, pediatrics, neonatology, and audiology), from different areas of service provision (direct service, administrative), and from different support levels (e.g., professional staff, support staff, and patients). One goal that should be shared by everyone involved is that the neonatal hearing screening program can be built within the existing routine and schedules. The program should be initiated with as little disruption and change as possible to the ongoing nursery activities. On occasion, persons may be reluctant to become involved with something new. It is important to explore their reasons for being hesitant and to address their concerns. Many of the concerns that are raised at the onset of the newborn-hearing screenings (or when existing programs are being modified) may impact the overall effectiveness and efficiency of the program. It is imperative that all of the personnel in the neonatal unit to which the screening program will be added are supportive; they have a thorough understanding of the current procedures and in the system. Their concerns regarding the addition of a hearing screening program often arise from their insight to potential problem areas. Further, involving them in the planning stages allows them to develop a sense of ownership through direct participation in the program.

It is also important to meet with key administrators from each department involved in neonatal care and to provide supportive documentation and address the feasibility of the program. Information should be presented as completely and concisely as possible. Many of the *whats, wheres, whys, whos, hows,* and *whens* (Table 11–5) should be addressed. It is important to describe what TEOAEs are, what screeners will "do" to the neonates, what support is needed, what the program wants; where screenings are to be performed, where data will be kept; why the program is proposed, why the facility should participate; who is responsible, who is in charge, who will perform the initial screenings, the rescreens, referrals, scheduling, tracking, and documentation of policies and policies; how the administration can help, how the program is to be financed; and when the program will start.

Equipment and Instrumentation Issues

Beyond the initial purchase, there are several other areas that should be considered regarding the EOAE equipment, including additional acquisitions, calibration, and maintenance. Of the six commercial devices for measuring EOAEs that are available at this time, the United States Food and Drug Administration (FDA) allows five DPOAE units to be marketed for clinical purposes (Virtual Corporation Model 330, Grason-Stadler GSI-60, Madsen Celesta, Biologic, and Etymotic Research CUBᵉDIS) and one for TEOAEs (Otodynamics ILO88). Although Otodynamics

Table 11–5. Administrative Considerations: Questions to Be Answered

What:
  are EOAEs?
  departments are involved?
  is done to the neonates?
  support is needed from the facility?
Where:
  will the screenings be performed?
  will rescreens be performed?
  will the equipment be kept?
  will data be kept?
Why:
  is universal hearing screening being proposed?
  should this facility undertake this activity?
How:
  will the program be financed?
  can the administrators help?
Who:
  is responsible?
  is in charge?
  will perform the EOAE screenings?
  will interpret the results?
  will do the rescreens? referrals? scheduling? tracking? data management?
  will document the policies and procedures?
When:
  will can the program begin?
  will the screeners be trained?
  will the program be self-sufficient?
  will third party reimbursement become a reailty?

also has a DPOAE unit available, FDA authorization allowing the ILO92 to be used for clinical purposes is pending. The use of TEOAEs has been more thoroughly explored than DPOAEs, particularly regarding neonatal hearing screening programs. Each program must decide which equipment will best serve their unique needs. Programs that will use EOAEs solely for neonatal screening may find that TEOAE instrumentation better suited for their purpose. Programs that will conduct research and do more in-depth testing of OAEs may wish to purchase instrumentation for measuring both TEOAEs and DPOAEs.

The initial purchase of EOAE instrumentation typically includes the necessary computer hardware, software, and peripheral equipment; probe assemblies; probe tips of various sizes; daily calibration-check equipment; and documentation. The purchase of several additional items will also benefit: discs or tapes for backing up and storing data; a system for tracking neonates and managing data; a surge protector; a spare or "back up" probe assembly; and a mobile computer cart or case. It also is wise to purchase and install a virus protection program on the hard drive of the computer. Ongoing expenses that should be anticipated include annual equipment calibration, probe tips, probe assemblies, and computer supplies. Upgrades of computer hardware or software may also be useful because of the rapid expansion of technology.

Because all EOAE systems are computer-driven, it is wise to ensure that someone is available to answer questions about the software being used and the computer hardware, to troubleshoot computer-related problems, and to be responsible for maintaining the computer in a good working condition. It is also important to have someone available to load software upgrades, transfer data files, and back up the data regularly. It is not unusual during the initiation of a new EOAE hearing screening program to have more than half of the calls for support and assistance be related to routine computer operations rather than to screening itself.

Maintenance of the EOAE probe assembly is another concern. Experience with the Otodynamics equipment with the initial probe design suggested that, depending on who is using the equipment and how well they have been trained, a probe may need to be replaced after screening about 1500 babies. Although there is a new probe design that should reduce the rate of replacement, information is not available regarding the durability of the new style. Similarly, there is not enough experience in large scale programs with the various types of DPOAE units to estimate how often those probes will need to be replaced. However, it is clear that because of the highly sensitive nature of the probes assemblies, a program should plan on some replacement costs, regardless of the equipment being used.

As with any other delicate electronic equipment, proper use and care of the probe assembly will extend its life. The probe assemblies should be stored carefully when they are not in use because they are easily knocked onto the floor. Screening neonates just prior to discharge will also assist in prolonging the life of the probe because many neonates have debris (e.g., vernix caseosa, amniotic fluid, blood) in their ear canals. The debris may enter the open ports of the probe assembly. Proper use of the probe tips designed to fit on the end of the probe assembly may also assist in prolonging the life of the probe assembly. It is suggested that as a probe tip becomes soiled, the tip be removed from the probe before cleaning the tip. Attempting to wipe the tip clean while it is in place on the probe assembly may cause debris to enter the ports. If the probe tip is covered with debris, it should be discarded, and a new one should be used. Although some programs recommend that used or soiled probe tips be cleaned in an ultrasonic cleaner in an effort to save money, they may find that improperly cleaned probe tips actually damage probes. A used tip may have debris remaining in the small holes even after being cleaned or may still have some of the liquid cleaning solution in the holes. Such a tip may clog the ports, or fluid may enter the electronic components at the base of the tubes on the probe assembly; replacing a probe assembly is more expensive than a supply of probe tips.

If the ports do become clogged in the use of the older style of probe assemblies (the newer versions have disposable ports), it is necessary to clear the debris from probes with extreme care. One way to clean the probe assembly is as follows: (a) removing soiled probe tips from probe assembly before cleaning the probe tip or the ports; (b) visually inspecting the ports, and if they are clogged using a semi-flexible, thin wire to remove debris from open ports in probe assembly, taking great care not to push the debris further into the tube or to push the wire deeper than the projection of the tubes (extending the wire deeper than the depth of the projection of the tubes may allow the wire to contact the electronic components and may further damage the probe assembly); (c) and selecting a clean tip before continuing the screening. One optional precaution to take when screening a neonate with debris remaining in the ear is to cover the probe tip with an acoustically transparent shield, such as an Ad*Hear Wax Guard, before initiating the EOAE screening. The shields may be placed on the probe tip to effectively cover the open ports without significantly changing EOAE measurements (Culpepper, Henderson, & Shelton, 1994). While EOAE measurements are not directly affected, attaching the shields on top of the probe tip may affect probe fit, which may affect the measurement. Using the shields with every neonate, therefore, is not advisable.

Clinical Issues

There are several key issues regarding the establishment of a universal neonatal hearing screening program is beyond the scope of this chapter. For instance, the JCIH 1994 Position Statement defines a hearing loss as 30 dB HL or greater in speech-frequency region, whereas the NIH Consensus statement suggests that programs identify neonates and infants with a moderate loss or greater, but fails to define *moderate* or the *critical frequency range*. One example of a purpose developed for Logan Regional Hospital's program (Table 11–6) is, "to identify children with significant congenital hearing impairment before 12 months of age. The program will ensure that all live births at the hospital are screened for peripheral auditory

Table 11–6. Policies and Procedures Developed
for the Logan Regional Hospital Newborn Hearing Screening Program

Purpose

> To identify children with significant congenital hearing impairment before 12 months of age. The program will ensure that all live births are screened for peripheral auditory pathology using transient evoked otoacoustic emissions.

Departmental Involvement

Utah State University:	
Logan Regional Hospital:	Nursery
	Department of Physical Medicine and Rehabilitation

Responsibilities

Utah State University	1. Provide qualified audiologists to conduct the training for transient evoked otoacoustic emissions.
	2. Provide qualified audiologist for the Skills Test administration.
	3. Provide educational pamphlet regarding normal development of hearing, speech, and language behaviors.
Logan Regional Hospital	1. Provide trained personnel for screening and interpreting TEOAE results.
	2. Provide referrals for auditory brainstem response measurement, immittance and/or behavioral audiometric testing for infants who fail the rescreening.
	3. Coordinate data management for neonatal hearing screening.
	4. Equipment maintenance.
	5. Perform standard hospital preventive maintenance program on equipment.

pathology using transient evoked otoacoustic emissions (TEOAEs)." The terminology selected in the first sentence reflects Healthy People 2000 goal 17.16, and the second sentence reinforces the fact that EOAEs are not a measure of true hearing, which implies some degree of central processing, but rather reflect a healthy cochlea and peripheral apparatus when present. Although the hospital does specifically not define the term *significant* in the Policies and Procedures document, all sensorineural hearing losses (including unilateral hearing losses) and chronic or permanent conductive hearing losses are considered significant. Neonates are not discharged from the program before passing the screening for each ear or until auditory status is determined.

Two other clinical issues that need to be addressed by each program relate to the areas of referral and follow-up. Although it is often not feasible for the screening facility to be responsible for the entire complement of necessary services, there is no point in screening without making efforts to ensure that the neonates identified as having congenital peripheral auditory dysfunction and their families receive the follow-up, diagnostic, support, and intervention services needed. It is often necessary to establish a network of local professionals, including pediatricians, neonatologists, pediatric audiologists, health departments, family care practitioners, early intervention programs, and other related professionals, to meet the needs of the infants, as dictated by the needs of each child. These and other clinical aspects of the screening program, such a patient demographics, the geographical and economical situation of the community, and available transportation for the infant and their family, should be considered when establishing a flow chart of services while in the organizational phase of developing a program.

Organization and Training

When establishing the foundation of a program, it is necessary to decide which departments, divisions, facilities, personnel, and clinics will be involved in the screening program. Personnel from each area involved should be invited to participate in the planning process, particularly in the portions of the program for which they are to be partially responsible. The organization and training phase consists of three primary components: (a) defining roles and responsibilities, (b) defining procedures, policies, and protocols, and (c) training personnel. Although not all contingencies can be anticipated, it is easier to have as much of the program established as possible before starting EOAE screening rather than continually modifying and changing an ongoing program. Several key points to keep in mind during the entire process include: (a) working within the existing system, (b) tailoring the program to coexist with and complement the ongoing schedule, and (c) disrupting the ongoing nursery activities as little as possible. It is beneficial to allow those who will be responsible for various attributes of the program to take an active role in defining the procedures, policies, and protocols, particularly since many of these persons are familiar with the ongoing activities of their department, division, or area.

Before delineating specific roles, responsibilities, protocols, policies, and procedures, a client-based flow chart that outlines the various stages and time lines of the screening, follow-up, and referral process must be created. Figure 11–3 illus-

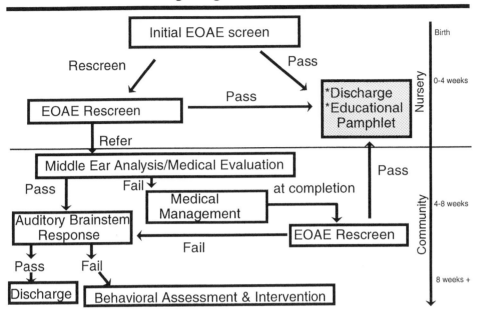

Figure 11–3. Flowchart for the Logan Regional Hospital Universal Neonatal Hearing Screening Program.

trates one such flow chart used at Logan Regional Hospital. The Logan Regional Hospital Hearing Screening Program begins by using TEOAEs to screen for peripheral auditory dysfunction prior the neonates' being discharged from the hospital. Neonates who pass the screening in both ears are discharged from the program and an educational brochure is provided for the parents. Neonates who do not pass the screening before they leave the nursery are referred for a TEOAE rescreen, also conducted within the nursery, preferably before 4 weeks of age (as infants get older, they become more active and more difficult to test quickly). If the infants pass TEOAEs bilaterally, they are discharged from the program and the parents are given an educational pamphlet. If the infant does not pass the second TEOAE screening, they are referred to their pediatrician for a middle ear analysis. Reports are sent to the infant's parents, the pediatrician, and the hospital audiologist.

The pediatrician may either make an immediate referral for an ABR or may delay further assessment temporarily if middle-ear dysfunction is present. Infants referred for ABR are initially tested with a screening ABR and moved immediately to a diagnostic ABR if they fail the screening ABR at 30 dB nHL in either ear. Infants who pass the ABR screening are discharged from the program while those who fail are immediately referred for audiometric assessment and early intervention (Utah's Parent Infant Program provides services for children with conductive hearing loss and their families, as well as children with sensorineural hearing loss).

One flow-chart modification to this program that is beneficial for several reasons is to complete an ABR screening (or diagnostic ABR when the screening is failed at 30 dB nHL) immediately after failing the TEOAE rescreen. This could potentially alleviate some parental concern by avoiding delays in diagnosis, reduce the number of extra appointments needed, and reduce the number of infants who do not return for follow ups.

Roles and Responsibilities

A well-designed program designates who is responsible for various portions of the program and assigns persons to specific duties. Each person and department within the program must understand their role in the program. Because the configuration of each program is unique, the division of roles and responsibilities varies. The Rhode Island Hearing Assessment Program's hospital-based universal screening program hired and trained personnel specifically to perform the initial TEOAEs, the rescreens (TEOAEs), and screening ABRs under the supervision of an audiologist (Johnson, Maxon, White, & Vohr, 1993). The audiologist is responsible for supervising and monitoring technicians, interpretation of TEOAEs and ABRs, and ensuring that audiological assessments and appropriate follow-ups are completed on all infants who fail the screening. The Rhode Island Hearing Assessment Program also employs a coordinator who is responsible for managing the various aspects of the program for the eight hospitals in the statewide system.

At Logan Regional Hospital, which has approximately 2000 births per year, both the Nursery and the Department of Physical Medicine and Rehabilitation-Division of Audiology are involved in the program. In addition, personnel from Utah State University (USU) are responsible for training the screeners (Table 11–6). To facilitate communication among the participants, a Hearing Screening Program Coordinator position was developed in the Nursery. A Policies and Procedures document has been prepared and filed at the hospital according to hospital regulations and a contract between USU and Logan Regional Hospital has been written delineating the roles and responsibilities of each for maintaining the universal TEOAE hearing screening program.

Training

USU is responsible for ensuring that all screeners in the Nursery develop and maintain the information and practical skills necessary to perform TEOAE screenings. Although information and TEOAE demonstrations about the program were provided to all Nursery personnel and pediatricians, only selected clerks and nurses went through an intensive training program. The lead nurse selected screeners based on their interest in the program, their existing schedules, aptitude, and work schedules. Due to short hospital stays (most healthy infants are discharged within 18–24 hours), at least one of the trained screeners must be available all week.

To document and maintain a desired level of competency in measuring TEOAEs, USU audiologists are responsible for developing and administering a skills test (Table 11–7). Each screener is required to pass the skills test annually and certificates are awarded to each individual who passes the test. Copies of the certificates are then filed in each screeners' personnel record.

Table 11–7.   Utah State University/Logan Regional Hospital TEOAE Skills Test

_____ 1. Turns on equipment
_____ 2. Selects appropriate hearing screening program
_____ 3. Follows appropriate sanitation protocols.
_____ 4. Picks up infant following nursery protocol.
_____ 5. Positions infant.
_____ 6. Selects and fits probe tip on probe assembly.
_____ 7. Inserts probe tip into infant's ear.
_____ 8. Enters infant data into computer.
_____ 9. Evaluates fit, makes adjustments.
_____ 10. Begins hearing screening.
_____ 11. Adjusts stimulus gain.
_____ 12. Adjusts noise bar appropriately.
_____ 13. Recognizes and trouble-shoots the following conditions:

      _____ a. Excessive noise
            _____ Adds low frequency filter.   _____ Repositions probe.
            _____ Checks probe for debris.   _____ Removes probe tip.
            _____ Cleans probe tip.   _____ Uses noise control.
      _____ b. Inadequate probe fit
            _____ Repositions probe.   _____ Changes tip size.
      _____ c. Inadequate stimulus
            _____ Adjusts stimulus gain.
            _____ Uses acoustically transparent shield.
      _____ d. Calms fussy infant
_____ 14. Collects data following designated protocol.
_____ 15. Checks for adequacy of data.
      _____ a. Appropriate # of low-noise samples
      _____ b. Appropriate stimulus
      _____ c. Recognizes adequate response (no further testing needed)
      _____ d. Recognizes inadequate test validity (needs repetition)
_____ 16. Saves data.
_____ 17. Completes hearing screening for other ear.
_____ 18. Completes documentation and prepares equipment for the next infant.
_____ 19. Returns infant according to nursery protocol.

Screening

Although several options were considered, clerks and nurses from the Nursery ultimately became responsible for the TEOAE screenings prior to discharge for each neonate born at the hospital (except for neonates who are transferred to the regional level III Neonatal Intensive Care Unit). Neonates who do not pass TEOAEs bilaterally before being discharged return to the Nursery for a TEOAE rescreen, preferably during the first 2 weeks of life. Neonates or infants who fail the rescreen are referred to the audiologist for a screening ABR and for diagnostic evaluations as needed.

Interpreting Results

All TEOAEs are interpreted by an audiologist (either the part-time audiologist employed by the hospital or an audiologist from USU). During the first three months of the program, records were reviewed at least once each working day and at least one day of the weekend by either the USU or Logan Regional Hospital audiologist. As the screeners have become more comfortable and proficient, records are now reviewed every 2 or 3 days. The Logan Regional Hospital audiologist is responsible for interpreting all test results obtained following the rescreening (e.g., ABRs, behavioral results).

Scheduling

All neonates who do not pass the initial TEOAE screening bilaterally (including those who are not screened prior to discharge) are scheduled to return to the Nursery for rescreening by the Hearing Screening Program Coordinator in the Nursery. Parents typically are asked to bring their newborns back to the Nursery after their first visit to the pediatrician. The audiology aide employed by Logan Regional Hospital is primarily responsible for scheduling ABRs and behavioral follow-up appointments for neonates who fail the rescreen. The secretarial and support staff of the Department of Physical Medicine and Rehabilitation also assist in scheduling appointments for infants who are to be seen by the Logan Regional Hospital audiologist.

Rescreening

When the program was initially established, rescreenings were scheduled to performed in Audiology facilities at Logan Regional Hospital during 30-minute time slots. However, several problems became apparent that prompted a change in the designed protocol. One of the problems depended on the Logan Regional Hospital audiologist working part-time in the afternoons. Ideally, a variety of times should be offered in attempt to accommodate the hectic schedules of new parents. Another problem was that there was only one piece of equipment for measuring TEOAEs at Logan Regional Hospital. Therefore, when the audiologist scheduled rescreenings, the Nursery did not have access to the equipment and infants were being discharged without being screened, and more babies needed to return for rescreens. Changing the site of rescreenings alleviated these problems. The Hearing Screening Program Coordinator contacts families with infants who have not returned for their schedule appointments. Because trained screeners are available in the nursery every day, parents may bring their infants in for rescreening at their convenience. If contact cannot be made with family members by telephone, letters are first sent to the family and then to the primary care physician in attempt to ensure follow-up for the rescreening.

Managing Data

The amount of data generated by a universal neonatal-hearing screening program may easily inundate even the most organized persons if a system to manage the data is not established at the onset of the program. Everyone involved in the TEOAE-screening program has some responsibility for documenting screenings and maintaining records. The Hearing Screening Program Coordinator has the primary responsibility for managing records and for determining ongoing program statistics. USU has provided the computerized tracking system and training necessary to use the system. To ease the burden of data management, the newest version of the TEOAE software includes not only the ILO88 software, but also an integrated program called HISCREEN. The HISCREEN program allows the screener to enter pertinent identifying information about all neonates born in the hospital into the computer at or before the time of screening, transfers pertinent data to the ILO88, records which neonates have been screened or need to be screened, and organizes files to streamline the scoring and tracking process. Audiologists score screening results from HISCREEN, then record the final status of each neonate. The scored and compiled data from HISCREEN may then be downloaded into HITRACK. HITRACK is a database software program that was developed to assist in managing the vast amounts of data that generated by newborn hearing screening programs. Using HITRACK, the status of each neonate may be tracked throughout screening, referral, diagnostic, and follow-up services. Screening and tracking information is readily available in a variety of report formats, including tickler files for infants who need follow-up as, well as program statistics (e.g., percentages of neonates screened, rescreened, missed, lost, and referred). HITRACK is individualized for each screening site and will accommodate screening programs using EOAEs, ABRs, or a combined screening approach. Also, it can automatically generate reports to parents or pediatricians with the results of auditory tests. Using HISCREEN and HITRACK saves time, increases the accuracy of information collected, and makes an overwhelming amount of data manageable. HITRACK is also capable of receiving information from different programs and different screening sites and provides a centralized system to coordinate and track children on a statewide or a regional basis.

Follow-Up

Ensuring that everyone understands the need to follow-up a newborn's hearing status is primarily the responsibility of the Logan Regional Hospital and USU audiologists, but is also a responsibility of the pediatricians, neonatologists, family practitioners, and all professionals involved in the program. In the Logan Regional Hospital program, neonates are referred to their pediatricians or family practitioners after failing the TEOAE rescreen for an assessment of middle ear status. When no middle-ear problem is found, the infants should be referred for an ABR. Because there are four places in the community where parents may take their infants for ABR, guaranteeing that proper follow-up services are received by all neonates is difficult at best and requires concerted effort on the parts of all involved. The tickler reports generated by the HITRACK program assists in determining the follow-up status of each newborn not yet discharged from the program.

Educating Others

Because of the relatively recent ability to screen all newborns for congenital hearing loss efficiently and effectively using EOAEs, education is a critical component of a universal screening program. Parents, caregivers, neonatologists, pediatricians, physicians, administrators, habilitative programs, and other associated professionals givers need to be advised about the program. Education may take many forms, including inservices, grand rounds, demonstrations, pamphlets, videotapes, informal and formal presentations, and workshops. USU has taken the lead role in the educational aspects of Logan Regional Hospital's Newborn Hearing Screening Program. Inservices and demonstrations have been held for all personnel associated with the Nursery. Workshops and presentations have been held for interested professionals, and all parents are given an educational pamphlet that describes TEOAEs, the importance of hearing, and milestones for hearing, speech, and language development. Parents are also cautioned that although their newborn child has passed the TEOAE screening, continued monitoring of their child's auditory status is necessary as hearing status may change. USU has also recorded a 3-minute videotape describing and demonstrating the TEOAE screening. The videotape immediately follows the breast-feeding videotape played on Logan Regional Hospital's closed-circuit instructional channel. The videotape is also shown during prenatal or parent preparation classes offered through the hospital prior to delivery. Showing the videotape during these classes has been beneficial because most infants are discharged within 24 hours of birth and many parents are occupied with things other than television during their brief time in the hospital. There is also a 15-minute videotape about the hearing screening that is available through the Nursery that goes into more detail for parents and families.

Procedures, Policies, and Protocols

Before training can be completed and the program can be implemented, the procedures, policies, and protocols that govern the program must be established. Besides the new documents for the universal screening program, there are typically others that must be recognized and incorporated. For instance, all programs should have procedures, policies, and protocols for infection control, documentation of services provided, and client confidentiality. Those used in the EOAE neonatal screening program cannot conflict with existing documents.

ILO88 Screen Description

Because the selection of pass-refer criteria is based on the information provided by the emissions unit, it is important to understand the data provided. In this chapter, the TEOAE information provided by the IL O88 after a screening is completed has been divided into six boxes (see Figure 11–4), and basic overview of the information provided in each box is discussed.

Box 1 (Stimulus) displays the stimulus waveform, which is measured in the initial click presentations during data collection. The tracing vertically displays the amplitude of the stimulus expressed in Pascals (0.3 Pa = 83.5 dB SPL) over time on the horizontal axis. Ideally, the stimulus waveform shows one positive and one negative deflection that quickly dampens to a flat line. It is common to observe slightly more oscillation in the stimulus waveform in neonates than in adults (Figure 11–1). Regardless of the ear being tested, however, no stimulus activity should continue past 2 ms. Increased oscillation is an indicator of a "ringing" stimulus, which may be the result of a poor probe fit, debris in the ear canal, or a stimulus level that is too intense.

Box 2 is divided into two sections. The upper section allows the neonate's name and medical records number (*Case*) to be entered. The date of the test is entered automatically. The lower panel provides information about software settings dur-

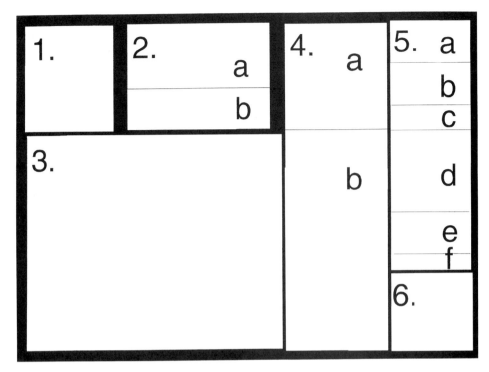

Figure 11–4.   TEOAE results obtained from the ILO 88 broken down into six boxes containing different information about a screening session.

ing the screening on the left side. The right side of the lower panel displays the amount of gain needed to reach the targeted stimulus level as compared to the reference gain of the system. For most screening sessions, the dB Gain reading will be within +3 dB.

Box 3 presents the *Response Waveform*. Time is displayed along the horizontal axis, and amplitude is shown on the vertical axis, although different scales are used as compared to the stimulus waveform (the stimulus scale displays a more intense measure). Two tracings, *A* and *B*, display averaged samples obtained for 12 ms after the stimulus onset. (The first 2.5 ms are omitted to reduce possible stimulus artifact). The ILO88 considers the correlated portions of the *A* and *B* tracings the response while the uncorrelated portions of the waveform are noise. High frequency information is focused towards the left of the waveform while lower frequency information is predominantly found to the right. In strong emissions, therefore, the *A* and *B* tracings will almost be superimposed on top of one another. The small box in the upper left hand corner of *Box 3* indicates that the low frequency filter, which helps reduce the detrimental effects of noise, was activated during the screening session.

In *Box 4* the upper panel (*a*) displays a Fast Fourier Transform (FFT) of the portions of the average *A* and *B* waveforms that are correlated. The FFT thus reflects those frequency regions in which the signal to noise ratio exceeds 0 dB (*Response*

SNR). The lower panel (*b*) presents a *Power Analysis* of the stimulus, response, and noise spectra. When the *Quickscreen* option is used, the bandwidths of interest for each of these displays is between 1000–4000 Hz. Although these two panels display similar information, you may notice that the noise floor displayed in the lower panel is zeroed out in the upper panel to present the amplitude of the emission above the noise floor.

Box 5 displays numeric rather than graphic information and has been subdivided into six different areas (*a* through *f*). Panel 5a (*NOISE Input*) displays the level of noise measured by the microphone in the ear canal during the quiet (averaged) samples; therefore, noisy samples (those that were above the noise reject level) are not included in this average. Although many neonates have emissions robust enough to overcome noisy test conditions, it is desirable to have a noise level below 40 dB. The second number displayed in this panel, *Rejection at*, is the dB level of the noise reject arrow at the end of the screening session. *Panel 5b* presents the number of quiet samples (samples included in the data) and noisy samples (those excluded from data analysis) in the upper and lower lines, respectively. Quiet samples are those that were below the noise reject arrow during the screening session while the noisy samples are those that were rejected for being above the noise reject arrow. The percentage of samples that were averaged and included in the response analysis during the screening session is presented to the right of the summed quiet samples.

The next area (*Panel 5c*) provides information about how the two response waveforms (*A* and *B*) compare to each other. The decibel level displayed by *A & B Mean* represents the amplitude of the correlated portions of the waveform, while *A-B Diff* displays the amplitude difference between the two response waveforms. Results from screening sessions with robust emissions and low noise will have *A & B Mean* amplitudes similar to the overall *RESPONSE* amplitude displayed in top row of *Box 6d*, which indicates the intensity of the emission. Neonates typically have responses that are more intense than adults. The next line, *Wave Repro[ducibility]* indicates how well the two tracings (*A* and *B*) of the response waveform overlap. Higher percentages indicate that the waveforms are highly correlated. Noise included in the averaged samples, particularly low frequency noise, interferes with the whole wave reproducibility and reduces the percentage displayed. The histogram to the right of the number displays the wave reproducibility over the duration of the screening session. The bottom two lines of numbers, *Band Repro[ducibility]* and *SNR* provide similar information for the response broken down into five frequency regions beginning at 800, 1600, 2400, 3200, and 4000 Hz. Band reproducibility is presented in the second to last row, where as the intensity of the response above the noise floor (the signal to noise ratio) for each bandwidth is displayed in the bottom row.

The peak *Stimulus* level is the first information given in Box 5e, which represents the intensity level at the peak of the stimulus spectrum. The stimulus *Stability*, expressed in a percentage, is an expression of the stimulus amplitude difference encountered between the stimulus represented in the check-fit procedure and the stimulus at the termination of the screening procedure. Thus, the information in this box does not display averaged data for the entire screening. The histogram to the right of the stability score, however, provides a visual representation of how consistent the click stimulus was in the ear canal at regular intervals throughout the screening session. Numeric information about stimulus peak and stimulus stability throughout data collection are available by pressing the P (Progress) key when viewing data from the computer. The last panel in *Box 5* (*f*) gives the time shows the elapsed time during the data collection portion of the screening session.

Box 6 provides information as to where files are stored on the computer.

Data Interpretation

Presence of TEOAEs suggests that hearing sensitivity is at least as good as or better than 25 to 30 dB HL (Hurley & Musiek, 1994). As with ABR, there are no universally recognized criteria for deciding what constitutes an EOAE pass. Each program must develop their own pass-refer criteria as dictated by the goals of the program. There are two factors that must be evaluated for the results of every EOAE screening: (a) the validity of the test and (b) the presence or absence of the designated response.

Test validity should be monitored for each EOAE screening. Suggested parameters for establishing test validity for TEOAEs are (a) stimulus stability measurement of 75% or greater; (b) peak stimulus targeted at 80 dBpk SPL (acceptable range 77–83 dBpk SPL; questionable from 84 to 85 dBpk SPL; unacceptable at or above 86 dBpk SPL); (c) stimulus spectrum across the desired frequency region (target at 40 dB SPL); and (d) a noise level of 40.0 dB SPL or less in the ear canal; and (e) at least 50 low noise samples. (Although no empirical data has been gathered, clinical experience suggests that collecting at least 50 low noise samples helps to ensure that "oddball" data are not misinterpreted as responses. Since noise is separated from signal by comparing correlated [signal or response] and uncorrelated [noise] portions of the response waveforms, screening with only a few samples increases the likelihood that the noise included in the measure may correlate at any given frequency.) While meeting all the criteria is desirable, the only mandatory criterion that must be met for test validity is having an acceptable peak stimulus. A TEOAE measurement with good test validity at Logan Regional Hospital is defined as having a stimulus peak within the acceptable region (<83 dB) and at least 50 low noise samples average. For DPOAEs, $2f_1 - f_2$ amplitudes should be two standard deviations above the noise floor and the two primary-tone stimuli should be within 3 dB SPL of their expected values.

Most universal screening programs are interpreting TEOAE responses in one of two ways—visually or numerically. Scoring with visual criteria is accomplished by inspecting the FFT generated from the response waveform. If a response is present at least halfway across each band in all of the designated frequency regions, the screening is scored as a "pass". Programs using the TEOAEs look for the presence of a response above the noise floor for three bandwidths, 1000 to 2000 Hz, 2000 to 3000 Hz, and 3000 to 4000 Hz. For DPOAEs, a visual pass would consist of the presence of the $2f_1 - f_2$ distortion product above the noise floor in each of the designated frequency regions.

For establishing numerical pass criteria for TEOAEs, there are several indexes that may be used in isolation or in combination. The indexes that may be included are overall response amplitude, whole wave reproducibility, response to noise ratio, TEOAE threshold, signal-to-noise (SNR) response amplitude by bandwidth, and reproducibility by bandwidth. Indexes for DPOAEs include amplitude for selected test frequencies, response to noise ratio, and DPOAE threshold.

For ease of illustration, the pass-refer criteria used at Logan Regional Hospital, which are the same as those suggested by the National Consortium on Newborn Hearing Screening (1995), will be used to interpret TEOAE screening results using examples of several different neonates. The Consortium has adopted a numerical pass criteria based on reproducibility by bandwidth. Using the *Quickscreen* option with the low frequency filter engaged, a neonate passes the screening if reproducibility is 50% or greater in the 1600 Hz bandwidth and 70% or greater in the 2400, 3200, and 4000 Hz bandwidths. The criteria are fairly conservative, and therefore will not miss neonates with peripheral auditory pathology, but may refer more neonates with normal auditory status that if a more liberal pass-refer system is adopted.

When interpreting the results of EOAE screenings, four possible outcomes exist (Figure 11–5): (a) a response with good test validity; (b) a response with poor test validity; (c) no response with good test validity; and (d) no response with question-

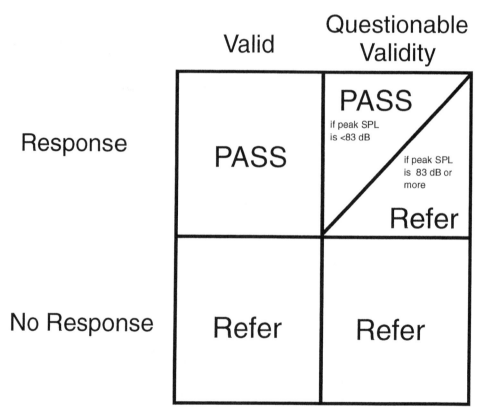

Figure 11–5. Interpretation matrix for outcomes of EOAE screenings.

able test validity. The first of these is the obviously preferred result and is unquestionably a *pass*.

Figure 11–6 presents the results of two neonatal ears with clear responses and good test validity.

Examples of the second potential outcome (response present, invalid test) are presented in Figure 11–7.

When the designated response is not present, whether test validity is good or poor, there is no question that the result of the screening is a *refer*. Figure 11–8 illustrates the absence of otoacoustic emissions under good and questionable test conditions.

Protocol for EOAE Screening

The basic steps followed at Logan Regional Hospital for EOAE screenings follow.

1. Set up the instrumentation. Turn on all equipment and ensure the equipment is functioning appropriately (calibration check or biological check).

2. Follow advised infection control or sanitation protocol.

3. Determine the neonate's state. As demonstrated by the Rhode Island Hearing Assessment Program, if the neonate is active or crying during screening, the chances of obtaining a passing response are reduced and the total time needed to complete the measurement is increased.

4. Enter identifying data for neonate. Along with the neonate's last name, it is advisable to enter additional identifying information, such as a medical record's number, social security number, or an *A*, *B*, or *C* in cases of multiple births. The need for this becomes readily apparent as the names of many neonates are changed during the infancy. As more information is recorded regarding each neonate, the possibility of mixing up case records is diminished.

5. Insert the probe into neonate's ear. One of the most important aspects of the entire EOAE screening process is the fitting the probe tip into the ear canal. Without a good probe fit, stimulus parameters may be faulty and ambient noise is more likely to interfere with the measurement of EOAEs. When screening neonates, it is often desirable to use the largest probe tip that, when inserted deeply into the ear canal, barely protrudes into the concha. Before inserting the probe tip into the ear canal, it is necessary to position the infant so that the screener has easy access to both the neonate and the instrumentation. Then while observing the neonates ear and angle of the ear canal, manipulate the ear by pulling outward and upward on the pinna with one hand while placing a finger of the opposite hand just in front of the tragus and pushing downward and slightly inward. This procedure will help separate collapsed canals (collapsed ear canals are more common for the ear which has been down on the mattress) and may assist in dislodging debris in the ear canal. Following this manipulation, again hold the pinna upward and outward and insert the probe gently but firmly into the ear canal with a slight twisting motion. The probe assembly cable should be positioned above neonates' head rather than across body (Figure 11–9).

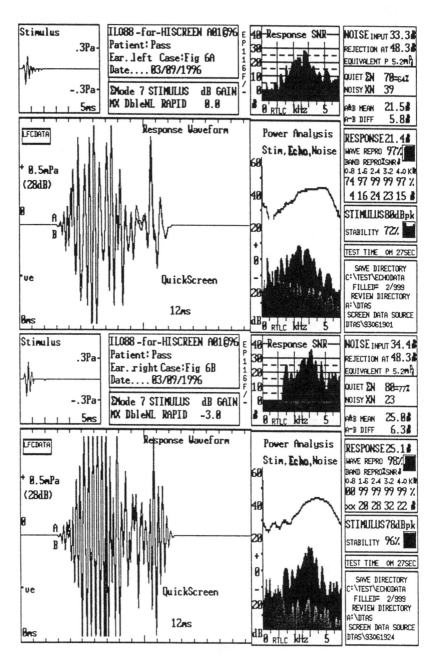

Figure 11–6. Examples of TEOAE screening results for two neonatal ears that passed the screening with good test validity. Note that each screening required only 27 sec to complete and that the robust responses leave little question as to the satisfactory status of the peripheral auditory mechanism.

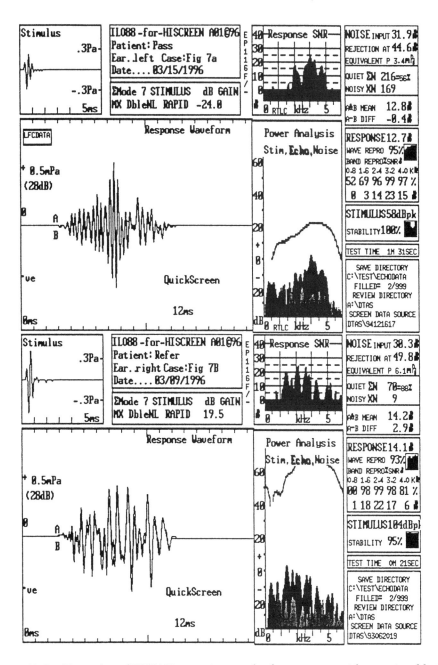

Figure 11–7. Examples of TEOAE screening results for two ears with questionable test validity. *A*: The peak stimulus (68 dBpk) is below the targeted intensity region. Nevertheless, this ear passes the screening because reproducibility exceeds the minimum criteria in all frequency bands. If the cochlea is able to overcome adverse test conditions and still present an acceptable response, the ear passes the screening. *B*: The result of a screening session that did not have an appropriate stimulus level (dBpk), and, therefore, the result is a refer. The acceptable peak stimulus region is exceeded. If this neonate had not been discharged, an attempt should be made to repeat the screening.

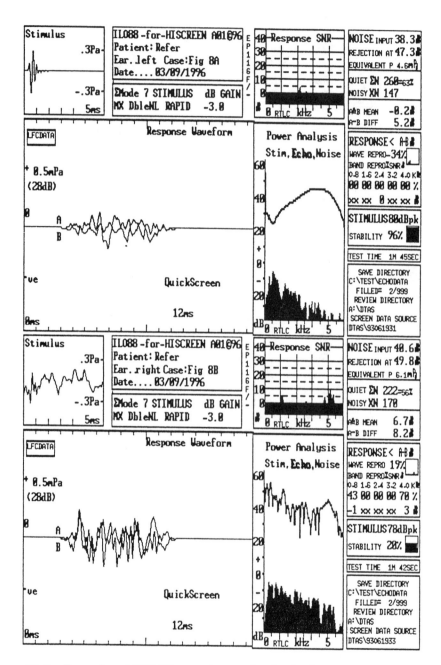

Figure 11–8. Examples of TEOAE-screening results that had no response and were referred. In the top panel (*A*) test validity was good, but in the lower panel (*B*) poor test validity leads one to question whether the ear was referred for lack of an emission or lack of the ability to measure an emission due to poor testing conditions. (Each of these ears need to be rescreened.)

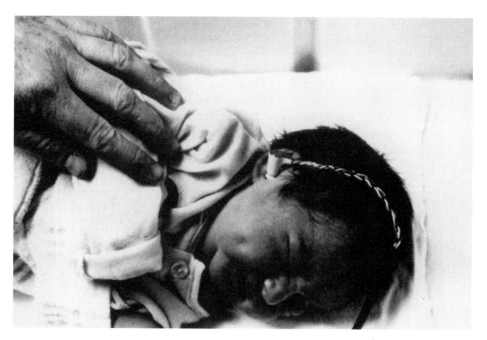

Figure 11–9. Illustration of proper positioning of the probe assembly and cord during EOAE neonatal hearing screening. Note that the neonate is tightly swaddled to reduce movement that would increase noise during the screening and that the probe tip is barely visible owing to deep insertion into the ear canal.

Proper insertion of the probe is perhaps the most difficult aspect of EOAE screening for some to learn, and a common problem area. Practice is necessary. There is a definite learning curve that each person must work through at her or his own pace.

6. Screen the neonate. When TEOAEs are being used to screen for congenital hearing loss, the *Quickscreen* test option is recommended rather than the Standard IL O88 test. Using *Quickscreen* reduces the total test time and decreases the effects of low frequency noise. The peak stimulus level should be targeted at 80 dB SPL. When DPOAEs are used, the suggested stimulus parameters are a frequency separation ratio of 1.22 and primary-tone stimuli at intensity levels of 65 dB SPL and 50 dB SPL for f_1 and f_2, respectively. Recording at two points per octave, although increasing the test time, may assist in reducing false positive rates.

7. Perform on-line review. Perform an on-line review of screening results, noting the adequacy of stimulus and response parameters and test validity. During the EOAE screening, it is necessary to monitor the progress of the test. When designated pass criteria have been met, the screening may be halted. It may be necessary to stop the screening test if the probe falls out of the ear, the neonate begins to cry, or the screening session is otherwise interrupted. It may also be necessary to remove and clean the probe tip, manipulate the ear canal, change

the size of the probe tip, reinsert the probe, change the angle of the probe in the ear canal, use the low frequency filter, improve neonatal state, or reduce the ambient noise levels. Figure 11–10 illustrates how screening results often improve by simply refitting and repositioning the angle of the probe assembly in the neonates' ear canal. A high frequency shift in the stimulus spectrum is another indicator of a poorly fit probe, which is apparent in both the stimulus waveform and the stimulus spectra. With a poorly fit probe, there is more oscillation in the frequency waveform because the stimulus is not locked into the ear canal. Stimulus stability may remain higher with appropriate probe fit as well.

8. Repeat steps 5 through 7 for the other ear.

9. Document the completion of screening.

10. Off-line interpretation. The supervising audiologist then interprets results.

One additional area regarding the screening process that should be addressed is noise control. There are two primary types of noise that must be considered in EOAE screenings—internal and external. Each of these terms refers to any unwanted acoustic energy that reaches the microphone in the probe assembly. Internal noise arises from the infant; external noise is generated from the neonate's environment. Eliminating or reducing sources of noise during EOAE screenings will not only improve the overall pass rate, but it will also reduce the amount of time needed to complete the screening.

The most effective means of controlling internal noise is accomplished by screening when the neonate is in a quiet state, preferably asleep. Additional measures that may increase the chances of reducing the fail rate include swaddling the neonate, ensuring that the cable from the probe assembly is positioned away from movement by either the neonate or the screener, and manipulating the infant's ear before inserting the probe tip. Attempting to hold the probe assembly in position typically adds noise to the measurement, but holding the cable away from noise sources may help to reduce noise. Although premature infants may be tested in the same manner as full-term infants, neonates requiring special care are typically noisier than healthy infants. To reduce some of the problems, it is recommended that special-care neonates be screened when they are medically stable, typically just before discharge. Neonates on ventilation rarely pass EOAEs because of high internal noise levels.

One way to reduce the negative influence of external noise on EOAE screening is to reduce ambient noise within the environment, such as turning off radios, nonessential equipment, and beeping monitors. Continuous noises (e.g., vents, motors) are more detrimental overall to the screening process than intermittent noises. As suggested earlier, a good probe fit in the ear canal greatly reduces the effects of ambient noise. Although it is not necessary to screen neonates in a sound treated environment (such as an audiometric booth), there are many measures that may be used to assist in sound control and improve the efficiency of the TEOAE screening process. At Women and Infants' Hospital of Rhode Island, neonates are sometimes screened in an Armstrong isolette (an older version of an incubator) while some are screened in their own bassinets. At Logan Regional Hospital, a sound shield made of plexiglass and a layer of a discarded lead apron was designed and used when necessary (Figure 11–11).

The TEOAE software has also been improved to assist in noise control since

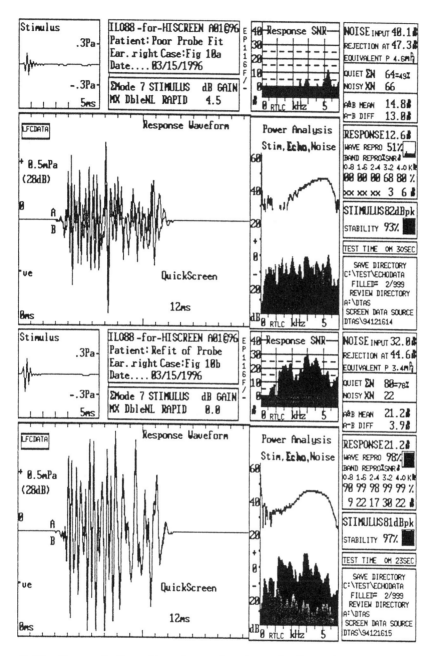

Figure 11–10. Demonstration of how improving the probe fit can improve screening results. In the top panel (*A*), there are several indicators that the probe was not set into the ear canal as deeply or firmly as desired. The noise floor spectrum is one of the best clues. When the probe is not inserted into the canal deep enough to seal out ambient noise, the noise spectrum essentially forms a flat spectrum from low to high frequencies. With a good fit as is seen in the lower panel (*B*), the noise spectrum slopes from a higher level in the lower frequencies (from internal noise) down to a lower level in the high frequencies. As might be expected, the overall noise in the ear canal with the poor probe fit (upper right corner) is 38.5 dB SPL, while the noise level is reduced to 34.9 dB SPL with an improved fit.

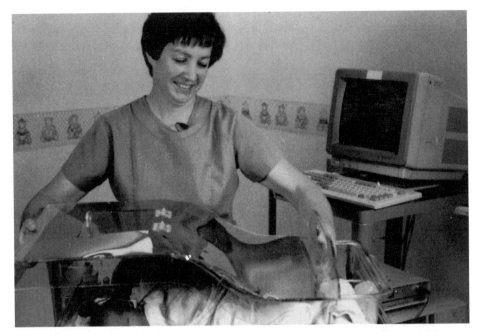

Figure 11–11. Plexiglass sound shield used to improve the efficiency of TEOAE screening.

the initial clinical trial in Rhode Island. The software options that assist in noise control include Quickscreen, the noise reject level, and the low frequency that is enabled in the *Check fit* menu.

Train Personnel

The final activities that must take place before implementing a screening program revolve around training the personnel who will conduct the program. There are several factors that need to be considered when scheduling training sessions. The first issue is to decide which people will be trained. Considerations of importance include work schedules and background experience. For instance, persons with some exposure to computers may be less intimidated by the instrumentation, persons unaccustomed to handling neonates need some additional training in moving, swaddling, and caring for the newborns they will be screening. The second factor to be considered during the training period concerns the instrumentation to be used. It is extremely beneficial to have hands-on experience throughout the training process. As such, it is often desirable to have additional units available to train more than two or three people at a time (training more than three screeners at a time on one unit is extremely difficult). As additional systems are borrowed to aid in the training process, the location of the instrumentation during the training sessions then becomes an issue. Most facilities use all available space for ongoing nursery activities and it becomes a challenge not to disrupt the ongoing nursery schedule. One final consideration to be addressed during the training phase of the program is the terminology that is used with the screeners. For programs using persons other than audiologists to complete the initial hearing screenings prior to discharge, the terms *pass* and *fail* are avoided because screeners typically are not qualified to interpret EOAE results. Owing to the number of false positives expected during the initial screenings, the word *fail* is avoided before the EOAE rescreening. *Rescreen* or *refer* is the accepted terminology and is less alarming to parents.

The training persons receive is dictated by their roles, responsibilities, and designated competency criteria (such as the Skills Test for screeners). Several items that need to be included in the training and an example of a training sequence are listed in Table 11–8. Monitoring individual screener progress and providing feedback is extremely useful during the training process and will improve the learning curve.

Implementation

After the planning, financing, organizing, and training have been completed, it is finally time to initiate the universal neonatal hearing screening program. For large programs, it may be necessary to begin with a targeted group of the neonatal population and gradually increase the number of neonates screened. At Logan Regional Hospital, which has a yearly birth rate of approximately 2000, universal coverage was possible at the programs' inception.

During the initial months of the program, it is often necessary to modify various aspects of the program. In addition, if data are kept regarding number of neonates screened, number passed, number referred, and so forth, the program coordinator is better able to evaluate the program's effectiveness. Of particular interest to most administrators are statistics regarding false positives and prevalence of hearing loss. For example, the initial refer rate at Women and Infants' Hospital of Rhode Island was 27% (White, Vohr, & Behrens, 1993). Since then, the monthly initial fail rate has decreased to as low as 5% (Robinette, 1994) and tends to fluctuate between 5–8% overall. Similar to many other hospitals in the nation, most neonates are

Table 8. Items to Be Included in a TEOAE Training Program and a Suggested Training Sequence

Items to be included	Suggested training sequence
Purpose and goals	Inservice
Computer hardware and software	Overview
Sanitation control	Demonstration
Probe fit	Identify interested persons
Stimulus adequacy	Initiate assignments
Response adequacy	Group Training
Screening validity	Hands on with adults
Troubleshooting	Hands on with neonates
Noise control	On-line training with neonates
Procedural items	Monitor individual screener progress
	Skills Test administration
	Skills Test updates

discharged within 24 hours of birth at this hospital. The statistics for the initial screening for first year (including the three-month training phase) of the Logan Regional Hospital program are presented in Figure 11–12. Overall, of the 1916 newborns, 19 were referred for further testing.

Quality Assurance

The final phase is to identify any existing gaps in any of the segments of the neonatal hearing screening program, including the initial screening, rescreening, referral, follow-up, and tracking components. One of the overall goals of quality assurance is to evaluate overall effectiveness and to improve the program. Persons establishing or modifying existing screening programs must work with the designated risk management or quality assurance personnel in their facility.

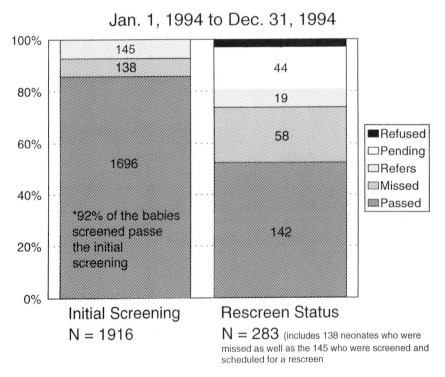

Figure 11–12. Summary statistics from the first year of Logan Regional Hospital's universal neonatal hearing screening program. *Panel A* shows the percentages of neonates who passed the TEOAE screening versus those referred for three reasons—they were screened and did not pass in each ear; they were discharged before they were screened; or they were screened, but were referred for technical reasons, such as invalid tests. *Panel B* shows the percentages of pass versus fail results for the TEOAE rescreens when infants were 2 to 6 weeks of age. The total number of rescreens includes infants who were missed, as well as those who did not pass the screening before discharge. Thus, about 1% of the newborn population was referred to receive an ABR screening.

Each phase of a program has different purposes, needs, and goals. It is difficult to use a single indicator to provide feedback about how well the system is functioning at all phases of the program. Areas in neonatal screening programs that need to be monitored for quality assurance are the number or percentage of neonates screened prior to discharge versus the number missed, overall pass and refer rates for individual screeners and for the overall program, parent satisfaction, personnel, administration, and facility acceptance of the program. Assuring that the screeners maintain designated proficiency levels, through continuing education, inservices, or skills test updates, also are a part of quality assurance. Regardless of the portion of the program being monitored, the information that is collected provides useful feedback to the persons associated with the program.

Other Issues

As with any screening program, there are many relevant issues surrounding the hearing screening for neonates. A universal neonatal hearing screening program cannot be viewed in isolation. It must be viewed as the first stage in a long-term process of identification, assessment, and intervention for infants with hearing loss and their families. The initiation of universal neonatal hearing screening programs requires change in the entire pediatric hearing health care system. Some necessary changes may be anticipated and others cannot. Audiologists may expect to be challenged by an increase in the number of referrals for pediatric auditory assessments. Obtaining audiograms for infants less than six months of age is difficult for even competent, experienced audiologists. Other electrophysiological measures

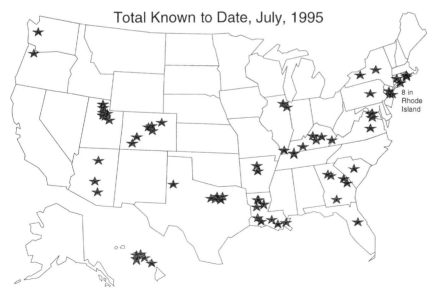

Figure 11–13.   Approximate locations of the more than 100 hospitals known to have existing universal neonatal hearing screening programs as of July, 1995.

(e.g., threshold ABR testing) generally is necessary. Early intervention programs, educational systems, and service coordination agencies will encounter increased demands. Caution must be exercised when screening results are interpreted for parents, pediatricians, and other professionals; they may be left with a false sense of security regarding the neonate's auditory status. Vigilance is necessary for identifying children with progressive or late onset hearing impairments when a neonate has passed a hearing screening.

Summary and Conclusions

Many discoveries regarding the clinical aspects of EOAEs as a tool for investigating the auditory status of neonates remain to be made. The clinical measurement of EOAEs are recognized as being objective, non-invasive, and sensitive to peripheral auditory dysfunction. They are repeatable, quickly recorded, frequency specific, and their measurement does not require highly trained personnel. At least 5% of the more than 4,000,000 babies born in the United States are having their hearing screened before they are discharged by hospitals operating universal (more than 85% of live births being screened) programs (Culpepper, 1995). Figure 11–13 denotes the approximate locations of the existing universal newborn hearing screening programs to date. EOAEs are extremely useful as a clinical tool for universal neonatal hearing screening, and they hold great promise for reducing the average age of identification of hearing loss.

References

Albright, K., Allen, L., Carlock, J., Wolters, C., & Finitzo, T. (1995, April). Universal hearing screening: Designing a successful program. American Academy of Audiology annual convention, Dallas, TX.

American Speech-Language-Hearing Association. (1994). ASHA task force recommends CPT Revisions. *Audiology Update, 13,* 12–13.

American Speech-Language-Hearing Association. Committee on Infant Hearing. (1989). Audiologic screening of newborn infants who are at risk for hearing impairment. *Asha, 31,* 89–92.

American Speech-Language-Hearing Association. (1991). Guidelines for audiologic assessment of children from birth-36 months of age. *Asha, 33* (Suppl. 5), 37–43.

Bess, F. H. (1993). Early identification of hearing loss: The whys, hows, and whens. *The Hearing Journal, 46,* 22–25.

Bess, F. H., & Paradise, J. L. (1994). Universal screening for infant hearing: Not simple, not risk-free, not necessarily beneficial, and not presently justified. *Pediatrics, 98,* 330–334.

Bonfils, P. (1989). Spontaneous otoacoustic emissions: Clinical interest. *Laryngoscope, 99,* 752–765.

Bonfils, P., Dumont, A., Marie, P., Francois, M., & Narcy, P. (1990). Evoked otoacoustic emissions in newborn hearing screening. *Laryngoscope, 100,* 186–189.

Bonfils, P., Uziel, A., & Pujol, R. (1988). Screening for auditory dysfunction in infants by evoked otoacoustic emissions. *Archives of Otolaryngology and Head and Neck Surgery, 114,* 887–890.

Brass, D., & Kemp, D. T. (1994). Quantitative assessment of methods for the detection of otoacoustic emissions. *Ear and Hearing, 15,* 378–389.

Bray, P. J. (1989). Click evoked otoacoustic emissions and the development of a clinical otoacoustic hearing test instrument. London University, Ph.D. thesis.

Burns, E. M., Arehart, K. H., & Campbell, S. L. (1991). Prevalence of spontaneous otoacoustic emissions in neonates. Abstracts of the Fourteenth Midwinter Research Meeting for the Association for Research in Otolaryngology, p. 66.

Culpepper, B. (1995). Universal newborn hearing screening with otoacoustic emissions in the United States of America. National Otoacoustic Emissions Study Day, University of Manchester Institute of Science and Technology, Manchester, England.

Culpepper, B., Henderson, B., & Shelton, T. L. (1994). Potential for using Ad*Hear Wax Guards for OAE probe assembly protection (abstract). *Asha, 36,* 131–132.

Elssmann, S., F., Matkin, N. D., & Sabo, M. P. (1987). Early identification of congenital sensorineural hearing impairment. *The Hearing Journal, 40,* 13–17.

Ewing, A. W. G., & Ewing, J. R. (1947). Opportunity and the deaf child. London: University of London Press.

Glattke, T. J., Pafitis, I. A., Cummiskey, C., & Herer, G. R. (1995). Identification of hearing loss in children and young adults using measures of transient evoked otoacoustic emissions. *American Journal of Audiology, 4*, 67–82.

Goldberg, B. (1993). Universal hearing screening of newborns: An idea whose time has come. *Asha, 35*, 63–64.

Hurley, R. M., & Musiek, F. E. (1994). Effectiveness of transient-evoked otoacoustic emissions (TEOAEs) in predicting hearing level. *Ear and Hearing, 5*, 195–203.

Johnsen, N. J., Bagi, P., Parbo, J., & Eberling, C. (1983). Evoked acoustic emissions from the human ear. IV. Final results in 100 neonates. *Scandinavian Audiology, 17*, 27–34.

Johnson, J. L., Mauk, G. W., Takekawa, K. M., Simon, P. R., Sia, C. C. J., & Blackwell, P. M. (1993). Implementing a statewide system of services for infants and toddlers with disabilities. *Seminars in Hearing, 14*, 105–119.

Johnson, M. J., Maxon, A. B., White, K. R., & Vohr, B. R. (1993). Operating a hospital-based universal newborn hearing screening program using transient evoked otoacoustic emissions. *Seminars in Hearing, 14*, 46–55.

Joint Committee on Infant Hearing. (1995). 1994 Position Statement. *Pediatrics, 95*, 152–156.

Kemp, D. T., Ryan, S., & Bray, P. (1990). A guide to the effective use of otoacoustic emissions. *Ear and Hearing, 11*, 93–105.

Kennedy, C. R., Kimm, L., Dees, D. C., Evans, P. I. P., Hunter, M., Lenton, S., & Thornton, S. D. (1991). Otoacoustic emissions and auditory brainstem responses in the newborn. *Archives of Diseases in Childhood, 66*, 1124–1129.

Koop, C. E., (1993). We can identify children with hearing loss before their first birthday. *Seminars in Hearing, 14*, Foreword.

Lafreniere, D., Jung, M. D., Smurzynski, J., Leonard, G., Kim, D. O., & Sasek, J. (1991). Distortion-product and click-evoked otoacoustic emissions in healthy newborns. *Archives of Otolaryngology and Head and Neck Surgery, 117*, 1382–1389.

Lasky, R., Perlman, J., & Hecox, K. (1992). Distortion-product otoacoustic emissions in human newborns and adults. *Ear and Hearing, 13*, 430–441.

Mahoney, T. USA models of early identification and follow-up. National Institutes of Consensus Development Conference, March 1–3, 1993.

Mauk, G. W., White, K. R., Mortensen, L. B., & Behrens, T. R. (1991). The effectiveness of screening programs based on high-risk characteristics in early identification of hearing impairment. *Ear and Hearing, 12*, 312–319.

Maxon, A. B., White, K. R., Behrens, T. R., & Vohr, B. R. (1995). Referral rates and cost efficiency in a universal newborn hearing screening program using transient evoked otoacoustic emissions. *Journal of the American Academy of Audiology, 6*, 271–277.

Meister, S. (1993). Emerging risk: Failure to detect hearing disability in newborns. The Problem: Lack of screening programs for "normal" newborns. *QRC Advisor, 10*, 1–4.

National Consortium for Newborn Hearing Screening. (1995, November 16–18). TEOAE-based universal newborn hearing screening. Georgetown University School of Medicine, Washington, DC.

National Institutes of Health Consensus Statement (1993, March 1–3). Early identification of hearing impairment in infants and young children. ii, 1–24.

Northern, J. L., & Hayes, D. (1994). Universal screening for infant hearing impairment: Necessary, beneficial and justifiable. *Audiology Today, 6*, 10–13.

Norton, S. J. (1994). Emerging role of evoked otoacoustic emissions in neonatal hearing screening. *The American Journal of Otology, 15* (Suppl. 1), 4–12.

Norton, S. J., & Widen, J. E. (1990). Evoked otoacoustic emissions in normal-hearing infants and children: Emerging data and issues. *Ear and Hearing, 11*, 121–127.

Picton, T. W., Kellett, A. J. C., Vezsenyi, M., & Rabinovitch, D. E. (1993). Otoacoustic emissions recorded at rapid stimulus rates. *Ear and Hearing, 14*, 299–314.

Plinkert, P. K., Sesterhenn, G., Arold, R., & Zenner, H. P. (1990). *European Archives of Otorhinolaryngology, 247*, 356–360.

Popelka, G. R., Karzon, R. K., & Arjmand, E. M. (1995). Growth of the $2f1 - f2$ distortion product otoacoustic emission for low-level stimuli in human neonates. *Ear and Hearing, 16*, 159–165.

Prieve, B. A. (1992). Otoacoustic emissions in infants and children: Basic characteristics and clinical application. *Seminars in Hearing, 13*, 37–52.

Robinette, M. (1994). Evoked otoacoustic emission screening for infant hearing impairment: Made simple, relatively risk-free, beneficial, and presently justified. *Pediatrics, 94*, 252–253.

Robins, D. S. (1990). A case for infant hearing screening. *Neonatal Intensive Care, 3*, 24–26, 29, 42.

Robins, D. S. (1991). New approaches to infant hearing screening. *Neonatal Intensive Care, 4*, 38–40, 46, 50.

Smurzynski, J. (1994). Longitudinal measurements of distortion-product and click-evoked otoacoustic emissions of preterm infants: Preliminary results. *Ear and Hearing, 15*, 210–223.

Smurzynski, J., Jung, M. D., Lafreniere, D., Kim, D. O., Kamath, M. V., Rowe, J. C., Holman, M. C., & Leonard, G. (1993). Distortion-product and click-evoked otoacoustic emissions of preterm and full-term infants. *Ear and Hearing, 14*, 258–274.

Stevens, J. C., Webb, H. D., Hutchison, J., Connell, J., Smith, M. F., & Buffin, J. T. (1989). Click evoked otoacoustic emissions compared with brain stem electric response. *Archives of Disease in Children, 64*, 1105–1111.

Stevens, J. C., Webb, H. D., Hutchison, J., Connell, J., Smith, M. F., & Buffin, J. T. (1990). Click evoked otoacoustic emissions in neonatal screening. *Ear and Hearing, 11*, 128–133.

Strong, C. J., Clark, T. C., Johnson, D., Watkins, S., Barringer, D. G., & Walden, B. E. (1994). SKI*HI home-based programming for children who are deaf or hard of hearing: Recent research findings. *The Transdisciplinary Journal, 4*, 25–36.

U.S. Department of Health and Human Services. Public Health Service. (1990). Healthy People 2000: National Health Promotion and Disease Prevention Objectives. Washington, DC.

Uziel, A., & Piron, J. P. (1991). Evoked otoacoustic emissions from normal newborns and babies admitted to an intensive care baby unit. *Acta Otolaryngologica, 482* (Suppl.), 85–91.

White, K. R. (1995). TEOAE-based universal newborn hearing screening: Past, present, and future. National Symposium on Hearing in Infants. Vail, CO.

White, K. R., & Behrens, T. R. (1993). The Rhode Island Hearing Assessment Project: Implications for universal newborn hearing screening. *Seminars in Hearing, 14*, 1–119.

White, K. R., & Maxon, A. B. (1995). Universal screening for infant hearing impairment: Simple, beneficial, and presently justified. *International Journal of Pediatric Otorhinolaryngology, 32*, 201–211.

White, K. R., Vohr, B. R., & Behrens, T. R. (1993). Universal newborn hearing screening using transient evoked otoacoustic emissions: Results of the Rhode Island Hearing Assessment Project. *Seminars in Hearing, 14*, 18–29.

White, K. R., Vohr, B. R., Maxon, A. B., Behrens, T. R., McPherson, M. G., & Mauk, G. W. (1994). Screening all newborns for hearing loss using transient evoked otoacoustic emissions. *International Journal of Pediatric Otorhinolaryngology, 29*, 203–217.

12

Evoked Otoacoustic Emissions in Evaluating Children

JUDITH E. WIDEN

Introduction

This chapter describes how evoked otoacoustic emissions (EOAEs) are being used or may potentially be used in evaluating children. Since the general concepts of EOAEs apply to children, as well as adults, this chapter then will focus on how children's EOAEs and the testing of children may differ from adults.

We began recording EOAEs in our clinic in 1989. Most of our early experience was with TEOAEs using the ILO88 Otodynamic Analyser. Only later did we begin measuring DPOAEs, also using the equipment of Otodynamics Ltd. Although our experience is thus slanted to the use of transients and limited by the use of one particular brand of equipment, the major points of this chapter should be applicable to all clinicians using EOAEs, no matter the type of EOAE or the type of equipment.

Selecting Candidates

Nearly every child seen in audiology clinics may be a candidate for EOAE testing. Infants too young for behavioral audiometry and who were not screened as newborns can be referred to rule out hearing loss. Infants and young children, who by definition are considered difficult to test, are prime candidates for EOAE testing to add to the audiometric information obtained through behavioral testing, evoked potentials, and immittance measurements. For other child referrals, EOAEs may provide diagnostic information or site of lesion data. And, finally, EOAEs may provide a means of monitoring changes in auditory function due to toxic agents such as chemotherapy.

Infant and Child versus Adult EOAEs

Numerous investigations have documented that in the absence of external and middle ear-pathology EOAEs are robust and broad-band in normally hearing neonates, infants, and young children. Their strength is so striking that we had T-shirts made up for our young subjects (Figure 12–1).

Prevalence of EOAEs in Neonates

Many of the studies of neonates focus on the prevalence (or the presence or absence) of TEOAEs in the neonatal population rather than on description of the

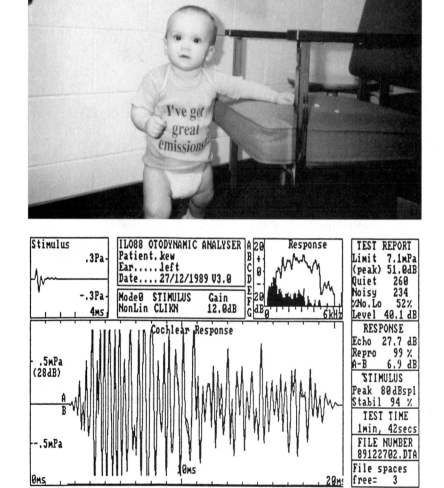

Figure 12–1. Infants typically have high-amplitude, broad-spectrum emissions. One of our first subjects shows off the shirt she earned for the TEOAE recording displayed below the photograph.

response characteristics. Johnsen, Bagi, and Elberling (1983) were the first to report "clearly observable responses comparable to adults" in each of the 20 healthy newborns they tested. Later they reported similar results for an additional 100 neonates (Johnsen, Bagi, Parbo, & Elberling, 1988). As investigators began experimenting with OAEs to screen newborns for hearing loss, similar findings of prevalent, robust emissions were reported for full-term healthy neonates, preterm infants, and graduates of neonatal intensive-care units (Stevens, Webb, Smith, Buffin, & Ruddy, 1987; Stevens, Webb, Hutchinson, Connell, Smith, & Buffin, 1989, 1990, 1991; Bonfils, Uziel, & Pujol, 1988; Bonfils, Dumont, Marie, Francois, & Narcy, 1990; Uziel & Piron, 1991; Smurzynski et al., 1993). Norton (1994) has a particularly good summary of newborn hearing studies that includes excellent tables delineating the details of each study published through 1992.

EOAE Amplitude

Although various means of measurement have been used and different criteria have been applied to determine the presence of emissions, most investigators have found that emissions of newborns are considerably larger than those observed in normally hearing adults. Most data indicate that babies' TEOAEs have greater amplitude than responses obtained from adults, by as much as 10 dB overall (Kemp, Ryan, & Bray, 1990; Norton & Widen, 1991; Lafreniere, Smurzynski, Jung, Leonard, & Kim, 1993). The difference is maintained over a wide range of intensities as seen in Figure 12–2 (Norton & Widen, 1991; Norton, 1993). Smurzynski et al. (1993) reported that neonatal TEOAE levels exceeded adults only at frequencies above 1500 Hz but acknowledged that the difference might be accounted for in the difference in the stimulus spectrum.

No large scale infant screening studies using DPOAEs have been reported, so there are fewer data on DPOAEs in neonates than on TEOAEs. With DPOAE recording, there are also more test parameters (e.g., frequencies, frequency ratio, levels, level ratio) to vary from study to study. Therefore, it is not surprising that the conclusions about adult-newborn differences in DPOAEs are still inconclusive. Some investigators have reported that newborn DPOAEs are comparable to adults. Lafreniere, Jung, Smurzynski, Leonard, Kim, and Sasek (1991) concluded that the DPOAE "audiograms" of their newborns were qualitatively similar to adults provided the same probe was used for recording. They found that the average DPOAE level of newborns was slightly higher (2.0–6.6 dB) than that of adults in the frequency region between 1 and 2.4 kHz, but lower (0.4–3.5 dB) than that of adults in the frequency region of 4.8 to 8 kHz. Although Lasky, Perlman, and Hecox (1992) concluded that their neonatal DPOAEs were comparable in amplitude to their adults, the neonates did not show the characteristic dip in the distortion product (DP)–gram between 1 and 3 kHz and in fact the amplitude of the neonatal DPOAEs in that region was significantly greater than adults. Bonfils, Avan, Francois, Trotoux, and Narcy (1992) reported that DPOAE amplitudes were 6 dB higher in neonates than in adults. Brown, Sheppard, and Russell (1994) using a low amplitude primaries (L1 = 55, L2 = 40) reported a mean DPOAE amplitude that was 10 dB higher in newborns than adults, but the variability was great enough that the differences were not statistically significant.

Smurzynski et al. (1993) showed a statistically significant correlation between

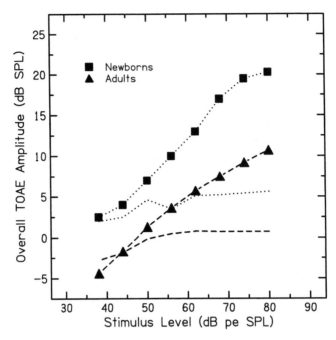

Figure 12–2. Mean overall TEOAE amplitude as a function of click stimulus level for a group of 27 fullterm newborns (21–54 hours of age) with no risk factors for hearing loss and a group of 20 young adults (21–25 years) with hearing levels of 10 dB or better. Mean noise levels are depicted with the *dotted line* for infants and *dashed line* for adults. (From Norton & Widen, 1991. Used with permission.)

DPOAEs and TEOAEs obtained between the same ears of infants, just as they had in adults (Smurzynski & Kim, 1992). They interpreted this finding to mean that a common mechanism underlies the generation of TEOAEs and DPOAEs in the human cochlea at different stages in development.

Noise

Another consistent finding of neonatal EOAE studies is that infant recordings are noisier than adults over the entire frequency region (Norton & Widen, 1991; Smurzynski et al., 1993). This difference is illustrated in Figure 12–2. The greater noise levels in infants affect the recording of DP emissions, as well as transient-evoked emissions. Both Lasky et al. (1992) and Brown et al. (1994) reported higher noise levels in infants than adults. Noise prevented Smurzynski et al. (1993) from collecting DPOAE data in the 1000 Hz range for many infants. Bonfils et al. (1992) reported that high noise levels precluded DPOAE testing below 1200 Hz.

EOAE Spectrum

With respect to the spectrum of the click-evoked EOAE, neonates typically show more high frequency energy than adults (Figure 12–3) (Kemp et al., 1990; Lafreniere

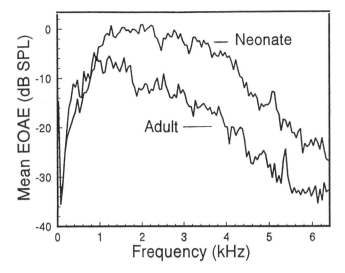

Figure 12–3. Mean TEOAE spectra for the group of neonates (*top line*) and adults (*lower line*) described in Figure 12–2. Click level was 80 dB peSPL. (From Norton & Widen, 1991. Used with permission.)

et al., 1991; Norton & Widen, 1991; Uziel & Piron, 1991; Smurzynski et al., 1993). There are two extrinsic factors that may contribute to this effect. One is that the higher noise levels may obscure low frequency emissions. This is the case with both TEOAEs and DPOAEs. A second factor for TEOAE recording is that the spectrum of the click in the neonatal ear canal is different than in adults' (Kemp et al., 1990; Lafreniere et al., 1991) with less low frequency energy for neonates than adults. This may be related to different resonance characteristics of the neonatal canal (Keefe, Bulen, Arehart, & Burns, 1993), as well as to the difficulties getting a good probe fit in the soft newborn canal.

Three primary questions emerge from the findings that newborn EOAEs differ from adults: (a) Why the difference between infants and adults? (b) When does the change occur? and (c) How do the differences affect our interpretation of test results? None of the questions has been answered yet. Speculations about *why* involve considerations of the differences in the size and resonance characteristics of the ear canal and middle ear (Lasky et al., 1992). Properties of the input imped-ance of the eardrum, middle ear, and cochlea may be unique to the neonatal ear (Keefe et al., 1993). Possible differences in cochlear function have not been ruled out. Are there differences in the mass and stiffness properties of the cochlear partition or changes in the properties of the stereocilia resulting in changed filter characteristics (Johnson, Parbo, & Elberling, 1989)? Maturation of the efferent system which regulates outer hair-cell motility may explain a portion of the differ-ence (Morlet, Collet, Salle, & Morgon, 1993; Ryan & Piron, 1994).

Changes with Age

CHANGES IN THE FIRST WEEK

A closer look at the changes that occur with age shows that babies at one week of age have higher amplitude emissions than when they were newborns. Several investigators have reported that neonatal TEOAEs are more likely to be present and have greater amplitude if testing is delayed until the second to fourth day of life (Kok, van Zanten, & Brocaar, 1992; Kok, van Zanten, Brocaar, & Wallenburg, 1993). The same is true with DPOAEs (Marco et al., 1995). The assumption, which has not yet been documented by otoscopy, is that the changes are related to the clearing of vernix from the ear canal and fluid from the middle ear. Chang, Vohr, Norton, and Lekas (1993) found that canal debris and canal collapse may account for failures within the first day or two of life.

However when Thornton, Kimm, Kennedy, and Cafarelli-Dees (1993) compared tympanometric data with TEOAE data in the first three days of life they concluded that other mechanisms must account, in part, for the improvement in the evoked emission as the infant matures.

CHANGES IN THE FIRST MONTHS

Bonfils, Francois, Avan, et al. (1992) found that EOAEs were present in 93% of preterm infant ears, with a mean overall amplitude of 23.3 dB SPL. There were no statistically significant variations in EOAE amplitude with gestational age from 32 to 41 weeks. Smurzynski (1994) reported that preterm infants born at 24 to 33 weeks gestational age and tested at 33 to 43 weeks gestational age tended to have TEOAEs and DPOAEs at the 90th percentile for normal full-1 term neonates. They speculated that the maturation of the auditory periphery followed a different time-course in premature versus full-term neonates. In a longitudinal study of full-term neonates, Widen and Norton (1993) found the overall amplitude of TEOAEs to be greater amplitude at one month than at 1-to-2 days of age (Figure 12–4). It is possible that the increase in amplitude can be attributed to post natal changes in the middle-ear transmission characteristics. The changes may occur as a result of exposure to the environmental conditions outside the womb. In that case the premature infants in the study by Smurzynski et al. had been exposed to standard atmospheric conditions longer than the full-term infants at the time of testing.

Engdahl, Arnesen, and Mair (1994a) successfully recorded TEOAEs in 192 ears of 100 consecutive full-term neonates on the third or fourth day of life, and then followed up those recordings when the children were 3, 6 and 12 months of age. They found that amplitudes were largest at 3 to 4 days of age. Some decrease in high frequency energy was noted at the older ages, but the changes were not systematic with increasing age. Widen and Norton (1993) also found that the changes from one month to 7 or 9 months were minimal.

OLDER INFANTS AND CHILDREN

There are many more published reports of newborn EOAEs than of older infants and children. Norton and Widen (1990) analyzed TEOAE data from normally hearing subjects from a few weeks to 30 years of age and found a statistically

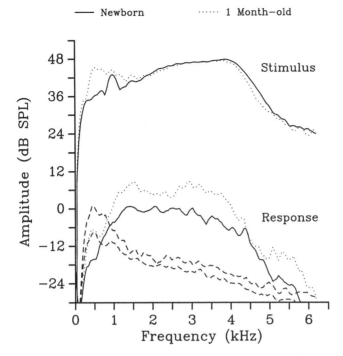

Figure 12–4. Mean TEOAE stimulus and response spectra for normal newborns tested at 1–2 days of age (*solid line*) compared to a group of one-month old infants (*dotted line*). The lower dashed lines in the response spectra depict the noise floor. (From Widen & Norton, 1993. Used with permission.)

significant decrease in EOAE amplitude as a function of age group despite a great deal of variability across individuals. Figure 12–5 illustrates these findings. When they compared the overall TEOAE amplitude of neonates with adults as a function of stimulus level (Figure 12–2) they found that the greater amplitude of neonates was maintained for all stimulus levels (Norton & Widen, 1991). Later Norton and Harrison (1993) added the data from a group of normally hearing children aged 4 to 13 years (Figure 12–6). At every stimulus level adults have lower overall EOAEs than children and children have lower amplitudes than neonates.

Subsequent studies of normal hearing children have not shown such large differences across age, as the Norton and Widen study did (Spektor, Leonard, Kim, Jung, & Smurzynski, 1991; Nozza & Sabo, 1992; Glattke, Paritis, Cummiskey, & Herer, 1995). Details of the studies are shown in Table 12–1. Figure 12–6 suggests that the mean EOAE amplitude of the 4- to 13-year-old subjects is approximately 15 dB SPL, falling between the values from Norton and Widen and the studies of Spektor et al., Nozza and Sabo, and Glattke et al. Although the studies varied from one another in some aspects, possible reasons for the differences are not readily apparent. Click level was approximately the same for all of the studies. Normal hearing was defined as 10 or 20 dB HL or better for each. The Norton and Widen

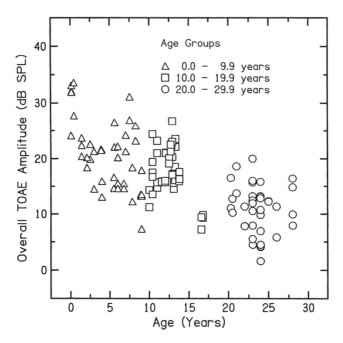

Figure 12–5.   Overall TEOAE amplitude to 80 dB peSPL clicks as a function of age from newborn to 30 years. (Adapted from Norton & Widen, 1990.)

(1990) and Norton and Harrison (1993) studies may have contained fewer children with history of ear disease since many of their subjects were recruited specifically for studies of normal hearing. Nozza and Sabo tested in a school and Glattke et al. selected their subjects from a speech and hearing clinic. Norton and Widen's high amplitudes may reflect the fact that their youngest group included many younger

Table 12–1.   TEOAEs in Normally Hearing Children

Study	Age in Years		Number of Ears	Overall Amplitude in dB SPL		Repro in %	
	Range	(Mean)		Mean	(SD)	Mean	(SD)
Norton and	0–9.0	(5.4)	32	20.0	(5.4)	90.4	(12.3)
Widen, 1990	10–19.9	(12.6)	37	17.0	(4.2)	90.6	(10.4)
	20–29.9	(23.7)	38	10.9	(4.3)	83.4	(14.8)
Spektor et al.,	4–10	(7.5)	13	13.5			
1991	22–29	(26)	11	9.1			
Nozza and	5–10		56 right	13.5	(4.4)	73.3	(22.1)
Sabo, 1992			56 left	12.9	(4.1)	71.4	(20.8)
Glattke et al.,	0–10		277	12.5		75	
1995	10–20		93	10.1		80	
	20–30		6	11.8		85	

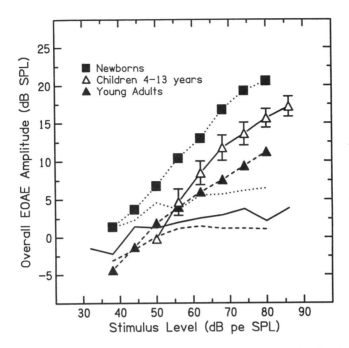

Figure 12–6.   Mean overall TEOAE amplitude as a function of click stimulus level for 3 different age groups. The newborn and adult data are the same as that described in Figure 12–2. The *open triangles* represent the mean TEOAE amplitude (the *bars* = 1 standard deviation) from 43 normally hearing children reported by Norton & Harrison, 1993. (Courtesy of Susan Norton.)

infants than the other studies did. That does not explain though their considerably larger and more reproducible OAEs in the 10-to-19-year age range.

With respect to DP emissions, many of the data from children have been case examples (Ohlms, Lonsbury-Martin, & Martin, 1990; Lonsbury-Martin, Martin, McCoy, & Whitehead, 1994; Lonsbury-Martin, McCoy, Whitehead, & Martin, 1994). In the large study from the Boys Town National Research Hospital approximately half the subjects were children, but the data were not analyzed with respect to age (Gorga et al., 1993a, 1993b). In their small sample, Spektor et al. (1991) reported that the differences seen in TEOAEs between children and adults (Table 12–1) showed up only at 1300 and 6000 Hz on the subjects' DP-grams.

Regarding longitudinal changes beyond the newborn period, 20 (Johnsen et al., 1983) were retested at 4 years of age to determine if their emissions had changed (Johnsen, Parbo, & Elberling, 1989). Only 10 of the 20 had normal otoscopy at the time of retest. Nine of the remaining children could be tested with pure-tone audiometry and tympanometry. Hearing threshold levels were 20 dB or greater (i.e., better) at 250, 1000, and 4000 Hz. Their TEOAE amplitudes and latencies were reported to be "essentially the same at 4 years as in the newborn period"; however, the investigators reported a change in frequency content with the dominant part of the emission at lower frequency at four than at birth. They postulated that this shift in frequency mapping occurs in the inner ear during development owing to change in the mass and stiffness of the cochlear partition or to changes in the properties of the stereocilia resulting in changed filter characteristics.

Interpretation of Child-Adult Differences

For clinical purposes audiologists need to know if the procedures designed for and tested on adults are also appropriate for children. For example, is the 80 dB peSPL click level typically used to test adults appropriate for children as well? This default level was initially chosen because it separated normal from impaired hearing in adults. If children as a group have more robust emissions then is another stimulus level more appropriate for them? Some investigators have questioned whether the 80 dB peSPL click stimulus level is too high a level to distinguish normal hearing from impaired hearing in children (Norton & Widen, 1991; Norton, 1993). One reason for this concern is that some children with sloping audiograms display TEOAEs with amplitude and reproducibility values within the range of normal hearing adults. With these children the amplitudes of their TEOAEs diminish more rapidly with reduction in click level than do normal ears. Figure 12–7 illustrates two such cases. This observation has led to the practice of testing at two levels rather than one. Usually we use the default screening level and another at least 6 dB (a halving of pressure) or 10 to 12 dB lower. In a normal ear, the emission

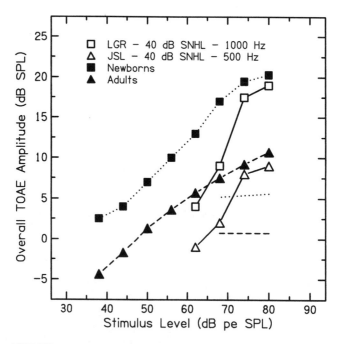

Figure 12–7. TEOAE input-output functions for two children with sensorineural hearing loss are compared with the mean functions for newborns and adults. L.G. is a 10-year old boy with 40 dB hearing loss at 1000 Hz and below. J.S. is a 5-year old girl with 40 dB hearing loss at 500 and 1000 Hz in her left ear.

will still be present at the lower level. If EOAEs are present at the higher level, but not the lower, a mild hearing loss is suspected, until corroborating information proves otherwise. The additional information may be either pure tone thresholds at some critical frequencies, a comparison of acoustic reflex thresholds to tones versus noise, or ABR thresholds.

Using ROC analyses Norton and Harrison (1993) sought to determine the click level (74, 80, and 86 dB peSPL) that best differentiated average hearing losses of 15, 30 and greater than 30 dB in children between 4 and 13 years of age. They reported that using an 80-dB peak SPL click as the evoking stimulus and an overall EOAE amplitude criterion of 3 dB, children with PTAs (1, 2, 4 kHz) greater than or equal to 30 dB could be accurately separated from children with PTAs greater than 30 dB. In the study, 80 dB differentiated losses of 30 dB and greater from hearing levels better than 30, but an 86 dB peak click level did not.

The levels used for DPOAE testing are at least as big a concern as click level for TEOAEs (Popelka, Karzon, & Arjamand, 1995; Brown, Sheppard, & Russell, 1994). Typically, the primary tones used to evoke DP-grams in adults have been 70 to 75 dB SPL, which is considerably higher than the spectrum level of the click in any one frequency region. The non-linear behavior of interest in OAE testing is associated with outer hair cells at low stimulus levels. At high levels a passive response of mechanical structures may also be generated. Stimulus artifact from over driving the microphones may also interfere (Brown et al., 1994). DPOAEs can be successfully recorded at lower levels in neonates, even in nursery settings (Popelka et al., 1995; Brown et al., 1994; Bergman, Gorga, Neely, Kaminski, Beauchaine, & Peters, 1995). The effects of stimulus level on DPOAEs in older children and on hearing-impaired children have not yet been reported. If DP emissions are to be used for hearing screening, the levels that effectively separate normal-hearing loss from mild-hearing loss must be known.

When it comes to test interpretation, not only is level a concern, but also frequency is. In many of the early clinical reports "presence" of EOAEs was undefined. Many investigators assumed that a valid emission was present if the reproducibility value on the ILO88 equipment exceeded 50%. It is important to remember that this 50% criterion was based on early studies of adults (Kemp, Brey, Alexander, & Brown, 1986) and that Bray and Kemp (1987) originally advised that the bandwidth of the TEOAE, as well, as its overall level should be considered when devising pass-fail criteria. Both TEOAEs and DPOAEs provide frequency-specific information concerning cochlear status. Whereas the stimuli used to evoke DPOAEs have narrower spectra than a click or tone pip have, the emissions evoked at a particular frequency by a click or tone pip are frequency specific in that they arise from the place within the cochlea tuned to their frequency (Norton, 1992, 1993, 1994; Kemp & Ryan, 1993).

There are several ways to get frequency specific information from click-evoked OAEs. For example with the ILO88, one of the specific function keys magnifies the fast Fourier transform (FFT) spectrum and allows the examiner to determine the frequency components in the response. This option is shown in the second panel of Figure 12–8. Newer versions of the software allow the examiner to examine TEOAE amplitude and noise in a variety of band-widths. The amplitude of the emission, the noise, and the emission-to-noise ratio is calculated for each band. The

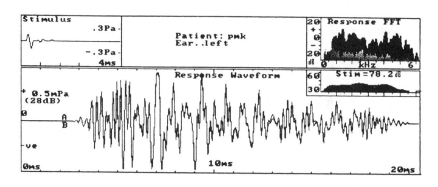

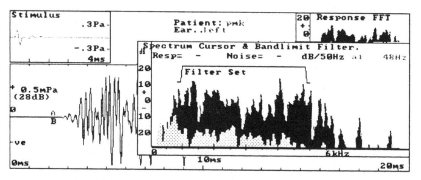

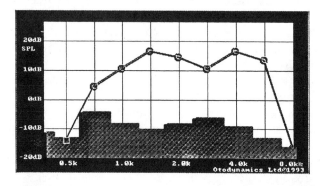

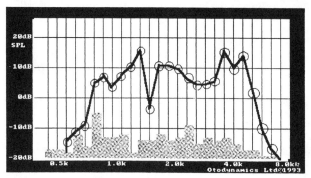

Figure 12–8. *Top panel*: The output screen of the IL 088 Otodynamic Analyser typically shows the emission waveform in the *lower left* section and the response spectra in the *upper right* box. An option which allows closer scrutiny of the frequency components of the response is shown in the second panel. Another option is to replace the response waveform with a power analysis. The third and fourth panels illustrate one-half octave and one-sixth octave analyses respectively.

third and fourth panels of Figure 12–8 show examples of half-octave and one-sixth octave analyses, respectively.

When the detail of the TEOAE is given fine definition, the result looks more like the DPOAE. The bands are not necessarily comparable to the DPOAEs in frequency— that is, TEOAE amplitude at 1k Hz frequency band cannot be expected to equate with DPOAE amplitude at 1K Hz. Not only is the emission amplitude calculated for slightly different area of the basilar membrane, the stimuli that evoked them were different. And the stimuli may be considerably different in terms of level (i.e., an 80-dB peSPL click does not have the same energy at 1000 Hz that an 80-dB SPL tone does) (Norton & Stover, 1994).

If one has the ILO88 and no access to DPOAE test equipment, he or she might get the kind of concentrated energy wanted (as in DPs) if a tone pip is created. However, Norton and Harrison (1993) found that tone pips did not improve performance over clicks except at 500 Hz. And Prieve, Gorga, Schmidt, et al. (1993) and Gorga et al. (1993a, 1993b) have found that neither TEOAEs nor DPOAEs were particularly effective in detecting hearing loss at 500 Hz.

Given that the EOAEs of infants and children differ from adults in terms of amplitude and spectrum, can adult norms be applied to children? Because emissions change with age, can neonatal norms be used to judge older children? The answers to these questions are not yet available. However, most clinicians assume that children are normal hearing if their EOAEs are as good as those of adults.

A few investigators have suggested criteria for interpretation based on data from children. The most often used comes from data collected by the Infant Hearing Project at Women and Infants Hospital in Rhode Island (White, Vohr, & Behrens, 1993; White, Vohr, Maxon, Behrens, McPherson, & Mauk, 1994). The criteria have evolved as the project database grows, but as of 1995, a neonate's test was considered a "pass" if the response spectrum contained 3 dB or more power than the noise spectrum in each of 3 1000-Hz frequency bands centered at 1500, 2500, and 3500 Hz. A pass was considered indicative of hearing sensitivity of 30 dB HL or better at those frequencies.

Smurzynski et al. (1993) used the 10th percentile of the half-octave RMS TEOAE level to establish the pass and fail criteria for screening newborns. They suggested that any ear with RMS TEOAE levels below the 10th percentile in at least two half-octave bands should be called a failure. This recommendation needs to be validated with behavioral audiometry.

The Glattke et al. (1995) study of 260 subjects from 20 months to 23 years of age is the most comprehensive analysis of children's EOAE to date. TEOAE data from 374 normal ears and 130 impaired ears were analyzed with respect to nearly every measure available on the ILO88. They found that the group with thresholds poorer than 20 dB HL fell below the 15th percentile of the normal group on overall amplitude and below the 10th percentile on reproducibility. In addition the difference between the ILO88's two measures of overall amplitude (*Response*, or the SPL of the correlated portion of the waveform, and $A + B$, the overall level of the response and noise) was the most distinguishing measure between the normal group and the hearing loss group. Of equal importance was their analysis of the reproducibility scores in the five frequency bands from 1000 to 5000 Hz. The 2000-Hz reproducibility score was the most efficient of all measurements in separating normal and impaired ears, regardless of the frequencies affected. The results from the Glattke et al. study are comparable to those of Prieve et al. (1993), whose sample included adults as well as children.

Gorga et al. (1993b) compared to DPOAEs of a large sample of normal and impaired ears in children and adults, but did not analyze them with respect to age. For DPOAE screening and evaluation of neonates, infants and young children, pass-fail criteria with validating measures of hearing sensitivity have not been determined.

Practical Considerations

Although pertinent to testing of all ages, there are several considerations that are particularly critical when testing children. They include controlling the effects of noise, accommodating a wide range of ear canal sizes, understanding the effects of middle ear problems, and deciding when the test is valid.

Controlling the Effect of Noise

Both external and internal noise is often reported to be a limiting factor in neonatal TEOAE measurements. It continues to be a problem with older infants and children. With respect to external noise, the ambient noise level in the test room as well as the fit of the probe in the child's ear can play a role.

TEST ENVIRONMENT

To keep environmental noise, such as voices, fans, and footsteps, to a minimum, a sound-treated audiometric test booth works well. In the nurseries at the University of Kansas Medical Center, we use an isolette as a portable sound booth of sorts to reduce the noise. But our clinic is quiet enough that the isolette is unnecessary. Testing is done in a quiet room of the clinic. We have a comfortable rocking recliner that can be used by parents who hold their children for the testing. An older child can sit back with firm but comfortable support (Figure 12–9). Room lights are controlled by a rheostat so the room can be darkened to induce sleep.

PEDIATRIC SIZE PROBES AND PROBE TIPS

Another way to minimize external noise is to select a probe tip that achieves maximal seal of the child's ear canal. A poorly fitting probe allows environmental noise to interfere. It also causes loss of low frequency energy of the stimulus. Personally when noise levels are high during recording the first thing I check is the probe fit. If re-fitting the probe doesn't solve the problem, other size probe tips may be used. The ILO comes with three different sizes of baby probe tips. Other sizes can be fashioned out of immittance probe tips of any type provided the intended stimulus spectrum is not altered.

Even when the test room is quiet and the best probe fit is obtained, the greater source of noise is the physiological noise that is generated within the patient. It seems that the younger the patients, the noisier they are.

SCHEDULING AND SEDATION

Careful scheduling of pediatric patients when they can be quiet and relaxed can make the difference between a successful and unsuccessful evaluation. We usually

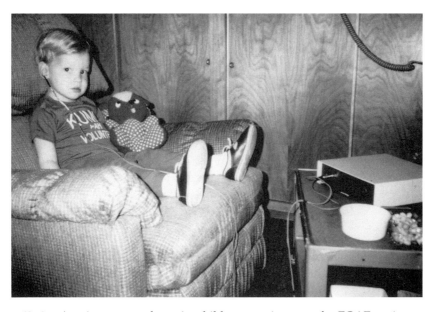

Figure 12–9. A quiet room and a quiet child are requirements for EOAE testing.

try to schedule infants under 6 months of age at a regular nap time. With older children the parents are asked to come prepared for sedation if necessary. Because EOAEs do not require preparing the skin for electrodes, the clinician may find that it is possible to do EOAE testing in situations where ABR testing would not be possible. We often judge the likelihood of success with EOAEs by the child's tolerance of tympanometry. If EOAEs are present and robust, they can often be recorded in a minimal amount of time, sometimes in seconds. It is the child whose EOAEs are low in amplitude who will require more averaging and thus the longer test time. There is no way to know who that is until the testing is done.

Sedation for EOAE testing is no different than for ABR testing. Usually if a child is to be sedated for evaluation, we plan to do EOAEs with the evoked potential and even immittance testing. In our facility this is done in the Pediatrics Clinic, by nurses who administer the prescribed medication (usually chloral hydrate [Noctec]) and who check the child upon awakening and prior to discharge from the clinic.

Many older children can be persuaded to sit quietly while they watch the activity on the monitor. Explanation of the noise reject monitor and how the child needs to be so quiet that "the purple line stays below the arrow" has worked for some youngsters. Usually giving the child a book or toy causes too much movement to get a good test. Some people use video tape cartoons, with the sound off, to keep the child mesmerized long enough for a good recording (Glattke et al., 1995).

Even when children are sleeping they can be noisy. The noise generated in children with conditions such as upper respiratory congestion and allergies can be a major factor in unsuccessful EOAE testing. There are several techniques for controlling the noise that remain after we have done the best we can in terms of environment, probe fit and activity level.

Noise rejection is one of the most important aspects of pediatric EOAE recording. With noisy patients, we rely on the visual feedback we see on the screen for judging the probe fit and setting the noise reject level. We have learned that the best strategy for getting a good emission recording is to keep the noise reject level as low as possible (usually at a point just above the median take level). If a child is breathing noisily or sucking on a pacifier the monitor may drop below the specified level only once every few seconds, but with patience a valid recording may ultimately be obtained. This capability of monitoring the on-line noise is so important in pediatric testing that practitioners should be advised to consider it carefully when purchasing equipment for clinical use with children.

Noisy patients may require more *averaging* to bring the emission up out of the noise. As with ABR each 3 dB of noise reduction requires a doubling of the summation time (or number of accepted sweeps). If the ILO88 typical default value of 260 averages is not sufficient, continued averaging may improve the emission-to-noise ratio.

Techniques developed for screening help in the clinic, too. The ILO *Quickscreen* shortens the typical response window from 20 to 12 milliseconds which allows the click stimuli to be presented more rapidly. The effect on the response, however, is to reduce the click stimuli (and thus lower frequency) portion of the response. If one plans to record emissions in the frequency region below 1000 Hz, then the Quickscreen should not be used. The ILO88 also has a low-cut filter option. The option should be used when noise precludes recording altogether and when the low frequency information can be sacrificed for the sake of getting some information. Noise can affect the recording of DPOAEs just as it does TEOAEs; in noisy patients the examiner may have to skip the lower frequencies.

Details about each of these features has been described by Kemp and Ryan (1993). Manuals for specific brands of equipment delineate how each can be achieved.

Accommodating a Wide Variety of Ear Canal Sizes

One challenge in testing children is the wide variation in the size of ear canals. The variation was noted earlier with respect to fitting probe tips. Another related difficulty is setting the gain of the instrument so that proper stimulus level can be achieved. Clinicians who see patients of all ages for TEOAE testing should be equipped with baby, junior, and adult probes. The baby probe has 20 dB of attenuation built into it to account for the small volume of the newborn ear canal. In my experience children quickly grow out of the baby probe, that is the maximum gain allowed by the equipment is less than the 80 dB per SPL required for screening at the default value. The adult probe may be too large. Otodynamics has responded to this problem by developing a junior-size probe that is the size of the baby probe but with less attenuation.

Middle Ear Problems

Another difficulty which clinicians frequently encounter when recording EOAEs in children is middle ear problems. Because middle ear problems are so prevalent in the pediatric population, a few comments and examples are also included here.

As a general rule, middle ear effusion precludes detection of EOAEs (Owens, McCoy, Lonsbury-Martin, & Martin, 1992, 1993). The absence of emissions by itself is uninterpretable. Corroborated by other findings, such as air-bone gap and abnormal tympanometry, the absence of EOAEs can indicate conductive hearing loss and middle-ear dysfunction. The amount of audiometric air-bone gap related to the effusion has been correlated with the reduction in EOAE amplitude (Prieve, 1992). Smurzynski et al. (1993), Kemp et al. (1990), and Bonfils, Francois, Avan et al., (1992) reported that only high frequency emissions were present in ears with middle ear effusion or flat tympanograms. However, there are numerous cases in which emissions are absent in ears with effusion despite normal hearing thresholds. One case (that of M.W.) is presented in Figure 12–10. Despite hearing thresholds that are similar for the two ears, EOAEs are present in M.W.'s right ear with the normal tympanogram but essentially absent at the left ear, which shows a flat tympanogram. EOAEs are absent at D.S.'s (Figure 12–10) left ear despite normal high frequency thresholds. His right ear serves as a good normal comparison. L.L.'s (Figure 12–10) illustrates the effect of negative middle ear pressure in reducing EOAE amplitude, a finding that has been reported by others (Naeve, Margolis, Levine, & Fournier, 1992; Hauser, Probst, & Harris, 1993; Owens et al., 1993; Trine, Hirsch, & Margolis, 1993).

Ears with patent p-e tubes will usually yield emissions with good amplitude and reproducibility if hearing thresholds are within normal limits (Owens et al., 1992, 1993). How the emission response spectrum is influenced by the tube is not known. In our clinical sample, we found a tendency for the emission to look like it had been band-passed filtered with only the mid-frequencies remaining. Examples are shown for J.B.'s left ear, L.L.'s right ear, and E.N.'s right ear in Figure 12–10. However, this is not always the case. For example A.F. (Figure 12–10d) has broad spectrum emissions despite her tubes and an audiogram similar to the others. E.N. (Figure 12–10f) illustrates the differences in emission recording between two ears, the right with a patent p-e tube and the left with a blocked tube.

The examples in Figure 12–10 also demonstrate another common observation when attempting to record emissions in children with middle ear pathology; that is, difficulty obtaining the recommended flat stimulus spectrum. Note the differences between the stimulus spectra of abnormal ears compared to normal ears for the cases in Figure 12–10. Changes in the resonance of the ear canal and middle ear often influence the stimulus spectrum which in turn can affect the resulting emission.

Because a normal middle ear is critical for the recording of EOAEs, it is prudent to do tympanometry prior to EOAE measurement in all patients. The probable status of the middle ear should be considered at the time the appointment is made to try to maximize the chances of seeing the child for EOAE testing when the middle ears are clear. The otolaryngologists at our medical center often request EOAE testing for difficult-to-test children on the first office visit after p-e tubes are inserted.

Test Validity

Neonatal screening programs have adopted a two-tiered approach to test interpretation. That is, there is first a determination of whether the test was valid; only

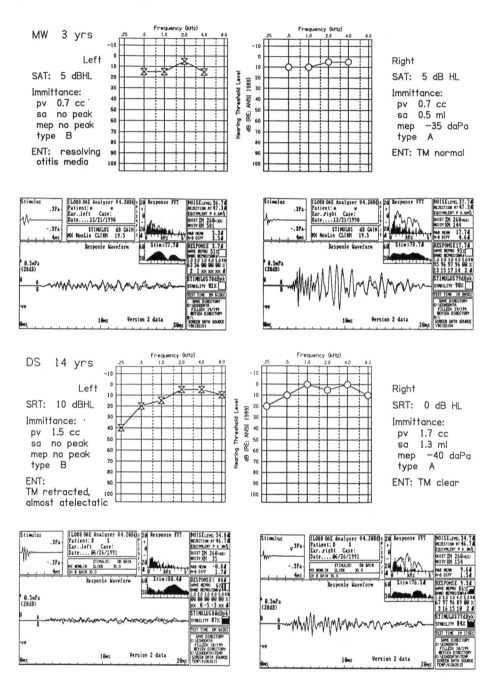

Figure 12–10. Audiograms and EOAE test results for six children from Cleft Palate Clinic. Each child's initials and age are shown at the upper left. Speech Awareness Thresholds (SAT) or Speech Recognition Thresholds (SRT) are given for left and right ears, respectively. Under Immittance, the following tympanometric values are listed when appropriate: *pv*: physical volume, *sa*: static admittance, *mep*: middle ear pressure and tympanogram type. A summary comment from the otologist's examination is given after ENT. ILO88 print-outs are shown for left and right ears respectively. (Figure continued on next two pages.)

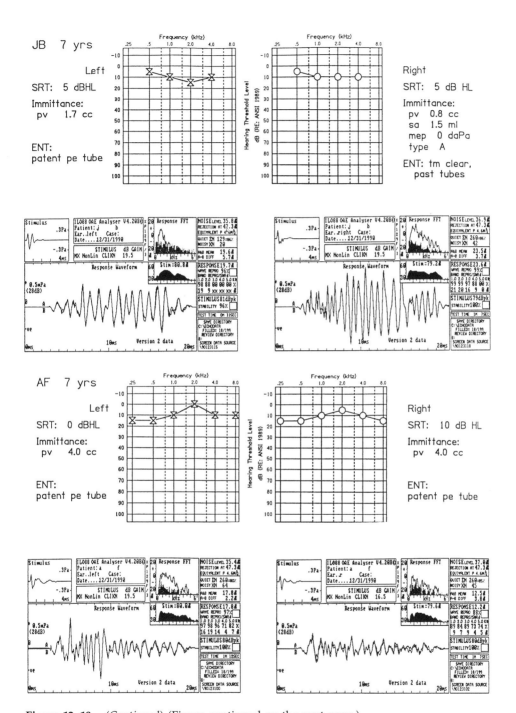

Figure 12–10. (*Continued*) (Figure continued on the next page.)

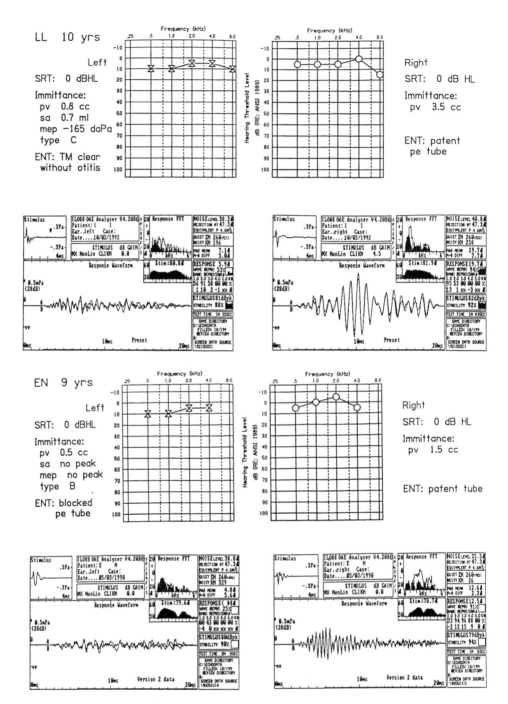

Figure 12–10. *(Continued)*

then, the valid tests are interpreted as "pass" or "fail". This approach is also advised in the clinic as well, especially when patient activity may have interfered with the recording session (a likely scenario with children). We always consider the stimulus stability, number of averages, and the stimulus level and spectrum in the process of making our interpretation of the results (Vohr, White, Maxon, & Johnson, 1993).

Testing Success and Testing Time

A fact of clinical life in a pediatric population is documented in the longitudinal study by Engdahl et al. (1994). They found that as the infants got older, they became more difficult to test. The average TEOAE test time systematically increased with an increase of age from 3 to 12 months. It will come as no surprise to practicing clinicians that data from large groups of normal-developing two-year olds is nonexistent.

Case Examples

There are several possible purposes for EOAE testing in the pediatric population. The following describes case examples taken from our clinic and how the EOAE results contributed to answering the referral questions.

Screening for Hearing Loss

Universal screening of newborns is not the norm. Many infants will not receive a hearing screening test prior to discharge from the newborn nursery. They may, however, be referred to outpatient clinics for the screening test. At our medical center, the Department of Family Medicine endeavors to refer all newborns for hearing screening. If the baby is not screened before discharge from the hospital, the parent is given a half-hour Audiology Clinic appointment that coincides with their first follow-up appointment at the Family Medicine Clinic, usually within a week or two of birth. At that age, the likelihood of the child sleeping for EOAE testing is high. The test is done in the clinic and follows the recommendations of the Rhode Island Hearing Assessment Project. The time required for a simple screen (click-evoked OAE recording with the IL 088 default parameters for each ear) is approximately that required for middle-ear–immittance measurements and is charged accordingly under the CPT Code 92587.

There are some advantages to screening neonates on an outpatient basis. First of all, fullterm babies are discharged from many hospitals at 24 hours of age when the chance of emissions being absent or of low amplitude is greater than if testing is delayed several days. Delaying the testing allows time for the absorption of vernix, clearing of canal debris, and the clearing of fluid from the middle ears—the presumed reasons for the changes that have been noted in the first four days of life (Chang et al., 1993; Kok et al., 1992).

There may be a second advantage to screening on an outpatient basis when parents are present for the test, which is not usually the case in nursery screening programs. The parents' effort to keep the appointment and their involvement in the test may enhance their understanding of the importance of hearing to their child's development.

Screening older infants and toddlers with EOAEs is also a possibility. Considering the lack of consensus about how best to screen toddlers outside the audiology clinic, EOAEs may be a promising alternative provided equipment is developed that is portable, quick, and interpretable by non-audiologists. Nozza and Sabo (1992) broached the subject of screening older children when they compared EOAE screening to standard audiometric and tympanometric screening in elementary school age children.

Filling in Audiogram Gaps

Although the relation between EOAE amplitude and hearing threshold level is poor, the presence of EOAEs across the audiometric frequency range can add considerably to confidence about the hearing status of children for whom valid, reliable, or complete audiograms are unobtainable.

Numerous other case examples using EOAEs for pediatric cross-check purposes have been reported in the literature (Gravel & Stapells, 1993; Stach, Wolf, & Bland, 1993). In addition, some clinicians have found EOAEs to be helpful documentation of pseudohypacusis (Musiek, Bornstein, & Rintelmann, 1995). Caution must be taken when interpreting such cases at the risk of declaring normal hearing sensitivity in the presence of an abnormality central to the outer hair cells.

CASE 1

By the time 14-month old P.M.K. (Figure 12–11) arrived in the Audiology Clinic after his developmental evaluation, he was tired and cranky. We were unable to elicit his cooperation for Visual Reinforcement Audiometry (VRA), so we settled instead for Behavior Observation Audiometry (BOA). Although minimum response levels to warbled pure tones of 30 to 40 dB HL did not allow us to rule out a mild hearing loss, the presence of normal tympanograms and robust, broad spectrum emissions (recorded when he fell asleep) suggested to us that the behavioral responses were not threshold and that hearing sensitivity was probably within the normal range. Subsequent successful VRA testing confirmed the impression of normal hearing sensitivity.

CASE 2

Likewise, the testing of a developmentally-delayed preschooler W.S. (Figure 12–12) yielded sound field VRA thresholds of 15 dB HL at 500 and 4000 Hz before she habituated to the reinforcers. The presence of emissions at the middle frequencies filled in the gap.

CASE 3

The absence of EOAEs in a 9-year-old multiply-handicapped student (Figure 12–13) in a classroom for the deaf-blind supported the impression of moderate sensorineural hearing loss that had been based solely on the previously-obtained ABR thresholds of 60 dB nHL and normal tympanometry. M.B. had never given conditioned behavioral responses to sound. Minimum response levels to behavior observation audiometry had ranged from 30 to 80 dB HL for a variety of signals over several test dates. Prior to EOAE testing, normal tympanograms were obtained for M.B. While he slept sedated in the Pediatrics Clinic, no EOAEs were

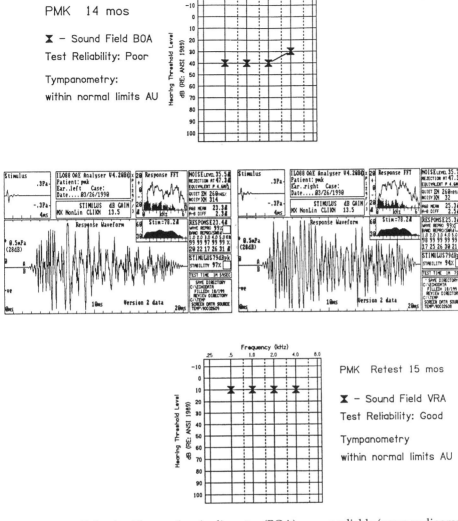

Figure 12–11.   Behavior Observation Audiometry (BOA) was unreliable (*upper* audiogram) for 14-month-old P.M.K., but the high-amplitude, broad-spectrum TEOAEs obtained for left and right ears (*middle* panels) suggested normal hearing sensitivity which was verified by later Visual Reinforcement Audiometry (VRA) (*lower* audiogram).

recorded for either ear using click stimuli or 1000 and 2000 Hz tone bursts (Figure 12–13). The results were consistent with previous results indicative of a moderate sensorineural impairment.

CASE 4

The presence of EOAEs at some frequencies and the absence at other frequencies may guide the audiologist in estimating the configuration of the hearing loss for children that do not cooperate for a full audiogram. D.T. was the 11-month-old

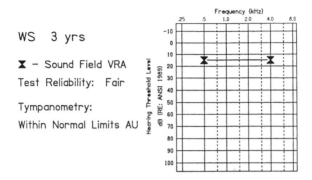

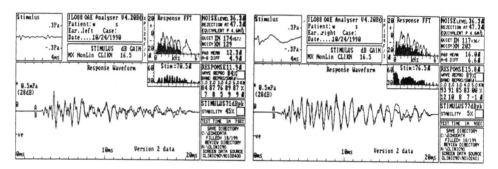

Figure 12–12. Audiometric (*top*) and TEOAE (*bottom*) results for 3-year-old W.S. led to the impression that hearing sensitivity was within normal limits from 500 through 4000 Hz. Note that the EOAEs were present despite poor recording conditions (poor stimulus waveform, spectrum and level, poor stability and fewer than 260 averages).

daughter of deaf parents whose newborn, and 4-month ABR were consistent with severe-to-profound hearing loss at the left ear (no ABR) and normal or near normal hearing at the right (ABRs down to 30 dB nHL). Behavioral responses to sound revealed minimum response levels of 35 to 40 dB HL, suggestive of possible mild hearing impairment. She was referred to our clinic for OAE testing by her audiologist who hoped that EOAE testing would supplement his previous ABR and behavioral test results and help determine the extent of hearing in the right ear. The IL 092 Otodynamic Analyser was used to test for both click-evoked and DPOAEs while D.T. slept sedated in an examining room of the Pediatric Clinic. At the left ear no EOAEs were recorded using click stimuli nor using tonal stimuli at octave intervals from 700 to 6000 Hz (Figure 12–14). At the right ear both transient-evoked and distortion product emissions were present, above the noise floor, at 1000 through 6000 Hz. In addition emissions could be evoked with clicks at lower levels. The following were our impressions:

1. The absence of emissions at the left ear suggests that there is a sensory impairment greater than 30 dB HL and supports the earlier diagnosis of severe-to-profound hearing impairment.

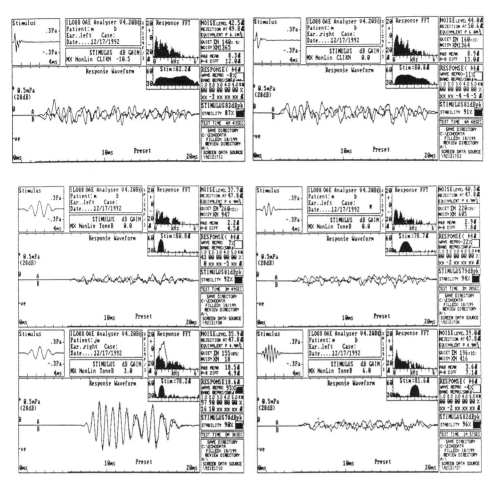

Figure 12–13. *A*: EOAEs were absent for both left and right ears of 9-year old M.B. His noisy breathing interfered with easy EOAE recording. Note the high number of rejected samples in the second box from the top in right panel under *Noisy* and the long test time in the second box from the bottom. Because we could not be sure that EOAEs might have emerged with more averaging, attempts were made to evoke OAEs with tone bursts. *B*: The upper left recording shows that M.B. had no response to a 1000 Hz tone burst. His recording is compared to the response from a normal-hearing ear at the lower left. At the right are recordings using 2000 and 3000 Hz tone bursts, neither of which show EOAEs.

2. The presence of emissions at the right ear suggests that hearing levels, at least for frequencies 1500 through 6000 Hz, are better than 30 dB HL. The presence of click-evoked emissions over a range of stimulus levels (in this case, 80 down to 54 dB peSPL) further supports the impression that hearing sensitivity is within normal limits for that frequency range.

3. At 2 years 11 months D.T. gave a reliable audiogram which is shown in Figure 12–14. It is now apparent that the absence of emissions below 1000 reflected 35

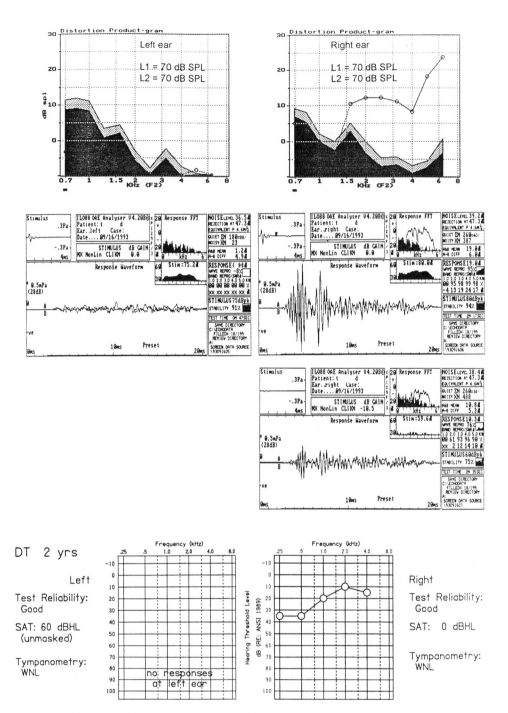

Figure 12–14. DPOAE (*top*) and TEOAE (*middle*) results for 11-month old D.T. were consistent with her earlier ABR findings of a severe-to profound loss at the left and normal-or-near-normal hearing at the right ear. Recordings were made at two click levels in an attempt to differentiate normal (better than 20 dB HL) from mild (20–40 dB) hearing loss. The ultimate audiogram (*below*) obtained with conditioned play audiometry showed a low frequency hearing loss at the right ear, which can account for the absence of emissions below 1000 Hz.

dB hearing thresholds at 250 and 500 Hz. Our impression of hearing levels better than 30 dB at higher frequencies turned out to be correct.

Separating Sensory from Neural Impairment

The potential use of EOAEs in differential diagnosis is one of the most fascinating because it gives a glimpse at the cochlea that was not previously available. This use may also be one of the most important in audiologists' work with children who cannot tell us about what they hear. Once EOAEs began to be used in conjunction with ABR, reports began to surface about persons who have normal EOAEs but either absent or significantly elevated ABR thresholds (Lutman, Mason, Sheppard, & Gibbin, 1989; Prieve, Gorga, & Neely, 1991; Norton, 1993). In these cases it is presumed that the site of lesion is central to the outer hair cells, in the inner hair cells, the eighth cranial nerve, or the functional unit between the two. A new term, *auditory neuropathy*, has been used to refer to a subset of the cases that, in addition to the normal EOAEs and absent ABRs, have mild-to-moderate elevation of pure tone air and bone-conduction thresholds, inordinately poor word recognition ability with respect to the audiogram, absent ipsilateral and contralateral acoustic reflexes, and other auditory deficits of the eighth cranial nerve or lower brainstem (Sininger, Hood, Starr, Berlin, & Picton, 1995). The presence of such disorders, as rare as they are, is justification for the use of EOAEs in combination with ABR when evaluating young children, especially those at risk neurologically. Either procedure used alone could provide inadequate information about auditory system status and lead to inappropriate diagnosis and treatment. Based on ABR alone, a child could be labelled hearing impaired and fitted with hearing aids when, in fact, cochleas are normal but the auditory nervous system is impaired. Based on EOAEs alone, a child could be declared normal hearing, but have auditory problems that affect language, speech, and auditory behavior.

The 9-year-old deaf-blind child whose EOAEs (or the lack of them) are shown in Figure 12–13 is a rather typical referral for EOAE testing for diagnostic purposes (i.e., multiply handicapped) when behavioral hearing testing may be limited and interpretation may be complicated by possible involvement of more than one auditory site. His long-standing objection to using amplification caused his audi-

Table 12–2.   Simplified Guide for EOAE Interpretation

If middle ear is OK and EOAEs are present	→ cochlea and middle ear are functioning
If middle ear is OK and EOAEs are present and no ABR	→ lesion central to outer hair cells
If middle ear is OK and NO EOAEs and elevated ABR	→ sensorineural hearing loss

ologist to consider the nature of the loss and whether or not the outer hair cells were functioning. The results of his evaluation supported cochlear or outer–hair-cell abnormality. They did not, however, rule out a neural abnormality.

CASE 5

T.H. (Figure 12–15) was another youngster with multiple abnormalities, including development delay, chronic pulmonary disease, seizure disorder and cleft lip and palate. She was seen in our clinic as a part of her multi-disciplinary evaluation through the Cleft Palate Clinic. Earlier evaluation at a clinic in her own community

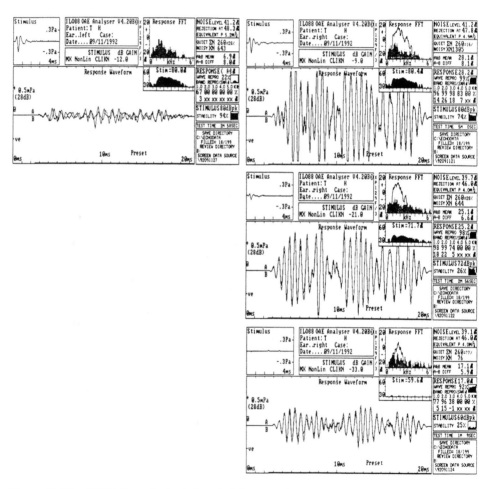

Figure 12–15. TEOAE results for left and right ears of T.H., who had been diagnosed with moderate sensorineural hearing loss and had been fitted with hearing aids. No emissions were present at the left ear. High amplitude, mid-frequency OAEs were evoked with 80 SPL clicks (*top*), 70 (*middle*), and 60 (*bottom*) SPL clicks. P-e tubes were patent at the time of testing.

had resulted in the diagnosis of mild-to-moderate hearing loss, "probably sensorineural in nature", based on click-evoked ABR thresholds of 45 dB nHL for the left ear and 55 dB nHL for the right ear. She had also been treated for persistent otitis media and currently had p-e tubes. Based on the ABR she had been fitted with binaural BTE hearing aids. Although the ABR remained unchanged after the placement of p-e tubes the parents reported that she objected to using the hearing aids in noisy places and that they had reduced the volume setting on the aids. Their observations of T.H.'s behavior led them to believe that even without the hearing aids she responded to sound and speech of low and normal loudness levels.

Otoscopy tubes were patent on the day of her clinic visit. Her EOAEs are shown in Figure 12–15. At the left ear, EOAEs were absent. At the right ear TEOAEs were present over a 20 dB range (80–60 dB peSPL). At the screening level of 80 dB peSPL, emissions ranged from 830 Hz to 4003 Hz. The reason for the absence of emissions 3000 Hz is unknown, as it might reflect the lack of stimulus energy in that region, a filtering effect of the tube, or a high frequency cochlear abnormality. Nonetheless, based on the presence of emissions in a significant portion of the speech range, coupled with the parents' observations of her behavior and her learning needs in an individualized special education program, we felt that the hearing aid for the right ear was not appropriate at this time.

Monitoring

A final possible purpose for EOAE testing in the pediatric population is monitoring for changes in cochlear status (Probst, Harris, & Hauser, 1993; Zorowka, Schmitt, & Gutjar, 1993). Little has been published about this, especially in children. There are still many questions to be answered before correct interpretation is assured. The spectrum of EOAEs has been shown to be remarkably consistent within individual ears (Kemp, 1978, 1988), and studies of normally-hearing adults suggest that amplitude of EOAEs recorded from day to day or week-to-week generally varies by no more than 1 to 2 dB (Harris, Probst, & Wenger, 1991; Vedantam & Musiek, 1991; Franklin, McCoy, Martin, & Lonsbury-Martin, 1992; Engdahl, Arnesen, & Mair, 1994b). Preliminary data from neonates suggest that infant TEOAE test-retest reliability is about as tight as adults (Krishnan and Widen, 1994). With children, especially the very young ones, the question is how much change can be expected due to normal developmental changes in external canal size, middle ear, and cochlear status? If audiologists are to use EOAEs as a monitoring tool in children, they must first separate the changes due to normal growth and development, before they can make assumptions about changes that may be due to medication, trauma, or treatment. With this caveat in mind, the following case illustrates how EOAE testing might be used in the future.

CASE 6

T.M. was diagnosed with a primary right hemispheric neuroblastoma of the cerebrum at 3 months of age. A ventricular-peritoneal shunt was placed to prevent hydrocephalus. Prior to initiation of chemotherapy with cis-platin, baseline ABR and TEOAEs were recorded. Click-evoked ABRs were recorded down to 10 dB nHL for right and left ears; wave V latency was more prolonged at the right than at

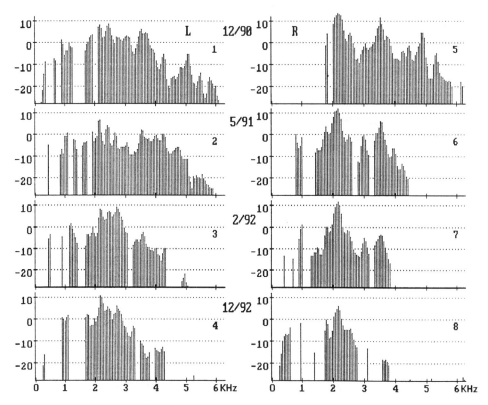

Figure 12–16. TEOAE spectra for left and right ears of T.M., who was monitored for possible changes in her hearing while receiving cis-platin treatments. Dates of the recordings span two years.

the left. The TEOAE spectra shown in Figure 12–16 for 12/90 represent the baseline recordings for each ear. The TEOAEs were of good amplitude and present out to 6000 Hz in each ear, although noise obscured recording of low frequencies. Subsequent tests were done prior to each new regimen of chemotherapy, approximately every 3 to 4 months. The first changes in ABR and TEOAEs were noted in May 1991 when ABR thresholds were obtained at 20 dB nHL and the right ear EOAEs showed a loss of high frequency emissions.

T.M. first conditions behavioral test was attempted in September 1991 (Figure 12–17) but was limited to an SAT of 10 dB HL in the sound field and screening at 20 dB HL for mid-frequencies which was generally consistent with the earlier ABR and EOAE results. No higher frequency information was obtained. In December 1991 ABR thresholds were established at 30 dB nHL and a sound-field VRA audiogram suggested a hearing loss at 6k Hz. OAE testing in February 1992 suggested that the emissions were no longer present above 4000 Hz in either ear. Further loss of high frequency hearing was confirmed with the audiogram of

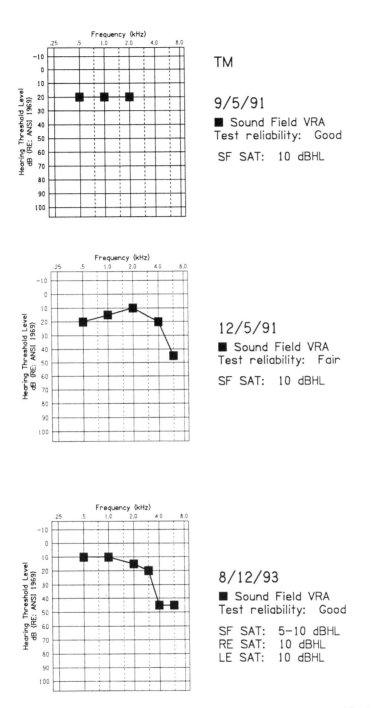

Figure 12–17.   Audiograms for T.M. obtained over her 2-year treatment with cis-platin.

August 1993 when sound field VRA thresholds showed a loss at 4000 Hz as well as 6000 Hz.

Cautious Interpretation

The point about cautious interpretation of changes in emissions over time is illustrated with the examples from two normally-hearing children shown in Figure 12–18. Although they showed less loss of high frequency energy than T.M., a reduction in overall amplitude and some high frequency components from first to second tests is nonetheless apparent and presumably reflects the changes that occur naturally in the first few years of life.

Reporting Results

As with many audiologic procedures, the presence of a response is usually more meaningful than the absence of response. With EOAEs alone, absence simply

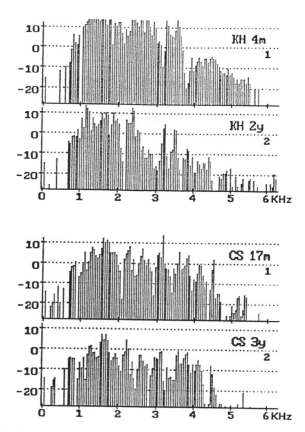

Figure 12–18. TEOAE spectra for two children with normal hearing and negative otologic histories. K.H. (*top*) was tested at 4 months and 2 years of age. C.S. (*bottom*) was tested at 17 months and 3 years.

means that there is some kind of abnormality that requires further assessment. For example, EOAEs could be absent with a deaf child; a child with middle ear effusion, flat tympanograms but audiogram within the normal range; a child with 40 dB hearing loss; or a child with 70 dB hearing loss. However, the absence of emissions can mean something when combined with other audiologic information, such as behavioral responses, evoked potentials, and immittance measures, including acoustic reflex thresholds.

We are generally comfortable stating that the presence of EOAEs is consistent with hearing levels better than 30 to 40 dB HL range and that the absence of EOAEs is consistent with hearing thresholds poorer than 30 to 40 dB HL (provided the middle ear is normal). We specify as precisely as possible the frequency region tested (e.g., "click-evoked OAEs were absent for the right ear at the screening level of 80 dB peSPL throughout the frequency range 500–5000 Hz"). We also report the frequency region where EOAEs were present (e.g., "EOAEs were present in the frequency range from 2800–4000 Hz." or "Hearing sensitivity [at least through the range of 1000–5000 Hz where we tested] is likely to range from normal to no poorer than 30 dB HL").

Regarding emission testing at different levels, the presence of click-evoked emissions over a range of stimulus levels further supports the impression that hearing sensitivity falls within the normal range.

If the site of lesion is in question, we are generally comfortable saying that "the presence of EOAEs suggests that there are functioning outer hair cells in the frequency region where they were recorded and that the absence of EOAEs implies a sensory (inner ear, specifically outer hair cells) site of lesion, provided the middle ear is normal."

In view of what is not known, especially about what is normal for hearing impaired infants and children, we are cautious in stating our interpretation. We often preface our comments with "Although clinical interpretation of emissions data is not yet fully understood,..." Likewise, when there are known outer or middle ear abnormalities, such as p-e tubes, we often state that "the influence of middle ear status and tubes on the resulting evoked emissions is not fully understood at this time."

We leave out mention of the specific stimulus level in the *impressions* section of the report because uninformed readers often interpret the mention of a decibel level as threshold. Thus, if one reads that OAEs were present at the default screening level of 80 dB peSPL, they have incorrectly assumed that 80 dB was the hearing threshold level.

Summary and Conclusions

Evoked otoacoustic emissions hold great promise for pediatric auditory evaluation. Accumulating data indicate that their role in screening is assured. They have already been helpful in supplementing limited audiometric information in the clinic. They are providing clinicians a new view of cochlear function and they may provide a sensitive tool for monitoring its change. There are many questions yet to be answered. Current estimates of sensitivity and specificity are tentative and have not yet been determined for each emission type and its numerous parameters. The time course of EOAE changes throughout childhood is unknown. Data from the most difficult-to-test children (i.e., toddlers and preschoolers) is lacking. The number of children with auditory neuropathy is unknown as are its effects on development and its appropriate treatment. Meanwhile, clinicians should keep careful records of their clinical cases and treat them as clinical trials. Clinicians should be intelligent and cautious in their interpretation and seek final diagnoses and audiometric outcomes whenever possible. Clinicians and researchers should share what is learned through presentation and publication of both group data and case reports. Finally, audiologists should keep careful watch for new data, from both the laboratory and the clinic, that give insight to the unanswered questions.

References

Bergman, B. M., Gorga, M. P., Neely, S. T., Kaminski, J. R., Beauchaine, K. L., & Peters, J. (1995). Preliminary descriptions of transient-evoked and distortion-product otoacoustic emissions from graduates of an intensive care nursery. *Journal of the American Academy of Audiology, 6,* 150–162.

Bonfils, P., Avan, P., Francois, M., Trotoux, J., Narcy, P. (1992). Distortion-product otoacoustic emissions in neonates: Normative data. *Acta Otolaryngologica, 112,* 739–744.

Bonfils, P., Dumont, A., Marie, P., Francois, M., Narcy, P. (1990). Evoked otoacoustic emissions in newborn hearing screening. *Laryngoscope, 100,* 186–189.

Bonfils, P., Francois, M., Avan, P., Londero, A., Trotoux, J., Narcy, P. (1992). Spontaneous and evoked otoacoustic emissions in preterm neonates. *Laryngoscope, 102,* 182–186.

Bonfils, P., Uziel, A., and Pujol, R. (1988). Evoked oto-acoustic emissions from adults and infants: clinical applications. *Archives of Otolaryngology (Stockholm), 105,* 445–449.

Bray, P., Kemp, D. T. (1987). An advanced cochlear echo technique suitable for infant screening. *British Journal of Audiology, 21,* 192–204.

Brown, A. M., Sheppard, S. L., Russell, P. T. (1994). Acoustic distortion products (ADP) from the ears of term infants and young adults using low stimulus levels. *British Journal of Audiology, 28,* 273–280.

Chang, K. W., Vohr, B. R., Norton, S. J., Lekas, M. D. (1993). External and middle ear status related to evoked otoacoustic emission in neonates. *Archives of Otolaryngology–Head and Neck Surgery, 119,* 276–282.

Engdahl, B., Arnesen, R., Mair, I. (1994a). Reproducibility and short-term variability of transient evoked otoacoustic emissions. *Scandinavian Audiology, 23,* 99–104.

Engdahl, B., Arnesen, A. R., Mair, I. W. S. (1994b). Otoacoustic emissions in the first year of life. *Scandinavian Audiology, 23,* 195–200.

Franklin, D. J., McCoy, M. J., Martin, G. K., Lonsbury-Martin, B. L., (1992). Test/retest reliability of distortion-product and transiently evoked otoacoustic emissions. *Ear and Hearing, 13,* 417–429.

Glattke, T. J., Pafitis, I.A., Cummiskey, C., Herer, G. R. (1995). Identification of hearing loss in children and young adults using measures of transient otoacoustic emission reproducbility. *American Journal of Audiology, 4,* 41–87.

Gorga, M. P., Neely, S. T., Bergman, B. M., Beauchaine, K. L., Kaminski, J. K., Peters, J., Jesteadt, W. (1993a). Otoacoustic emissions from normal-hearing and hearing-impaired subjects: distortion product responses. *Journal of the Acoustical Society of America, 93,* 2050–2060.

Gorga, M. P., Neely, S. T., Bergman, B. M., Beauchaine, K. L., Kaminski, J. K., Peters, J., Schulte, L., Jesteadt, W. (1993b). A comparision of transient-evoked and distortion-product otoacoustic emissions in normal-hearing and hearing-impaired subjects. *Journal of the Acoustical Society of America, 94,* 2639–2648.

Gravel, J. S., Stapells, D. R. (1993). Behavioral, electrophysiologic, and otoacoustic measures from a child with auditory procesing dysfunction: case report. *Journal of the American Academy of Audiology, 4,* 412–419.

Harris, F. P., Probst, R., Wenger, R. (1991). Repeatability of transiently evoked otoacoustic emissions in normally hearing humans. *Audiology, 30,* 135–141.

Hauser, R., Probst, R., Harris, F. P. (1993). Effects of atmospheric pressure variation on spontaneous, transiently evoked and distortion product otoacoustic emissions in normal human ears. *Hearing Research, 69,* 133–145.

Johnsen, N. J., Bagi, P., Elberling, C. (1983). Evoked acoustic emissions from the human ear. III. Findings in neonates. *Scandinavian Audiology, 12,* 17–24.

Johnsen, N. J., Bagi, P., Parbo, J., Elberling, C. (1988). Evoked acoustic emissions from the human ear. IV. Final results in 100 neonates. *Scandinavian Audiology, 17,* 27–34.

Johnsen, N. J., Parbo, J., Elberling, C. (1989). Evoked acoustic emissions from the human ear. V. Developmental changes. *Scandinavian Audiology, 18,* 59–62.

Keefe, D. H., Bulen, J. C., Arehart, K. H, Burns, E. M. (1993). Ear-canal impedance and reflection coefficient in human infants and adults. *Journal of the Acoustical Society of America, 94,* 2617–2638.

Kemp, D. T. (1978). Stimulated acoustic emissions from within the human auditory system. *Journal of the Acoustical Society of America, 64,* 1386–1391.

Kemp, D. T. (1988). Development in cochlear mechanics and techniques for noninvasive evaluation. *Advanced Audiology, 5,* 27–45.

Kemp, D. T., Bray, P., Alexander, L., & Brown, A. M. (1986). Acoustic emission cochleography—practical aspects. *Scandinavian Audiology* Supplement, *25,* 71–95.

Kemp, D. T., Ryan, S., Bray, P. (1990). A guide to the effective use of otoacoustic emissions. *Ear and Hearing, 11,* 93–105.

Kemp, D. T., Ryan, S. (1993). The use of transient evoked otoacoustic emissions in neonatal hearing screening programs. *Seminars in Hearing, 14,* 30–45.

Kok, M. R., van Zanten, G. A., Brocaar, M. P. (1992). Growth of evoked otoacoustic emissions during the first days post-partum—a prelimariny report. *Audiology, 31,* 140–149.

Kok, M. R., van Zanten, G. A., Brocaar, M. P., Wallenburg, H. O. S., (1993). Click-evoked oto-acoustic emissions in 1036 ears of healthy newborns. *Audiology, 32,* 213–224.

Krishnan G., Widen, J. E. (1994). Repeatability of click-evoked otoacoustic emissions in neoantes. *Abstracts of the Association for Research in Otolaryngology, 17,* 50.

Lafreniere, O., Jung, M. D., Smurzynski, J., Leonard, G., Kim, D. O., Sasek, J. (1991). Distortion-product and click-evoked otoacoustic emissions in healthy newborns. *Archives of Otolaryngology—Head and Neck Surgery, 117,* 1382–1389.

Lafreniere, D., Smurzynski, J., Jung, M., Leonard, G., Kim, D. O. (1993). Otoacoustic emissions in full-term newborns at risk for hearing loss. *Laryngoscope, 103,* 1334–1341.

Lasky, R., Pearlman, J., Hecox, K. (1992). Distortion-product otoacoustic emissions in human newborns and adults. *Ear and Hearing, 13,* 430–441.

Lonsbury-Martin, B. L., Martin, G. K., McCoy, M. J., Whitehead, M. L. (1994). Otoacoustic emissions testing in young children: middle-ear influences. *American Journal of Otolaryngology, Supplement No. 1,* 13–20.

Lonsbury-Martin, B. L., McCoy, M. J., Whitehead, M. L., & Martin, G. K. (1993). Clinical testing of distortion-product otoacoustic emissions. *Ear and Hearing, 14,* 11–22.

Lutman, M. E., Mason, S. M., Sheppard, S., Gibbin, K. P. (1989). Differential diagnostic potential of otoacoustic emissions: A case study. *Audiology, 28,* 205–210.

Marco, J., Morant, A., Caballero, J., Ortells, I., Paredes, C., Brines, J. (1995). Distortion product otoacoustic emissions in healthy newborns: normative data. *Acta Otolaryngologica (Stockholm), 115,* 187–189.

Morlet, T., Collet, L., Salle, B., Morgon, A. (1993). Functional maturation of cochlear active mechanisms and of the medial olivocochlear system in humans. *Acta Otolaryngologica, 113,* 271–277.

Musiek, F. E., Bornstein, S. P., Rintelmann, W. F. (1995). Transient evoked otoacoustic emissions and pseudohypacusis. *Journal of American Academy of Audiology, 6,* 293–301.

Naeve, S. L., Margolis, R. H., Levine, S. C., Fournier, E. M. (1992). Effect of ear-canal pressure on evoked otoacoustic emissions. *Journal of the Acoustical Society of America, 91,* 2091–2095.

Norton, S. J. (1992). Cochlear function and otoacoustic emissions. *Seminars in Hearing, 13,* 1–14.

Norton, S. J. (1993). Application of transient evoked otoacoustic emissions to pediatric populations. *Ear and Hearing, 14,* 64–73.

Norton, S. J. (1994). The emerging role of evoked otoacoustic emissions in neonatal hearing, screening. *American Journal of Otolaryngology, 15 Supplement 1,* 4–12.

Norton, S. J., Harrison, W. A. (1993). Transient evoked otoacoustic emissions in normally-hearing and hearing-impaired children. *Abstracts of the Association for Research in Otolaryngology, 16,* 44.

Norton, S. J., Stover, L. J. (1994). Otoacoustic Emissions: an emerging clinical tool. In J. Katz (Ed.), *Handbook of Clinical Audiology* (pp. 448–462). Baltimore, MD: Williams & Wilkins

Norton, S. J., Widen, J. E. (1990). Evoked otoacoustic emissions in normal-hearing infants and children: Emerging data and issues. *Ear and Hearing, 11,* 121–127.

Norton, S. J., Widen, J. E., Otoacoustic emissions in infants and young children. Presented at the International Symposium on Otoacoustic Emissions: Theory, Application, and Technique. Kansas City, MO, May 1991.

Nozza, R. J., Sabo, D. L. (1992). Transiently evoked OAE for screening school-age children. *Hearing Journal, 45,* 29–31.

Ohlms, L. A., Lonsbury-Martin, B. L., Martin, G. K. (1990). The clinical application of acoustic distortion products. *Otolaryngology—Head and Neck Surgery, 103,* 52–59.

Owens, J. J., McCoy, M. J., Lonsbury-Martin, B. L., Martin, G. K. (1992). Influence of otitis media on evoked otoacoustic emissions in children. *Seminars in Hearing, 13,* 53–66.

Owens, J. J., McCoy, M. J., Lonsbury-Martin, B. L., Martin, G. K. (1993). Otoacoustic emissions in children with normal ears, middle-ear dysfunction, and ventilating tubes. *American Journal of Otolaryngology, 14,* 34–40.

Popelka, G. R., Karzon, R. K., Arjamand, E. M. (1994). Growth of the $2f_1$–f_2 distortion product otoacoustic emission for low-level stimuli in human neonates. *Abstracts of the Association for Research in Otolaryngology, 17,* 51.

Prieve, B. A. (1992). Otoacoustic emissions in infants and children: Basic characteristics and clinical application. *Seminars in Hearing, 13,* 37–52.

Prieve, B. A., Gorga, M. P., Neely, S. T. (1991). Otoacoustic emissions in an adult with severe hearing loss. *Journal of Speech and Hearing Research, 34,* 379–385.

Prieve, B. A., Gorga, M. P., Schmidt, A. R., Neely, S. T., Peters, J., Schulte, L., Jesteadt, W. (1993). Analysis of transient-evoked otoacoustic emissions in normal-hearing and hearing-impaired ears. *Journal of the Acoustical Society of America, 93,* 3308–3319.

Probst, R., Harris, F. P., Hauser, R. (1993). Clinical monitoring using otoacoustic emissions. *British Journal of Audiology, 27,* 85–90.

Ryan, S., Piron, J. P. (1994). Functional maturation of the medial efferent olivocochlear system in human neonates. *Acta Otolaryngologica (Stockholm), 114* 485–489.

Sininger, Y. S., Hood, L. J., Starr, A., Berlin, C. I., Picton, T. W. (1995). Hearing loss due to auditory neuropathy. *Audiology Today, 7(2),* 11–13.

Smurzynski, J. (1994). Longitudinal measurements of distortion-product and click-evoked otoacoustic emissions of preterm infants: preliminary results. *Ear and Hearing, 15* 210–223.

Smurzinski, J., Kim, D. O. (1992). Distortion-product and click-evoked otoacoustic emissions of normally-hearing adults. *Hearing Research, 58,* 227–240.

Smurzynski, J., Jung, M. D., Lafreniere, D., Kim, D. O., Kamath, M. V., Rowe, J. O., Holman, M. C., Leonard, G. (1993). Distortion-product and click-evoked otoacoustic emissions of preterm and full-term infants. *Ear and Hearing, 14,* 258–274.

Spektor, Z., Leonard, G., Kim, D. O., Jung, M. D., Smurzynski, J. (1991). Otoacoustic emissions in norman and hearing-impaired children and normal adults. *Laryngoscope, 101,* 965–976.

Stach, B. A., Wolf, S. J., Bland, J. (1993). Otoacoustic emissions as a cross-check in pediatric hearing assessment: case report. *Journal of the American Academy of Audiology, 4,* 392–398.

Stevens, J. C., Webb, H. D., Hutchinson, J., Connell, J., Smith, M. F., Buffin, J. T. (1989). Click evoked otoacoustic emissions compared with brain stem electric response. *Archives of Diseases of Childhood, 64,* 1105–1111.

Stevens, J. C., Webb, H. D., Hutchinson, J., Connell, J., Smith, M. F., Buffin, J. T. (1990). Click evoked otoacoustic emissions in neonatal screening. *Ear and Hearing, 11,* 128–133.

Stevens, J. C., Webb, H. D., Hutchinson, J., Connell, J., Smith, M. F., Buffin, J. T. (1991). Evaluation of click-evoked otoacoustic emission in the newborn. *British Journal of Audiology, 25,* 11–14.

Stevens, J. C., Webb, H. D., Smith, M. F., Buffin, J. T., Ruddy, H. (1987). A comparison of otoacoustic emissions and brain stem electric response audiometry in the normal newborn and babies admitted to a special care baby unit. *Clinical Physical and Physiological Measurements, 8,* 95–104.

Thornton, A. R. D., Kimm, L., Kennedy, C. R., Caferelli-Dees, D. (1993). External- and middle-ear factors affecting evoked otoacoustic emissions in neonates. *British Journal of Audiology, 27,* 319–327.

Trine, M. B., Hirsch, J. E., Margolis, R. H. (1993). The effect of middle ear pressure on transient evoked otoacoustic emissions. *Ear and Hearing, 14,* 401–407.

Uziel, A., Piron, J-P. (1991). Evoked otoacoustic emissions from normal newborns and babies admitted to an intensive care baby unit. *Acta Otolaryngologica* Supplement, *482,* 85–91.

Vedantam, R., Musiek, F. E. (1991). Click evoked otoacoustic emissions in adult subjects: standard indices and test-retest reliability. *American Journal of Otolaryngology, 12,* 485–442.

Vohr, B. R., White, K. R., Maxon, A. B., Johnson, M. J. (1993). Factors affecting the interpretation of transient evoked otoacoustic emission results in neonatal hearing screening. *Seminars in Hearing, 14,* 57–72.

White, K. R., Vohr, B. R., Behrens, T. R. (1993). Universal newborn hearing screening using transient evoked otoacoustic emissions: results of the Rhode Island hearing assessemnt project. *Seminars in Hearing, 14,* 18–29.

White, K. R., Vohr, B. R., Maxon, A. B., Behrens, T. R., McPherson, M. G., and Mauk, G. W. (1994). Screening all newborns for hearing loss using transient evoked otoacoustic emissions. *International Journal of Pediatric Otorhinolaryngology, 29,* 203–217.

Widen, J. R., Norton, S. J. (1993). Changes in otoacoustic emissions as a function of age, birth through 7 months. Presented at the International Congress on Otoacoustic Emissions, Lyon, France, May 1993.

Zorowka, P. G., Schmitt, H. J., Gutjar, P. (1993). Evoked otoacoustic emissions and pure-tone threshold audiometry in patients receiving cisplatinum therapy. *International Journal of Pediatric Otorhinolaryngology, 25,* 73–80.

13

General Recording Considerations and Clinical Instrument Options

T. Newell Decker

Introduction

The methods of recording otoacoustic emissions (OAEs) are complicated by many factors. First, OAEs are divided into two major classes (spontaneous and evoked) and the recording methods for each are different. Second, different instruments for recording OAEs accomplish their measurement routines in different ways. Some of the ways are proprietary in nature, making it difficult to acquire complete information from the manufacturer. Finally, the clinicians and researchers using and investigating these responses do not agree on which methods and procedures are the best. Despite these problems, some common elements are involved in recording OAEs. (Table 13–1 provides a list of current manufacturers of OAE instruments and details some of the characteristics of each system.)

Overview of Measurement Methods

Otoacoustic emissions are audio frequencies that are transmitted from the cochlea to the middle ear and into the external ear canal (Kemp, 1986). Four types of OAEs have been measured: spontaneous OAEs (SOAEs), transient evoked OAEs (TEOAEs), intermodulation distortion product OAEs (DPOAEs), and stimulus frequency OAEs (SFOAEs). Figure 13–1 shows a representation of the emission recording process.

In general, the detection and measurement of all types of emissions requires that a sensitive, low-noise microphone be placed in the external ear canal. The microphone then records the sound present in the external ear canal and includes the sound source (for evoked emissions) and the audio frequencies transmitted from the inner ear. Probe assemblies are now commercially available that contain both the sound source and the measurement microphones. Depending on the type of emission being recorded, recovery and analysis of the emission require some signal averaging in the time or the frequency domain.

Table 13–1. Equipment Available for Purchase in the United States[†]

Manufacturer	Tests Performed	Features
CUBᵉDIS Mimosa Acoustics Mountainside, NJ	Distortion product emissions DP-grams Input/output (I/O) functions*	Allows for automated finding of optimum f2//f1 amplitude and frequency ratio. Contains a basic audiometer. Software is IBM compatible.
GS160 Grason-Stadler Milford, NH	Distortion product emissions DP-grams I/O functions*	Allows for single or multiple pair primary presenations. Operates in DOS and Windows environment.
ILO88 and ILO92 Otodynamics, Ltd. Hatfield, Hert UK	ILO88 System: Transient evoked emissions Spontaneous emissions ILO92 System: Transient evoked emissions Distortion product emissions DP-grams I/O functions* Spontaneous emissions	Allow for click or tone burst stimuli. Operates with IBM compatible platforms Same as above with addition of pure tone stimuli for DPOAEs.
Model 330 Virtual Corporation Portland, OR	Distortion product emissions DP-grams I/O functions* Spontaneous emissions	Operates on Macintosh platform. Can be integrated with Model 310 Immittance Bridge and Model 320 Audiometer.
Celesta 503 Madsen Electronics Minnetonka, MN	Spontaneous emissions Distortion product emissions	Lightweight ergonomic probe. External signal processing unit operates with IBM compatible platforms.
Scout OAE Bio-Logic Systems Corp. Mundelein, IL	Distortion product emissions	Primary stimuli sweep from high to low. On-line adjustment of artifact rejection level. Battery powered microphone preamp. Can be configured with evoked potential system Operates on IBM compatible platform.
Ranger OAE Bio-Logic Systems Corp. Mundelein, IL	Distortion product emissions	Simplified version of the Scout system. Fewer user options. Operates on IBM compatible platform.

[†]Available as of June 1996.

*Note: The Food and Drug Administration (FDA) has not approved the I/O function as a test procedure.

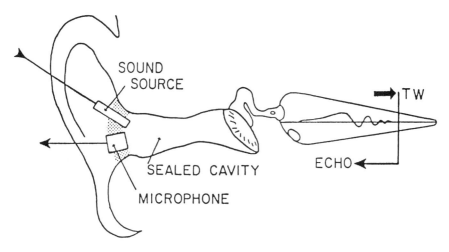

Figure 13–1. General scheme of a typical emission recording set-up. The sound source and recording microphone are held in ear canal by a rubber cuff. Sound travels through middle ear to the cochlea and the emission returns to the recording device.

Methods for SOAE

SOAEs are low-level acoustic signals measured in the ear without external stimulation (Kemp, 1979). They occur in approximately 40 to 60% of healthy ears at frequencies peculiar to each ear (Kemp, Ryan, & Brey, 1990), and are typically detected between 1000 and 5000 Hz (Bonfils, 1989).

The basic instrumentation needed for obtaining SOAEs includes a low-noise microphone with a foam tip coupled to the ear canal. No external stimulation is required. The noise characteristic of the microphone is extremely important: The average level of the SOAE is usually less than 20 dB SPL. The microphone output is led to a low-noise amplifier and then routed to a signal-spectrum analyzer that can provide real-time fast Fourier transforms (FFT) analysis of the signal. A specified frequency range (e.g., 20–20,000 Hz) can then be analyzed for SOAEs by analysis of discrete frequency bandwidths. Usually, several samples of the energy in a given bandwidth are submitted to averaging procedures to resolve the emission from the background noise. Spontaneous emissions can then be defined as the discrete peaks that are repeatable and are at some specified level above the noise floor of the instrumentation. Figure 13–2 shows a general recording scheme for SOAEs and a typical emission response.

Methods for TEOAEs

These emissions were described by Kemp (1978), have been called *Kemp echoes*. They seem to be in nearly all healthy ears to some degree, but are generally not observed in ears where threshold shifts as small as 30 dB HL have occurred (Kemp, 1978). TEOAEs have been most frequently measured between 500 and 4000 Hz (Elberling, Parbo, Johnson & Bagi, 1985; Probst, Coates, Martin, & Lonsbury-

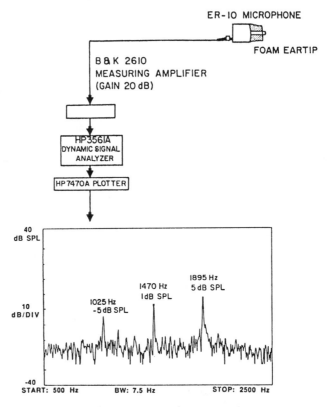

Figure 13–2. Schematic diagram of instrumentation for measuring spontaneous otoacoustic emissions (SOAEs) and examples of SOAEs at three different frequencies. The spectrum analyzer was set to track across a frequency range from 500 Hz to 2500 Hz. This was done using a 7.5 Hz bandwidth for analysis. Three clearly identifiable peaks in the spectrum are seen at 1025, 1470, and 1895 Hz. Provided that these peaks in the spectrum are above the criterion noise floor, they are identified as spontaneous emissions.

Martin, 1986), and have decreasing latencies with increasing stimulus frequency (Norton & Neely, 1987).

As with the spontaneous emissions, a probe is securely positioned in the external auditory canal. However, in the measurement of TEOAEs the probe serves two purposes: First, it delivers the stimulus. Second, it receives the meatal sound pressure, which is a combination of stimulus and emission. The stimulus is a brief, "flat" acoustic-spectrum pulse presented to the external canal at a relative low intensity (e.g., 0–50 dB SPL). The stimulus is presented repeatedly, and the input to the probe is amplified and the signal is averaged. The duration of each sample is typically 20 to 40 ms. The averaged response is then analyzed by FFT to obtain a frequency spectrum of the emission and confirm the presence of a response. TEOAEs can also be elicited with tone bursts. Again, the stimuli are presented at relatively low intensity levels, but the tone burst frequency can be altered. Figure 13–3

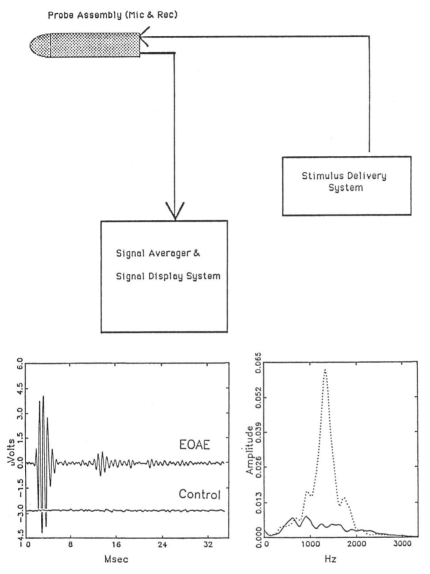

Figure 13–3. Typical recording schematic for Transiently Evoked Emission (TEOAE) recovery. Example of TEOAE displayed in the time domain (left) and accompanying spectrum (FFT) to the right. TEOAE spectrum is shown as dotted line and noise floor, as solid line. The evoking stimulus in this case was a 1500 Hz tone burst. Notice the peak of energy present in the output spectrum centered at approximately 1500 Hz (dotted line). This represents the spectrum of the TEOAE after the stimulus spectrum has been removed. The control tracing (solid line) is a recording from the ear canal without stimulus present and so represents background noise only.

represents a recording schematic for TEOAEs, as well as the TEOAE displayed in the time domain and the accompanying FFT.

Methods for DPOAEs

DPOAEs are recorded when two stimulus tones (f_1 and f_2) are presented to the ear; amplitude distortion known as interference occurs and combination tones result. First-order combination tones are $f_1 - f_2$ and $f_1 + f_2$, and second-order combination tones are $2f_1 - f_2$ and $2f_1 + f_2$. The first of each pair is the difference tone, and the latter is the summation tone. The distortion product $2f_1 - f_2$ is of the most interest to researchers because it is believed that this distortion product emission comes from the second level of analysis at the peripheral level, i.e., outer–hair-cell bio-mechanics. It has been shown that the $2f_1 - f_2$ DPOAEs occur primarily in the frequency range of 500 to 8000 Hz, and its amplitude is dependent upon the frequencies and intensities of f_1 and f_2 (Martin, Probst, & Lonsbury-Martin,1990a). DPOAEs are normally measured in two ways: (1): distortion product (DP)–Grams and, (2) input/output functions.

DP-GRAMS

As with the other emissions, a probe must be sealed in the ear canal, but with DPOAEs the probe must contain two sound inputs to deliver the f_1 and f_2 stimuli (primaries) and a microphone to measure the SPL in the external ear canal. The oscillators presenting f_1 and f_2 step across frequencies, and the microphone is coupled to a phase-locked filter-analyzer, which records the amplitude of the $2f_1 - f_2$ distortion product, as well as the amplitude of f_1 and f_2. One manufacturer has developed a method whereby several groups of primaries can be presented at the same time (Painter, 1994). This innovation may help to reduce the time needed to administer the test.

The suggested suitable conditions for measuring DPOAEs are two stimuli pre-sented at equal intensities with a frequency ratio of approximately 1.2 to 1.3 (frequency spacing between f_1 and f_2) (Martin, Whitehead, Lonsbury-Martin, 1990a). Martin et al. point out that the frequencies of f_1 and f_2, the intensities of f_1 and f_2, and the frequency and level ratios may need adjustments to obtain the best DPOAE amplitudes in any given patient; however, additional investigation is needed. Figure 13–4 shows a recording schematic DPOAES and shows the DP and primary stimulus energy in a spectral plot. Figure 13–5 depicts a typical DP-gram from a normal, healthy ear. Because it often happens that the DPOAE will come very close to or intermingle with the noise-floor tracing, it is essential that the clinician adopt some reference signal to noise criteria that will allow for objective identification of the presence of the DP.

INPUT/OUTPUT FUNCTIONS

The input/output measure of the DPOAE is accomplished in a similar manner as the DP-gram. Unlike the DP-gram which measures across a range of several frequencies at a given SPL, the input/output test presents signals at several levels for a specific frequency. Input/output functions can be plotted for any frequency subject to the limitations of the equipment. The input/output test provides several potentially important bits of information including detection threshold, maximum

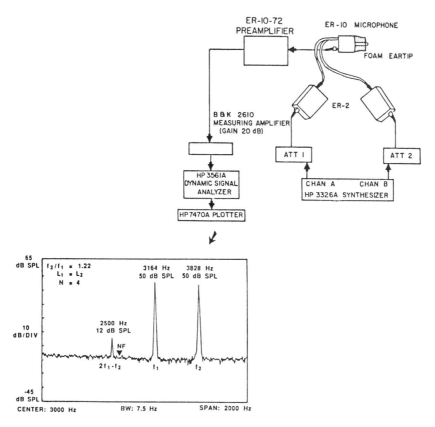

Figure 13–4.   Typical recording schematic for distortion product otoacoustic emission. Also shown is the distortion product (2500 Hz) and primary stimulus energy (3164 & 3828 Hz) in a spectral plot.

output level, and slope of the growth function. Figure 13–6 shows a typical input/output function.

Methods for SFOAEs

These emissions are similar to TEOAEs, but are evoked with continuous pure tones instead of click stimuli. They have not been studied as extensively as the other emissions, but SFOAEs can be primarily seen in the same frequency region as TEOAEs (Martin, Whitehead, & Lonsbury-Martin).

For SFOAEs, the eliciting stimulus is a low level continuous pure tone that is swept from a particular low frequency to a particular high frequency (e.g., 800–2800 Hz). As the stimulus is swept across frequencies, the energy from the ear canal can be tracked by a signal analyzer which spectrally averages the ear canal signal utilizing a narrow frequency bandwidth resolution. In this manner, any corresponding SFOAEs present in the ear canal will combine with the stimulus and result in an elevation of SPL of a particular frequency region. If no emission frequency component that corresponds to a particular stimulating frequency is de-

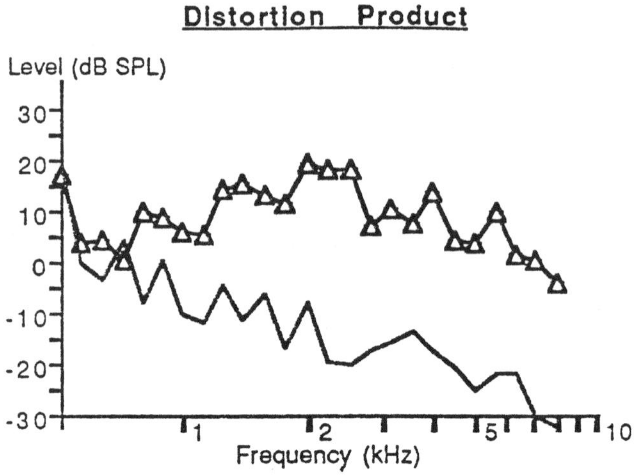

Distortion Product

Figure 13–5. Typical DP-gram recording showing OAEs as triangles above the background noise floor (*solid line*) for this listener. The upper tracing is the distortion product, and the lower tracing represents the noise floor.

tected in the ear canal signal, the level of the corresponding frequency-bandwidth SPL remains unchanged or may decrease, depending upon the phase relation produced by the ear-canal acoustics and eliciting signals. The SFOAE is typically represented by peaks and valleys superimposed upon the frequency response of the sound system. Two techniques may be used to separate the response from the stimulus.

The first process is a multilevel technique involves recording SFOAEs to high-level, swept pure tones, as well as to the low-level pure tones. Then the high- and low-level responses are scaled and subtracted. The subtraction cancels out any stimulus or resonance effects, but leaves the emission (Kemp & Chum, 1983). The second extraction process is a suppression technique. As with the multilevel technique, SFOAEs to the low-level, swept pure tones are recorded. Additional responses, however, are recorded in the presence of a tone near in frequency to the stimulus frequency. This "suppresser" tone serves to suppress or decrease the emission, but produces no changes in any stimulus or resonance effect. Subtraction of the suppressed and combined responses extracts the SFOAE, which remains in the difference trace (Kemp & Brown, 1983). This extraction process is more complex than with the transient evoked emission. Figure 13–7 displays necessary instru-mentation for recording SFOAEs and displays a representative emission response.

Preparation

As with any other procedure involving patients, it is wise to take some preliminary steps to insure that the equipment is in good working order. The extra effort will save valuable clinician and patient time.

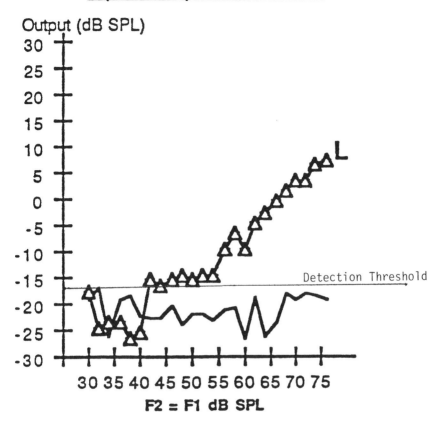

Figure 13–6. Typical DP input/output function. Detection threshold is shown where the OAE rises above noise floor by 3 dB. OAE amplitude is shown by triangles above the solid line noise floor.

Preliminary Precautions

Most clinicians have come to rely on the biological calibrations that they carry out routinely when they turn on the audiometric equipment each day. This is a procedure whereby clinicians compare their own expected auditory experience to those that they actually measure on a specific day. The same procedure works well for OAE equipment. It takes very little time for clinicians to test themselves each morning when they turn on the equipment.

Visual inspection of the patient's ear canal prior to testing is also an important preliminary step. A good examination will reveal any wax that might block the probe or any abnormalities that will prevent a good fit. The examiner can also make a preliminary determination of the size of the rubber cuff needed around the probe. It is also valuable to precede OAE measurement with immittance measurement. In order for the OAE procedure to work, the signal must be able to reach the

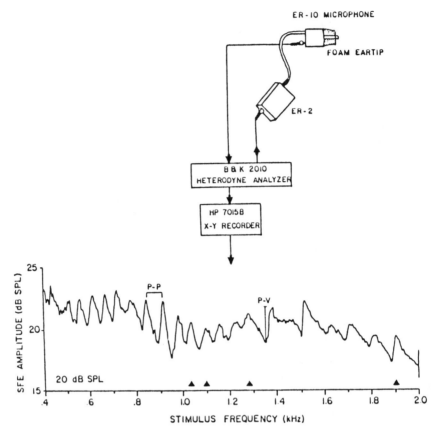

Figure 13–7. Schematic diagram of recording instrumentation for stimulus frequency otoacoustic emissions and representative example of the SFOAE.

inner ear and the emission must be able to return from the inner ear to the probe. Any transmission loss caused by middle-ear abnormalities will reduce or eliminate a measured OAE response.

Probe Examination

Careful examination of the probe assembly each day can prevent wasted time. The tubing that protrudes from the tip of the probe should be examined to insure that it is free of debris. In most cases, any debris will be visible, but sometimes the debris may become lodged in the tubing beyond view. To remove debris, the probe has to be carefully disassembled and the tube cleared with a fine wire or other suitable tool. Attention must be paid to ensure that the debris is not forced further up in to the tubing. Also, no liquid can be used in the cleaning operation because it will damage the transducers. At the conclusion of each test the transducer-probe assembly should be placed in a safe location.

Probe Placement

Fitting of the probe into the external ear canal is an important step to the successful completion of the test. The probe must fit tightly to exclude as much ambient noise as possible, but unlike immittance measurements, an air tight seal is not necessary. However, it is necessary to select a rubber probe tip that will allow the probe to be inserted approximately half way into the canal and provide for a secure and comfortable fit. Any appropriate size immittance probe tip will work. In many cases the soft sponge-rubber tips used for tubephone placement will work, but these tips are not as good at excluding ambient noise as the firm rubber tips. When placing the probe in the canal, care must be taken to insure that the tubing protruding from the tip of the probe is not crushed or pinched against the ear-canal wall and that the probe tip is facing the tympanic membrane. Fit seems to be more critical in the recording of TEOAEs than in other emissions recordings. Culpepper (Chapter 11) and Kemp, Ryan, and Bray (1990). provided a detailed report of tip placement.

PATIENT INSTRUCTIONS

For adult patients, instruction can be minimal. Aside from a brief description of what will take place and a caution against verbalization during the test, nothing is required. Dealing with the pediatric patient is another matter! It works well to tell the patient, "The machine is going to help the ear draw a picture". Children may watch and help their ears to draw the pictures by sitting as still and being as quiet as possible. The child is then allowed to watch the picture develop and usually finds the process of great interest. Of course, the occasional child comes along that will not sit still or will not stop talking, and the testing cannot be accomplished.

Organization of Patient Records

In most cases, all the data collected and the testing parameters in a testing session on a patient can be saved electronically on a diskette for later review. One important software-design consideration is the ability to save the patient data as a text file that may later be easily exported to a spreadsheet. (Equipments' operation manuals reveal if this feature is possible).

Equipment Considerations

Probes

Detailed discussion of probe design is beyond the scope of this chapter. However, it is important to note that the design of the probe is critical to obtaining a flat-frequency response in both the output and input spectra. Figure 13–8 shows one example of probe design. Output transducers are not always contained in the probe. For example, some manufacturers use tubephones outside of the probe with the tubes terminating inside of the probe. Thus, the output transducers are separate from the probe. (Examples of available commercial equipment are listed in Table 13–1.)

The miniature microphone system that has typically been used consists of four matched transducers that are mounted in mechanical opposition to one another.

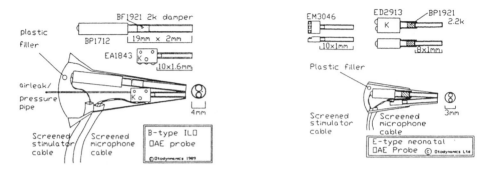

Figure 13–8. Construction details for a typical otoacoustic emission probe.

This insures that any vibration-induced output from the microphones will be in phase opposition and will cancel each other out. This arrangement produces approximately a 6 dB improvement in S/N ratio by reducing the internal noise by 6 dB (Killion & Stewart, 1986). In order to avoid acoustic coupling between the microphone and receiver, plastic tubing is attached to each and extends past the opening of the probe. The tubes are typically different in length by several millimeters to avoid the "proximity effect" described by Burkhard and Sachs (1977).

Drivers

Manufacturers use different types of output transducers and use them in different design formats. However, a good deal of information about OAEs has been collected using Etymotic Research ER-2 insert phones, which have a flat frequency response (0.2–10 kHz) and linear operation up to 112 dB SPL in the ear canal.

Computer Platforms

There are seven commercially available systems for measuring OAEs. Six of them use the IBM platform, and the other uses the Macintosh platform. For someone anticipating the purchase of OAE instrumentation, it would be wise to consider the types of computers used routinely in other aspects of one's clinical or research work. It is much easier to transfer files back and forth between Macintosh platforms and Macintosh applications or IBM platforms and IBM applications than it is to transfer from Macintosh to IBM or IBM to Macintosh. While this is a consideration now, it may not be in the future because the technology is rapidly changing. (For example, Apple has just produced the Power Macintosh computer [Power PC] that can recognize both Disk Operating System (DOS) and Macintosh applications. Nevertheless, now it is only possible to record TEOAEs on an IBM-compatible platform.)

Stimulus Considerations

Calibration

As in most other hearing-measurement procedures, OAE measurements should be made under conditions where the acoustic stimulation parameters have been carefully quantified with respect to calibration of probe-output intensity. This is not a trivial matter. It is well known that the very best place to make measures of sound pressure in the ear canal is at the plane of the tympanic membrane (TM). However most OAE probes do not reach all the way to the TM and, in fact, may terminate 2 cm or more lateral to the TM, depending on the insertion depth. This means that the probe measure is subject to the problems produced by standing waves in the ear canal. Standing waves are produced when there is overlap between the incident wave (traveling toward the TM) and the reflected wave (traveling toward the probe). Depending upon the phase relations at the point of overlap, there will either be reinforcement or cancellation at the probe microphone. The standing wave characteristics of the ear canal are difficult to predict because the specific geometry is critical. In general, it is known that as the distance between the probe end and the TM approach one fourth of the wave length of the target signal, the problem can become quite serious. Given the average length and shape of the ear canal, this means that particular calibration problems arise in the frequencies around and above 8000 Hz. The problem, therefore, is to try and deliver a constant signal to the ear canal in a system that is inherently nonlinear in its transfer function. Manufacturers have approached this problem in different manners.

One method employed is to attempt to level the ear canal SPL in much the same manner as is done in hearing-aid–test chambers. This compensation method attempts to keep the SPL at the probe microphone constant across frequency by raising or lowering the SPL to compensate for the ear canal resonance peaks and valleys. Although this insures a relatively flat response at the probe microphone, it does not necessarily allow for a flat response at the TM.

Another method is to carefully measure ear canal dimensions and acoustics and create a standard correction based upon the model. The dynamics of the model are then applied to all real ears. This method, of course, does not avoid the problems associated with individual ear characteristics and can reasonably be expected to lead to errors of 10 dB or greater, particularly in children. It is the same problem as predicting real ear hearing-aid gain from measures made in a standard 2 cc coupler.

A third method is to rely on a transducer in the probe that has uniform output characteristics and to disregard the peaks and valleys caused by standing waves. This method places a heavy emphasis on the fidelity of the output transducer.

Because each manufacturer accomplishes calibration of signals in the ear canal in a different way, clinicians should be familiar with the method used in their instrumentation. Calibration is important to validity and reliability, and attention should be paid to the instructions in the operations manuals. In addition, manufacturers use different methods for coupling the probe to the microphone of the calibrating instrumentation. For example, a manufacturer may use only a single calibration coupler in the process, whereas another may use a larger coupler volume for adults and a smaller volume for children. Indeed, the manufacturer may use two different probes, in which case two separate calibration files are maintained in the instrumentation.

Specific procedures for calibration are contained in the operations manuals. However, it is important that insofar as calibration involves high frequencies (e.g., 10,000 Hz) the clinician must be very careful with the coupling of the probe to the sound level meter. Minor variations in positioning can produce large variations in SPL. Clinical experience has shown that it is advantageous to begin with the higher frequencies and progress to calibration of the lower frequencies. This saves time when the clinician gets to the calibration of the higher frequencies and finds that the coupler was not positioned properly at the start.

In general, immediately after initiation of the test, the equipment makes two determinations using sound levels in the ear canal. First, the equipment calculates the effective ear-canal volume to tell the software how to compensate the level of the input signals. Second, the equipment usually makes some preliminary estimation of the ambient noise in the ear canal. The estimate is then used as a reference for the desired signal-to-noise ratio during the actual measurement.

Response-Recovery Considerations

Averaging

Because the SPL of emissions is low relative to the noise in the ear canal, signal averaging techniques must be used to recover the response. Readers familiar with signal-averaging techniques used in the recovery of auditory evoked potentials will recognize that the technique is similar to that for OAE recording. One item that can cause some confusion is the relation between time averaging and FFT averaging (or data point averaging). *Time averaging* refers to the number of times that the signal's time-domain root-mean-square (RMS) voltage is sampled and averaged for the purposes of noise reduction. The improvement in the S/N ratio will be equal to the square root of the number of times the signal is sampled and averaged. FFT or data point averaging involves repetitive summation in the frequency domain of the signal at one data point and is performed to provide an estimate of the standard deviation of the measurement. Some instruments performs both functions. Unfortunately, not all user documentation is careful to detail the processes by which any single instrument accomplishes data acquisition. (The user, therefore, may wish to query the manufacturer directly regarding this matter.)

Of the two functions, time averaging may be the more important because it has a direct effect on the level of the noise floor. While the signal to noise relationship is improved by the square root of the number of samples, it is necessary for the clinician to decide on an optimum number of samples to be taken so that the acquisition period is not too long for the patient. Ike and Krumm (1993) recorded DPOAEs with averages equal to 1, 4, 8, 16, 32, and 64 samples. They found that one and four averages yielded the highest DPOAE threshold values and that the other sampling values yielded lower and comparable DPOAE thresholds. The study suggested that eight averages would be sufficient to yield good threshold information. However, it is likely that the number of samples needed depends on the ambient-noise levels in the clinical setting. Therefore, it is necessary for clinicians to find the optimum number of samples for their circumstances.

Filtering and Spectral Analysis

All OAEs must be detected in the presence of the noise that exists in the ear canal. The noise is usually a composite of electrical and thermal noise in the equipment, ambient environmental noise, and physiological noise. With the exception of TEOAEs, OAEs are essentially pure-tonelike signals and the noise is typically broad-band. The S/N ratio must be improved by using small sampling segments (*bins*) of the total spectrum: The smaller the bins, the longer the test takes. Most equipment, therefore, uses bin widths of several Hertz (e.g., 10 Hz). In order to detect the presence of the OAE, the equipment must be able to determine that the measured SPL in a particular bin is greater than the expected SPL of the noise in that bin. The noise level is usually estimated by averaging across several adjacent bins because the noise in adjacent bins is likely to be approximately the same as the noise in the OAE bin. Numerous studies have shown that the noise levels range from -25 to -5 dB below the level of the OAE. The phenomenon is somewhat frequency-dependent, with lower noise levels occurring above 1000 Hz.

Artifact Reject

The *artifact* in OAE recordings is the acoustical energy that is not part of the response and needs to be controlled. There are several methods and procedures that reduce the amount of noise aside from relying on the equipment. The first and most obvious method involves the patient being quiet during the recording session. With children this may be difficult, but certainly the clinician's discussing the need for quiet with the child before the test will help. The second method involves a good position of the probe in the ear canal and a quiet room for the test, which will help reduce artifact. But because these steps alone often do not provide adequate control of artifact, manufacturers have provided for a system of automatic artifact reject in the instruments. Normally, this is accomplished by the software's being set to reject data samples that have an SPL value above some arbitrary level. Data entering the equipment is first sampled for its noise level; if it is above the set level, it is rejected and not added to the signal-averaging process that leads to the final response.

Noise Floor and Waveform Repeatability

With the advent of any new technique, there is a need to understand the issues that affect the presence or absence of a response. Two major concerns are (a) the relation between the response and the background noise and (b) the relation between the reliability and the repeatability of the response.

Decisions about the presence or absence of the response rely on the type of OAE measured and the equipment used. The presence or absence of both TEOAEs and DPOAEs is based primarily upon visual detection. For TEOAEs Kemp (1990) suggested that an autocorrelation or reproducibility factor of at least 50% was associated with the presence of an echo. It is important to point out that even with correlations of less than 50% an echo may be buried in the noise floor. In these cases an echo may be identified, if the clinician clearly sees some repeatable response rising above the spectrum for the noise. With SOAEs, SFOAEs, and DPOAEs, a common method for deciding the presence of an emission involves the looking for repeatable tracings at least 3 to 5 dB above the noise floor in the recording (Lonsbury-Martin, Harris, Stagner, Hawkins, & Martin, 1990). This method places importance on the collection and the display of the noise levels in the recording. Some instruments have the capability for keeping a running database consisting of noise measures made during sessions. The data base can then be used to display the noise-floor mean with a 1 or 2 standard deviation interval displayed around it.

Response Identification Methods

Some response recovery methods are specific to the type of emission being recorded, particularly the TEOAEs and DPOAEs.

TEOAEs

In human beings, the latency between the offset of the stimulus in the ear canal and the onset of the emission ranges between 4 and 5 ms for the high frequencies and 20 ms for the low frequencies. This separation helps identify the TEOAE in most circumstances. However, when a good-probe fit can not be assured, it is essential that one of the several more objective methods be used to determine the presence of the emission.

DIFFERENTIAL NONLINEAR RESPONSE (DNLR)

In this method first described by Bray and Kemp (1987), stimulus blocks consist of stimuli, i.e., transients or tone bursts, at two different levels that are balanced in intensity. A subaverage of the responses to stimuli does not contain any artifacts, such as stimulus ringing, because of their cancellation in the summation. The emission signal, however, is not canceled and is passed on to the signal averager. The procedure is illustrated in Figure 13–9. Every fourth stimulus is inverted and is three times larger in amplitude than the preceding three stimuli. With the procedure the ear canal response (linear system) is canceled by the summation of the four stimuli while the nonlinear portion (OAE) of the response is passed on to the signal averaging portion of the instrument and used in the final average. Kemp, Ryan, and Bray (1990) described four advantages of this method. First, it removes all middle ear artifacts that could be confused with the emission from the cochlea. Second, because all stimulus artifact is removed, it allows for the "trapping" of patient and ambient noise signals at lower levels than otherwise possible. Third, the stimulus-blanking period (i.e., the time during which the instrumentation ignores the response) can be shortened, which allows for the capture of the short-latency, high-frequency components of the echo. Fourth, because of more effective artifact handling, higher levels of stimulation can be used, which tends to increase the level of the emission.

Recently, Ravazzani and Grandori (1993) compared simple signal averaging of the entire TEOAE waveform (stimulus plus response) to the DNLR method. They found that with high intensities of stimulation the two methods were comparable with the added advantage that the DNLR method removes the stimulus artifact. However, with lower intensities they found that the detectability of the DNLR method was not as good as straight averaging. They concluded that if emissions are to be used in a response detection task, i.e., a screening, the DNLR technique appears to be the most suitable for recovering TEOAEs.

DECONVOLUTION

This method was described by Neely, Norton, Gorga, and Jesteadt (1988) and more fully explained by Grandori and Ravazzani (1990) Deconvolution is illustrated in Figure 13–10. In this method, a reference signal of a sufficiently high level (so that

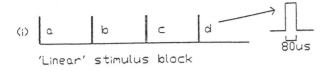

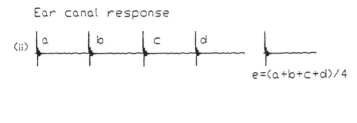

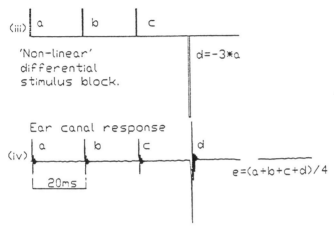

Figure 13–9. Differential nonlinear response example. *i, ii*: The ear can be stimulated by rectangular pulses of 80 ms with equal amplitude, and the ear canal responses can be averaged to increase visibility by reduction of noise. *iii, iv*: In the DNLR method, every fourth stimulus is inverted and three times larger in amplitude. The average of the ear-canal responses results in a cancellation of the stimulus portion of the response, which leaves a clear view of the portion of the response likely to contain the OAE.

the OAE component is negligible in its amplitude relative to the stimulus component) is presented to the ear. This signal is measured in the ear canal and is then compared with the original stimulus waveform to estimate the transfer function of the ear-canal–probe system. An inverse filter is then constructed with a band pass equal to the inverse of the estimated transfer function. This filter is then applied to each waveform, which effectively removes all the delay and dispersion of the stimulus component of the waveform due to the stimulus delivery system. The remaining waveform is passed to the signal-averaging portion of the system. Grandori and Ravazzani concluded that at low intensities (i.e., near threshold) the

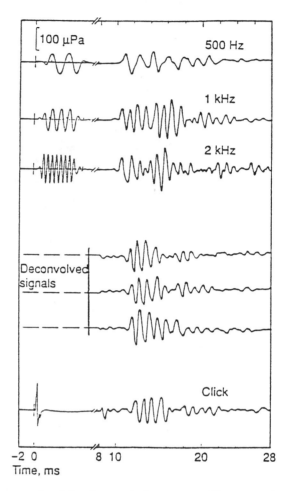

Figure 3–10. An example of the deconvolution process. The upper-three traces show the response to three different stimulus frequencies. The middle-three traces show the results of deconvolution of the upper-three traces. The bottom trace is the response to a click stimulus.

deconvolution-method waveform is easily identified, in part, because the method increases the magnitude of the threshold-level emission. Moreover, they indicated it would provide some advantages over the DNLR method.

MAXIMUM LENGTH SEQUENCES

Picton, Kellett, Vezsenyi, and Rabinovitch (1993) noted that stimuli used for evoking TEOAE's can be presented with as little as a 5 ms interstimulus interval (ISI). Shorter ISIs than this appear to cause suppression of the OAE evoked by the second click in the train. This suggested that presentation rates as high as 200/sec could be used in recovering TEOAEs. However, at that presentation rate the resulting waveform would be overlapping and distorted. Through the use of maximum length sequences (MLS), the overlapping responses could be disentangled. MLS has been used in a variety of ways, including the recording of auditory brainstem responses (Burkard, Shi, & Hecox, 1990). Figure 13–11 illustrates the process. Burkard, Shi, and Hecox showed that click-evoked OAEs can be recorded at rapid rates if the stimuli are presented using the MLS paradigm. They found that the size of the emission became smaller at the high rates, but that the amplitude reduction of the emission was offset by the increased number of stimuli that could be presented within a given amount of time. The increased number of total presentations had the effect of increasing the noise reduction and allowed reliable response identification of evenly reduced response amplitudes.

DPOAEs

FREQUENCY DOMAIN RMS AVERAGING

Because DP emissions are removed in frequency from the evoking stimuli, they have typically been recorded using standard RMS averaging in the frequency

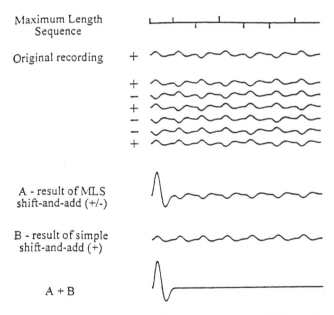

Figure 3–11. Schematic of the Maximum Length Sequence (MLS) method of response collection. The top portion of the figure shows the MLS with a length of 7. The next 7 waveforms show the original and 6 "shifted" response waveforms in either positive or negative polarity. The first shift and add process is accomplished according to the MLS sequence. This produces a waveform (A) with an initial response equal to 7 times the positive response. The B waveform is compose of a simple addition of the original response and all 6 of the shifted responses. The final (A + B) waveform is the result of adding together the A and B waveforms. (Picton et al., 1993).

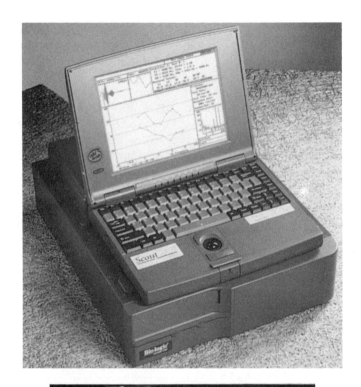

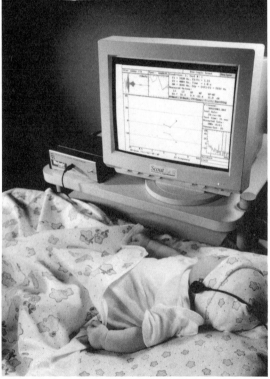

Figure 13–12. Photo of the Scout OAE System top and bottom. (Courtesy of Bio-Logic Systems Corp.)

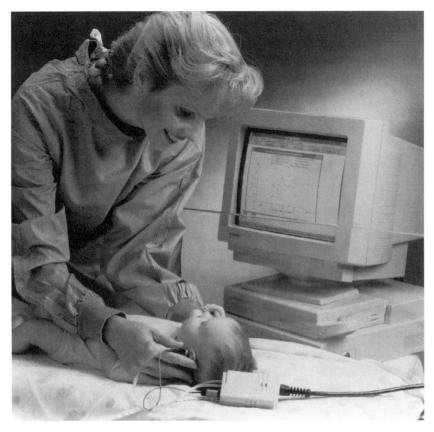

Figure 13–13. Photo of the GSI 60 DPOAE System. (Courtesy of Grason-Stadler, Inc.)

domain (FFT averaging). A set number of samples of the emission data are recorded in discrete frequency bandwidths (bins) and summed. Unlike time averaging, the process does not produce changes in the noise floor. To alter the noise floor when doing FFT averaging, one must narrow the frequency band width that contributes to the average. However, the narrowing of the bin results in an increase in the amount of time needed to acquire the average.

LINEAR TIME DOMAIN AVERAGING

Recently, Rasmussen and Oterhammel (1992) proposed "linear time-domain averaging", rather than frequency-domain averaging, with the use of a "special trigger circuit", which provided trigger signals to the A/D converter whenever the two stimulus signals (primaries) have a certain fixed phase relation. The proposal appeared guarded and probably represents some proprietary interest. They suggested, however, that linear time-domain averaging resulted in both an improved S/N ratio and a lowered-noise floor. They reported that the method enabled the recovery of responses at lower frequencies (500–750 Hz) where the responses are typically masked by residual physiological noise and external ambient noise. They

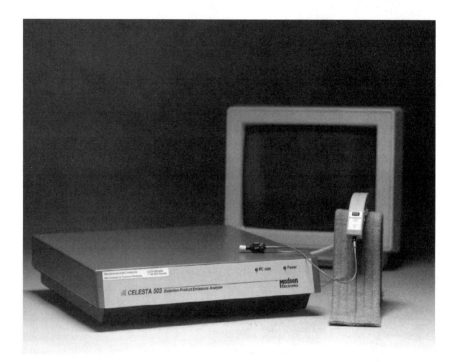

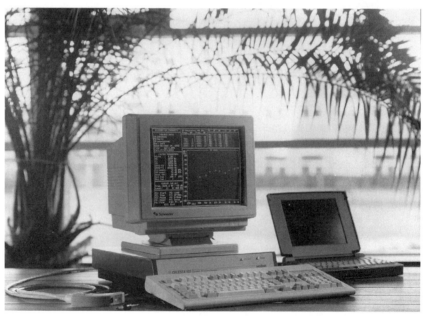

Figure 13–14. The Celesta 503 OAE Analyzer. (Courtesy of Madsen Electronics.)

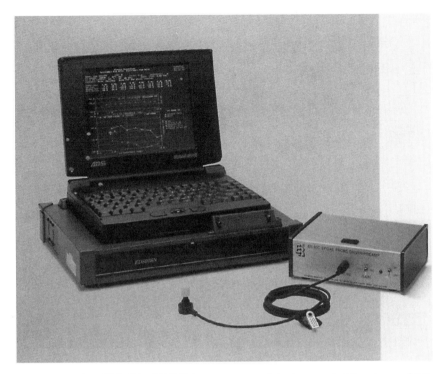

Figure 13–15. The CUB^eDis DPOAE measurement instrument. (Courtesy of Mimosa Acoustics.)

also reported that another benefit of linear time-domain averaging was the suppression of spontaneous OAEs due to the lack of a time-locked trigger signal.

Summary and Conclusions

This chapter has attempted to provide the reader with some basic understanding of the current recording methods. This is a dynamic arena in which a relatively new technique is finding a purpose. Manufacturers will likely provide us with rapid advances in equipment and in the methods by which the instrumentation systems evaluate and control the data collection. Interpretation of the data should be made easier by future instrumentation, but clinicians must always be familiar with the most current literature.

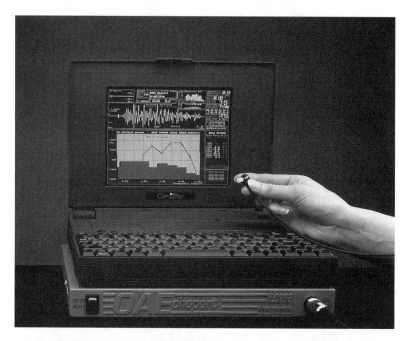

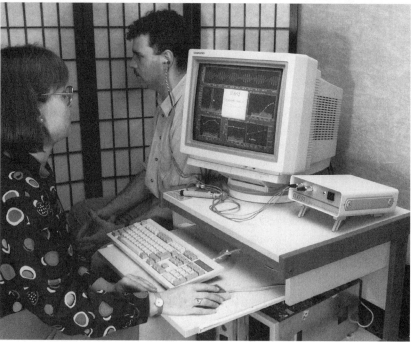

Figure 13–16. The ILO88 Echo Port TEOAE System (top) and ILO92 DPOAE System (bottom). (Courtesy of Otodynamics, Ltd.)

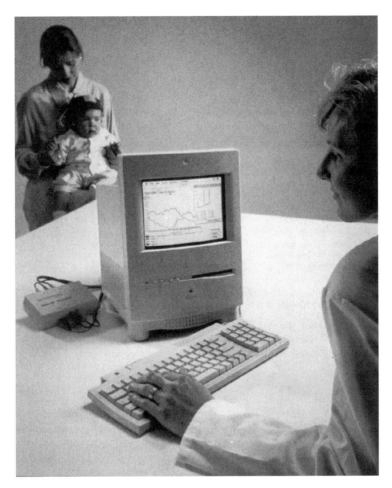

Figure 13–17. The Virtual Model 330 DPOAE System. (Courtesy of Virtual Corporation.)

References

Bonfils, P. (1989) Spontaneous otoacoustic emissions: Clinical interest. *Laryngoscope, 99*, 752–756.

Bray, P., & Kemp, D. T. (1987). An advanced cochlear echo suitable for infant screening. *British Journal of Audiology, 21*, 91–204.

Burkhard, M. D., & Sachs, R. M. (1977). Sound pressure in insert earphone couplers and real ears. *Journal of Speech and Hearing Research, 20*, 799–807.

Burkard, R., Shi, Y., & Hecox, C. (1990). Brainstem auditory evoked responses elicited by maximum length sequences: Effect of simultaneous masking noise. *Journal of the Acoustical Society of America, 87*, 1665–1672.

Elberling, C., Parbo, J., Johnsen, N. J., & Bagi, P. (1985). Evoked acoustic emission: Clinical application. *Acta Oto-Laryngologica, 421* (Suppl.), 77–85.

Grandori, F., & Ravazzani, P. (1990). Deconvolution of evoked otoacoustic emissions and response nonlinearity. In F. Grandori, G. Cianfrone, D. T. Kemp (eds.), *Cochlear mechanisms and otoacoustic emissions* (pp. 99–109). New York: Adv. Audiol. Basel, Karger.

Kemp, D. T. (1978). Stimulated acoustic emissions from within the human auditory system. *Journal of the Acoustical Society of America, 64*, 1286–1391.

Kemp, D. T. (1979). The evoked cochlear mechanical response and the auditory microstructure. *Scandinavian Audiology, 9* (Suppl.), 35–46.

Kemp D. T. (1986). Otoacoustic emissions, traveling waves, and cochlear mechanisms. *Hearing Research, 22,* 95–104.

Kemp, D. T., & Brown, A. M. (1983). An integrated view of cochlear mechanical nonlinearities observable from the ear canal. In E. deBoer and M. A. Viergever (Eds.), Fifth international symposium on hearing (pp. 75–82). The Hague, Amsterdam: Martinus Nijhoff.

Kemp, D. T., & Chum, R. A. (1983). Observations on the generator mechanism of stimulus frequency acoustic emissions: Two tone suppression. In G. van den Brink and F. A. Bilsen (Eds.), *Psychophysical, physiological, and behavioural studies in hearing* (pp. 34–42). Delft, Germany: Delft University.

Kemp, D. T., Ryan, S., & Bray, P. (1990). A guide to the effective use of otoacoustic emissions. *Ear and Hearing, 11,* 93–105.

Killion, M. C., & Stewart, J. K. (1986, May 12–16). Low Noise Microphone for Cochlear Emissions. Paper presented 111th meeting of the Acoustical Society of America, Cleveland, Ohio, Vol. 79, Suppl. 1.

Ike, S., & Krumm, M. (1993, November). The effect of time averaging on DPOAE threshold levels. Paper presented at American Speech Language Hearing Association Annual Convention, Anaheim, CA.

Lonsbury-Martin, B. L., Harris, F. P., Stagner B. B., Hawkins, M. D., & Martin, G. K. (1990) Distortion product emissions in humans: I. Basic properties in normally hearing subjects. *Annals of Otology, Rhinology and Laryngology, 99,* 3–14.

Martin, G. K., Probst, R., & Lonsbury-Martin, B. L. (1990a). Otoacoustic emissions in human ears: Normative findings. *Ear and Hearing, 11,* 106–120.

Martin, G. K., Whitehead, M. L., & Lonsbury-Martin, B. L. (1990b). Potential of evoked otoacoustic emissions for infant hearing screening. *Seminars in Hearing, 11,* 186–203.

Neely, S. T., Norton, S. J., Gorga, M. P., & Jesteadt, W. (1988). Latency of auditory brainstem responses and otoacoustic emissions using tone burst stimuli, *Journal of the Acoustical Society of America, 83,* 652–656.

Norton, S. J., & Neely, S. T. (1987). Tone burst evoked otoacoustic emissions from normal hearing subjects. *Journal of the Acoustical Society of America, 81,* 1860–1872.

Painter, J. (1994). Personal communication.

Picton, T. W., Kellett, A. J., Vezsenyi, M., & Rabinovitch, D. E. (1993). Otoacoustic emissions recorded as rapid stimulus rates. *Ear and Hearing, 14,* 299–314.

Probst, R., Coats, A. C., Martin, G. K., & Lonsbury-Martin, B. L. (1986). Spontaneous, click, and tone burst evoked otoacoustic emissions from normal ears. *Hearing Research, 21,* 261–275.

Rasmussen, A. N., & Oterhammel, P. A. (1992). A new approach for recording distortion product otoacoustic emissions. *Scandinavian Audiology, 21,* 219–224.

Ravazzani, P., & Grandori, F., (1993). Evoked otoacoustic emissions: Nonlinearities and response interpretation. *IEEE Transactions on Biomedical Engineering,* Vol. 40, No. 5.

14

Basic Instrumentation Issues in Acquiring Distortion Product Otoacoustic Emissions

JANICE E. PAINTER

Instrumentation Overview

Distortion product otoacoustic emission (DPOAE) systems generally consist of a uniquely designed probe assembly, a digital-signal processing (DSP) board, a series of floppy diskettes containing the operational software, and an isolation transformer for patient safety. A variety of accessories may also be included, such as a probe cleaning kit and a number of eartips for sealing the ear canal.

The probe assembly contains two miniature speakers and a low-noise microphone. It may even resemble an immittance probe as their purposes are very similar. Each speaker is dedicated to delivering a pure tone, either f_1 or f_2. The f_1 and f_2 tones (known as the *primary tone pair*) are kept separated from each other until they are inserted into the ear canal to minimize the possibility of instrumentation artifact interfering with the measurement of the biological response from the cochlea. The f_1 and f_2 tones are presented simultaneously to the ear canal so as to elicit a response from the cochlea known variously as the *distortion product*, the *intermodulation product*, and the *cubic-difference tone*.

The frequency-response curve of the microphone shows a roll-off beginning at 5k Hz, and the presence of biological and environmental noises make measurements below 500 Hz difficult. As a result, the frequency range available with the probe microphone is generally 500 Hz to 8K Hz. The microphone should have a low-noise floor so as not to introduce additional noise to the already noisy measured signal. The signals detected by the microphone include the primary tone pair; a series of intermodulation products; biological sounds, such as those associated with breathing, blood flow, and muscle movements; and room sounds. The challenge for the DPOAE system is to isolate the desired distortion product from the multitude of other frequencies present within the ear canal. This task is simplified by knowing mathematically the location of each disortion product (DP) frequency through the use of the formula for a specific DP, such as $2f_1 - f_2$. For example, if $f_1 = 1000$ Hz and $f_2 = 1200$ Hz, the DP frequency would be $2 \times 1000 - 1200$ or 800 Hz. Since only the frequencies in the immediate vicinity of the DP frequency have the potential of interfering with the measurement of the DP frequency, it is possible to examine only the amplitude of these frequencies when calculating the separation of the DP from the noise. Each manufacturer has a preset algorithm for the frequencies surrounding the DP frequency. One algorithm involves the examination of the average root-mean-square (RMS) value of the frequencies in the two frequency bins on either side of the DP frequency bin.

The probe assembly may also contain indicator lights to keep the operator informed of the test's status on data acceptance or rejection due to high-noise levels. Since the probe is inserted into the ear canal, it is possible for cerumen to migrate up into the probe tip. Therefore, it is important that the probe tip be (a) easily removable in case any cerumen build-up needs to be removed and (b) readily reassembled for reuse. Some manufacturers provide cleaning wires for the cleaning process.

Figure 14–1 is a sample DP-gram.

The DSP board is the command center for the DPOAE system. It contains a high-performance chip known as a *DSP processor*. This DSP chip represents the "brains" of the system because it is where signal generation, data acquisition, and averaging are controlled. The chip contains software known as *firmware*. Although several manufacturers may use the same DSP chip, the firmware written by each manufacturer determines how the system is unique.

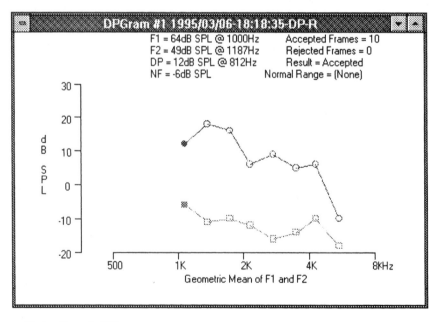

Figure 14–1. Sample DP-gram.

A fast Fourier transform (FFT) is performed on the raw data to transform (transfer) it from the time domain to the frequency domain. The transformed data is then averaged according to the test protocol used. Either complex-signal averaging (magnitude and phase) or time averaging techniques are used to improve the signal-to-noise ratio. The FFT contains a number of bins or data compartments to partition the frequency information measured by the microphone into equal size bandwidths for analysis. For example, the FFT may contain 256, 512, 1024, 2048, or even 4096 bins, depending upon the instrument design and test mode. The number of bins in the FFT, along with the sampling rate, has an impact on the bandwidth of the frequency information contained within each bin.

The DSP board may be packaged within a personal computer where it is inserted into an available Industry Standard Architecture (ISA) slot, or it may be placed within its own housing and then be attached to the serial or parallel port of a personal computer. Once the data analysis is completed for each DP point by the DSP board, the DP value is plotted on the personal computer screen.

Most personal computers are designed for nonmedical purposes. Therefore, it is necessary to isolate the patient from the possibility of a shock from the computer and its peripherals with the use of an external-isolation transformer. All system components, such as the computer console, monitor, and printer, must be plugged directly into the transformer, which is plugged directly into the AC outlet. Additionally, any personal computer that is used with a DPOAE system should meet the international standards for safety as they apply to information-technology equipment (ITE) (such as EN 60 950, IEC 950, UL 1950, and CSA 950). The software may operate in the Disk Operating System (DOS) or Windows environment. The purpose of the software is to provide a user interface to initiate a test session, to display the test results as they become available from the DSP board, and to store the test results for later retrieval. Database-management utilities improve the ease of data manipulation.

Stimulus Protocol Selection

The amplitude of the distortion product in dB SPL is influenced by the ratio of the f_2 frequency to the f_1 frequency (f_2/f_1) and the intensities of L1 (amplitude of f_1 frequency) and L2 (amplitude of the f_2 frequency). The most frequently used ratio is 1.2 or 1.22 because those ratios elicit the most robust DP at most frequencies. V. Prys (1995) suggested that a slightly higher ratio of 1.3 is more suited for the 500 to 1000 Hz and the 4000 to 8000 Hz regions. (In this instance, it would be necessary to set the ratio for measurements below 1000 Hz and above 4000 Hz to one value and those between 1000 and 4000 Hz to another value.)

A test protocol may require the L1 and L2 intensities to be equal in amplitude (e.g., L1 = L2 = 70 dB SPL), or it might require the L1 amplitude to be higher than that of L2 by 10 to 15 dB (e.g., L1 = 65 dB and L2 = 55 (or 50 dB SPL). The DPOAE system should provide flexibility in independently selecting intensity levels for L1 and L2 or L2 relative to L1 (Figure 14–2).

Even though the DPOAE system measures for the amplitude of the DP at the $2f_1 - f_2$ frequency, this is not the actual frequency generated within the cochlea as a result of the simultaneous presentation of the f_1 and f_2 frequencies. The $2f_1 - f_2$

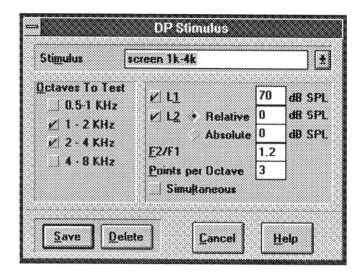

Figure 14–2. Stimulus protocol selection.

frequency merely acts as a marker for the presence of a DP. The actual site of the emission is influenced by the relation between the L1 and L2 intensities. When L1 equals L2 in intensity, it is believed that the geometric mean frequency (square root of $f_1 \times f_2$) more closely identifies the frequency region of the cochlea emitting the DP response because the traveling waves of f_1 and f_2 would overlap approximately midway between the two frequencies. However, when L1 is greater than L2, the region of overlap is probably at the site of f_2 because the traveling waves of f_1 and f_2 would overlap at the f_2 frequency point. In this instance, the x-axis of the DP-gram would be labeled f_2 (D. O. Kim, 1995).

While the ratio of f_2/f_1 and the intensities of L1 and L2 determine the amplitude of each DP value, the number of DP points collected in a DP-gram are determined by selecting the number of octaves and the number of points within each octave to be tested. Most instruments currently available allow the selection of one to four octaves for the DP-gram, i.e., 500 to 1000 Hz, 1000 to 2000 Hz, 2000 to 4000 Hz and 4000 to 8000 Hz. The particular octaves selected for the test depend upon the test's purpose. For example, a screening application may only investigate the mid-frequencies of 1000 to 4000 Hz or the octaves of 2000 Hz and above. A more complete evaluation of cochlear function may require the measurement of the entire frequency region from 500 to 8000 Hz. Finally, testing for drug toxicity might only require the analysis of the frequencies of 4000 to 8000 Hz.

The number of points per octave that are tested also depends upon the reason for the testing. For example, with a screening protocol, one might only be interested in two to four points per octave, whereas a researcher may be interested in more closely evaluating subtle changes along the cochlea and, thus, might want to measure more than six points per octave. The important point to keep in mind when selecting the number of octaves and the number of points per octave to test is that each additional DP value measured adds to the overall test time. It may be necessary to select fewer points to be tested in the interest of time, especially when testing a person who is unable to keep still or unable to keep quiet during the test.

Customizing the DP Stimulus Protocol

It is sometimes necessary to use a test protocol that allows the ratio of f_2/f_1, the frequencies of f_1 and f_2, the intensities of L1 and L2, and the number of points per octave to be varied from the standard computer-controlled sequence. In other words, it might be necessary to customize the stimulus presentation sequence to meet the specific needs of a particular patient. This versatility would allow the collection of DP values in the desired sequence. For example, when testing an active patient, such as an infant, it might be more productive to test from high frequencies to low frequencies to obtain as much information as possible before having to terminate the test session. Movement tends to interfere more with data collection at the lower frequencies (<1500 Hz) than the higher frequencies. Another example is the need to test only one or two points within some octaves, but more points within other octaves. An instrument which provides this degree of versatility makes the unit a more productive clinical tool.

Figure 14–3 presents an example of a custom DP-stimulus protocol.

Simultaneous Presentation of Multiple Primary-Tone Pairs

The collection of DP data is not time consuming (under a minute per ear with most protocols) when compared with the time spent in the clinic collecting an audiogram, a tympanogram with ipsilateral and contralateral reflex thresholds, or an auditory-brainstem response. However, when one considers the population being tested (newborns, infants, or critically ill patients), the length of the test becomes important.

Patrick Zurek and William Rabinowitz patented the use of simultaneous, multiple primary-tone–pair presentations while working on the development of a DPOAE system at Massachusetts Institute of Technology (MIT). Their technique allows the collection of multiple DP data points at the same time without impacting on test performance. The DP-gram that results from the presentation of multiple primary-tone pairs looks similar to the results collected when the same primary-tone pairs are presented one after the other. The important difference is in the time it takes to collect the data: In most instances, test time is reduced by at least 50%.

Test performance is maintained by simultaneously presenting primary-tone pairs that are at least one octave apart from one another. The spatial distance in frequencies avoids any interference from harmonics generated by the primary tones. Figure 14–4 a comparison of sequentially collected data with simultaneously collected data.

Impact of Sampling Rate

During DP testing, the primary tones are presented continuously, and the microphone within the probe tip constantly measures the frequencies from 500 to 8000

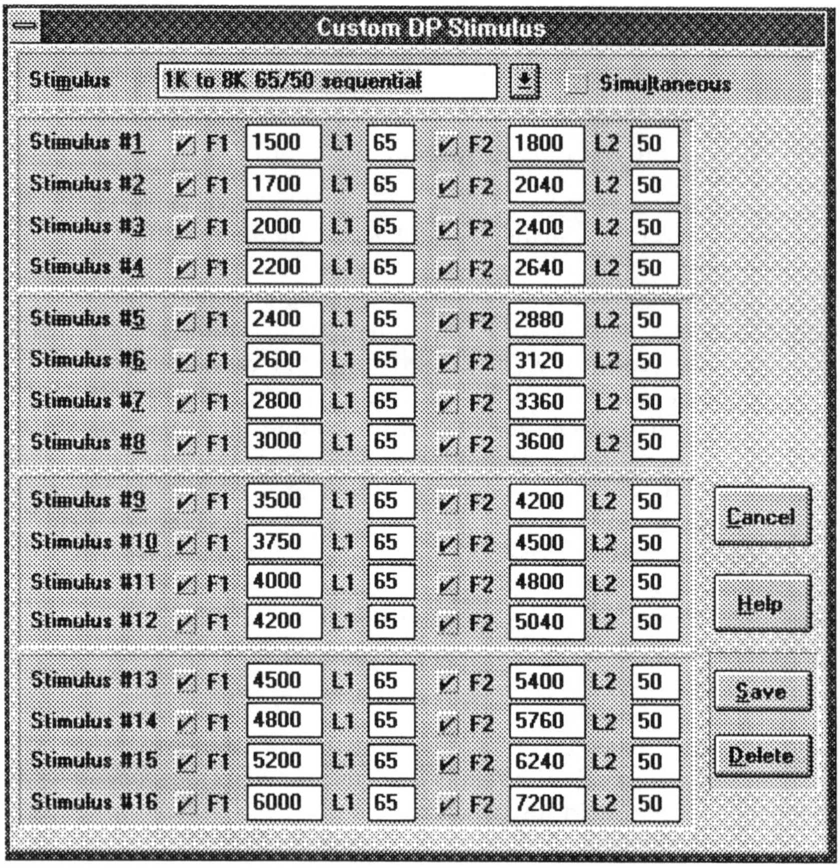

Custom DP Stimulus							
Stimulus	1K to 8K 65/50 sequential						Simultaneous

Stimulus #1	F1	1500	L1	65	F2	1800	L2	50
Stimulus #2	F1	1700	L1	65	F2	2040	L2	50
Stimulus #3	F1	2000	L1	65	F2	2400	L2	50
Stimulus #4	F1	2200	L1	65	F2	2640	L2	50
Stimulus #5	F1	2400	L1	65	F2	2880	L2	50
Stimulus #6	F1	2600	L1	65	F2	3120	L2	50
Stimulus #7	F1	2800	L1	65	F2	3360	L2	50
Stimulus #8	F1	3000	L1	65	F2	3600	L2	50
Stimulus #9	F1	3500	L1	65	F2	4200	L2	50
Stimulus #10	F1	3750	L1	65	F2	4500	L2	50
Stimulus #11	F1	4000	L1	65	F2	4800	L2	50
Stimulus #12	F1	4200	L1	65	F2	5040	L2	50
Stimulus #13	F1	4500	L1	65	F2	5400	L2	50
Stimulus #14	F1	4800	L1	65	F2	5760	L2	50
Stimulus #15	F1	5200	L1	65	F2	6240	L2	50
Stimulus #16	F1	6000	L1	65	F2	7200	L2	50

Cancel | Help | Save | Delete

Figure 14–3. Example of custom DP stimulus protocol.

Hz, along with their respective amplitudes present within the ear canal. To facilitate the transfer of data from the microphone to the digital circuitry, the spectral information from the microphone is captured in sweeps or distinct frames that cover a finite amount of time. (The transfer is comparable to the shutter speed on a camera.)

The time spent per sweep or frame of data is determined by the sampling rate and the number of bins or data compartments in the FFT. The sampling rate determines how frequently the microphone captures spectral data, and the number of bins in the FFT determines how many samples need to be collected before the desired spectral information is collected per sweep or frame of data. For instance, a sampling rate of 16,000 indicates that the microphone is capturing spectral information every 62.5 ms (1/16,000 = 0.0000625), whereas a sampling rate of 32,000 causes the microphone to sample spectral data every 31.2 ms (1/32,000 = 0.0000312). When a sampling rate of 16,000 is used with an FFT containing 512 bins, the time spent per sweep is 32 ms (512/16,000), and a sampling rate of 32,000 with an FFT

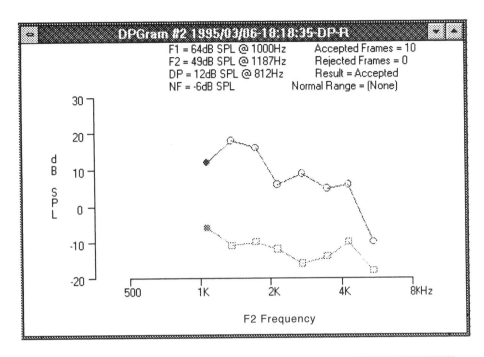

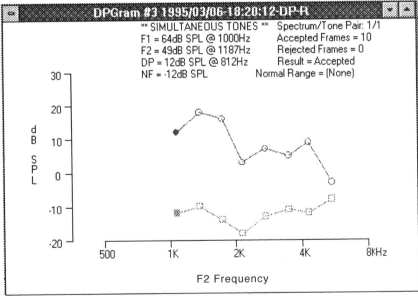

Figure 14–4.   A comparison of sequentially collected data with simultaneously collected data. Note that the DP-grams are similar, but the test times are different.

Time in milliseconds spent per frame based upon # bins in FFT					
Sampling Rate	256	512	1024	2048	4096
4000	64	128	256	512	1024
6000	43	85	171	341	683
8000	32	64	128	256	512
12000	21	43	85	171	341
16000	16	32	64	128	256
24000	11	21	43	85	171
32000	8	16	32	64	128

Figure 14–5. Sampling rate and test time per frame.

containing the same 512 bins yields a sweep or frame time of 16 ms (512/32,000). Figure 14–5 presents sampling rate and test time information.

In addition, the sampling rate has an impact on the maximum frequency that can be measured. The frequency is determined mathematically by dividing the sampling rate by 2.1. Therefore, the maximum frequency which can be measured reliably with a sampling rate of 16,000 is 7619 Hz. This means that the maximum f_2 frequency that can be presented is 7619 Hz. In this case, the maximum DP frequency which can be measured is 4871 Hz when the f_2 to f_1 ratio is 1.22 (i.e., $f_2 = 7619$; $f_2/f_1 = 1.22$; $f_1 = 6,245$; $2f_1 - f_2 = 4871$ Hz). If the DP is plotted as a function of the geometric-mean frequency, then the maximum DP value will be 6897 Hz (square root of $f_1 \times f_2$), or if the DP is plotted as a function of f_2, the maximum DP value will be 7619 Hz. There is an additional relation between the number of bins in the FFT and the sampling rate. The number of bins divided into the sampling rate determines the bandwidth of frequencies contained within each bin in the FFT. For example, when the FFT contains 512 bins and a sampling rate of 16,000 is used, the bandwidth per bin is 31.25 Hz (16,000/512 = 31.25 Hz) whereas a sampling rate of 32,000 used with a 512 bin FFT yields a bandwidth of 62.5 Hz (32,000/512 = 62.5 Hz).

Figure 14–6 presents sampling rate and bandwidth per bin in FFT.

The bandwidth within each bin is important when measuring the noise floor. For example, when an instrument evaluates the two bins of frequency information that

Bandwidth per bin based on # bins in FFT					
Sampling Rate H2	256	512	1024	2048	4096
4000	15.6	7.8	3.9	2.0	1.0
6000	23.4	11.7	5.9	2.9	1.5
8000	31.3	15.6	7.8	3.9	2.0
12000	46.9	23.4	11.7	5.9	2.9
16000	62.5	31.3	15.6	7.8	3.9
24000	93.8	46.9	23.4	11.7	5.9
32000	125.0	62.5	31.3	15.6	7.8

Figure 14–6. Sampling rate and bandwidth per bin in FFT.

surround the bin with the DP frequency, a bandwidth of 31.5 Hz per bin does not interfere with the DP measurement at low frequencies. However, it does interfere with the DP frequency measurement when the bandwidth is 62.5 Hz at low frequencies. This is particularly important if f_1 equals 500 Hz and f_2 equals 600 Hz ($2f_1 - f_2 = 400$ Hz). Two bins of information to the right of the DP frequency of 400 Hz would overlap with the bin containing the f_1 frequency if the sampling rate was 32,000 ($2 \times 62.5 = 125$ Hz; $400 + 125 = 525$ Hz), but would not cause a problem when the sampling rate is 16,000 ($2 \times 31.5 = 63$ Hz; $400 + 63 = 463$ Hz).

Data Acceptance and Rejection

If DPOAE systems could not reject certain frames or sweeps of data, all data measured by the microphone would be considered with equal weight in the FFT for averaging. This would unnecessarily add time to the averaging process because it is only possible to achieve a 3 dB SPL improvement in noise level for each doubling of the number of frames averaged. In other words, when 2 frames of data are averaged, the noise floor is improved by 3 dB over a single frame of data. An additional 3 dB improvement is achieved every time the number of frames is doubled. The DP amplitudes may vary in patients from around 20 dB SPL to -5 dB SPL or lower, whereas noise levels may be as high as 60 dB SPL depending upon environmental and physiological noise. In order to have confidence in the reliability of a DP measurement, it is necessary to improve the signal-to-noise ratio, i.e., the intensity difference between the amplitude of the DP and the noise level in the surrounding frequency bins.

Figure 14–7 presents rejection criteria.

An improvement in the signal-to-noise ratio can only be achieved through averaging owing to the 3-dB improvement effect. The task can take less time if frames of data that are too noisy are rejected. It is important to be able to select the dB SPL level above which a frame of data is rejected so as to prevent the noisy data from being averaged in with the preceding quieter data. An instrument which provides the ability to select a noise rejection criterion will make the DPOAE system usable in a variety of environments and reduce the overall test time.

Another criterion to consider when collecting frames of data is whether or not

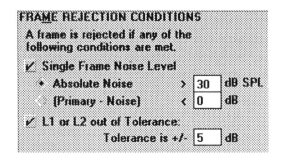

Figure 14–7. Selection of rejection criteria.

the f_1 and f_2 tones are actually presented at the intensity level specified in the test protocol. If the averaged frames of data are the result of varying intensity levels of f_1 and f_2, the DP measurement will be erroneous. Therefore, it is important to reject frames of data that are the result of f_1 or f_2 intensity levels that are outside a specified tolerance range, such as 2 to 5 dB. The ability to specify tolerance ranges for f_1 and f_2 gives reliability to test results because the DP is the result of a controlled intensity-level presentation.

Amount of Averaging

The purpose of averaging is to improve the signal-to-noise ratio between the DP frequency and the surrounding frequency bins (noise). Obviously, when there is a large difference between the amplitude of the DP and the noise floor, it is possible to place more confidence in the reliability of the test results. However, there is a point beyond which the additional improvement of the signal-to-noise ratio does not add much to the reliability of the results.

While room noise certainly has an impact on the amount of averaging required, the noise within the patient's ear may be even more significant. A signal-to-noise difference of 10 dB SPL can be achieved rather quickly in a quiet ear with a robust DP (10 frames or less), whereas it may require the averaging of 500 frames or more of data to achieve the same signal-to-noise difference in a noisy ear with a low-amplitude DP. A DPOAE system that allows the operator to select a desired signal-to-noise difference as a means of determining the number of frames of data to average provides greater clinical flexibility. It also allows the test time to vary depending upon the robustness of the DP response above the noise floor.

Establishing DP-Gram Templates

Since the DP amplitude varies by frequency, person, and test protocol used, it can be useful to overlay a template on the DP-gram result that is representative of the results obtained from a population where there is no cochlear disorder present. The template may provide visual feedback while the test is in progress or may be used after the DP-gram has been collected to assess cochlear status. The template may represent the dB SPL of the distortion product results from an otologically normal population, or it might represent the dB SPL range of results obtained from a group with a particular cochlear disorder.

An instrument that provides a facility to overlay multiple DP-grams from different persons makes it easier to determine the upper and lower boundaries of a particular population. The boundary values may be used directly to construct a template, or the individual values may be used to calculate the ± one standard deviation values for the boundaries.

Each template should be given a unique name that describes the population tested to ensure the use of the appropriate template with each person tested. A template should only be used as a visual aid on DP-grams obtained with the same test protocol because each template is developed through the use of a particular test protocol.

Spontaneous Emissions Testing

Distortion product otoacoustic emissions (DPOEAs) are classified as evoked emissions because a stimulus is used to elicit a specific type of response from the cochlea. When no external stimulus is presented by the DPOAE system, the signals measured by the probe microphone represent the spontaneous activity within the cochlea. The measurements of the on-going activity in the cochlea are classified as *spontaneous emissions testing*. In both tests, the probe microphone must have a sufficiently low noise floor so as not to compromise the measurement process. But unlike DPOAE testing, in spontaneous emissions testing the speakers in the probe are not used, and there is no way to predetermine the frequencies where a response needs to be measured. As a result, it is necessary to employ a different test protocol to measure these spontaneous emissions.

During spontaneous emissions testing, the ability to capture the entire frequency range available within the DPOAE system and average all frequencies measured at the microphone is necessary. Because noise is a random signal, i.e., the amplitude of the frequencies vary from frame to frame, the frequencies representing noise are averaged out if enough sweeps of data are collected. However, the actual frequencies generated by the cochlea are present throughout the measurement process and, thus, appear as "spikes" above the noise floor on the frequency spectrum. The amplitude of the frequency spike(s) does not vary during the measurement process.

Figure 14–9 provides an example of a spontaneous emission.

As with DPOAE measurements, in spontaneous emissions testing a combination of sampling rate and the number of bins present within the FFT determine the bandwidth of frequencies present in each bin of data. The bandwidth of frequencies in each bin during spontaneous emissions testing needs to be as narrow as possible so as to be able to detect the presence of any spontaneous activity. The ideal bandwidth to eliminate the possibility of interference from random noise appears to be 1 Hz. To achieve a bandwidth of 1 Hz, the test protocol would have to consist of a sampling rate of 4000 and the number of bins in the FFT would have to be 4096 (4000/4096 = 1). If the sampling rate is 4000 Hz, the maximum spontaneous frequency which could be measured is 1904 Hz (because the maximum frequency measurable by the DPOAE system is determined by the sampling rate divided by 2.1). This is a correct test protocol if there is no spontaneous activity from the cochlea above 1904 Hz; if there is activity above this frequency, it would not be detected owing to the protocol selected. Therefore, care should be taken in selecting a test protocol for spontaneous emissions testing.

Figure 14–8 outlines the maximum frequency detectable per sampling rate and can be used as a guide in developing the test protocol for spontaneous emissions testing.

By reviewing the maximum frequency that can be measured along with the frequency bandwidth per bin and the time spent per frame of data, it is possible to determine the most appropriate combination of sampling rate and number of bins in the FFT for testing. It is also important to be able to utilize an acceptance-rejection criterion for each frame of data to reduce the overall time needed for averaging.

Impact of sampling rate on maximum frequency detectable

Sampling Rate	Maximum Hz
4000	1902
6000	2859
8000	3812
12000	5718
16000	7625
24000	*9492
32000	*9500

*Note: the maximum calibration frequency
on the device is 9500 Hz

Figure 14–8. Determination of maximum frequency detectable.

Database Management

The ability to store and retrieve DP-gram results is a valuable feature as it allows the clinician to analyze and print test results at a later date. However, database integrity depends on good database management, such as making regular backups of the data files, deleting records that no longer need to be saved (sometimes called *purging the database*), cleaning up the hard drive on a regular basis, and archiving records that do not need to be readily available. How frequently the tasks are performed depends upon the user's evaluation of the risk, which includes the number of different users accessing the database.

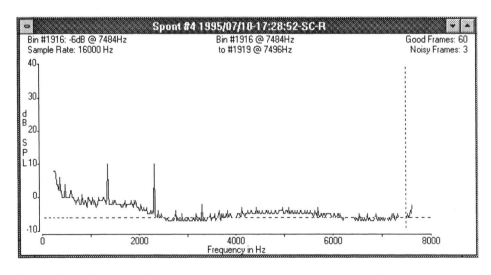

Figure 14–9. Example of a spontaneous emission.

If the test results stored in the computer's hard drive are never printed out or if the printout is forwarded to someone outside your department, the hard drive contains the only source of the test results. If the risk or the impact of hard drive damage is great, the files should be frequently copied. A backup can be made to floppy diskettes, to a different hard drive, or to a tape backup system.

Compression utility software programs reduce the amount of space that the backup data uses. Every database sets a fixed amount of space aside for each field in the database. However, not all data entries are large enough to fill this available space. A compression utility examines the number of characters occupying each field and temporarily eliminates the unused portions of each data field and allows the test data to be stored in a smaller amount of space. These compression utilities are particularly useful when storing the backup data onto floppy disks.

If the test results for a particular patient are no longer needed, it is good practice to delete the test results from the hard drive. This keeps the access time for needed records fast by keeping the database small.

A side effect of deleting unnecessary records from the database is that the stored records become fragmented on different portions of the hard drive. A fragmented database takes more time to access than a database which is more tightly packed. The practice of bringing related data closer together on a hard drive is called *packing the database*; it can easily be performed if a utility is included in the DPOAE program.

Record archiving is another good database management practice. The practice consists of deciding on a method for storing groups of patient records. When a database is new little thought is given to long-term storage of the results. However, over time, the hard drive is not large enough to store all patient records. Therefore, an archiving method should be used early to prevent future problems.

The archiving method should be simple to follow and be practical to maintain. In a busy clinic where patients are not expected to return regularly for follow-up testing, one archiving method is the storage of each day's records on separate floppy disk; each disk is labelled by date, and a log is kept of each disk. If a patient returns to the clinic for follow-up testing, the previous result is located by knowing the date of the last visit. The important point is not so much what the method is, but rather that a good method exists and that it is followed.

Some users may wish to transfer the test results from the DPOAE database to a spreadsheet or wordprocessing program. The easiest way to accomplish this is by converting the DP test result into an ASCII file (Figure 14–10). An ASCII file is recognized by most commercially available software packages and simplifies the challenge of transferring data from one program to another.

Summary and Conclusions

The accuracy of DPOAE testing depends upon the design of the instrument probe and the test protocol selected to collect data. The probe microphone needs to have a low-noise floor to prevent interference with the measuring. The sampling rate, the number of bins in the FFT, the number of averages performed, and the ability to specify a rejection criterion for each frame of data—all influence the degree of accuracy and the time spent collecting the data. When performing DPOAE mea-

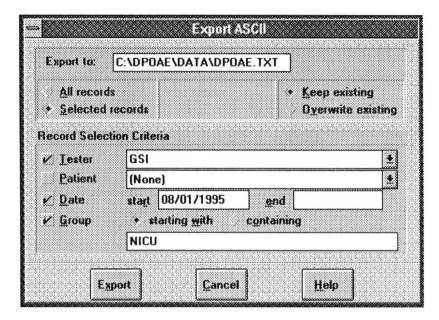

Figure 14–10. Exporting data as an ASCII file.

surements, the stimulus protocol selected influences the amplitude of the DP measurement and the number of data points collected. If a DP-gram template is used as a visual tool during DP measurements, it is important to use the same test protocol during data collection as was used to develop the template. A DP-gram may be collected in less time without impacting performance by presenting multiple primary-tone pairs simultaneously.

References

Kim, D. O. (1995). Personal communication.
Prys, V. (1995). Personal communication.

Index

Acetylcholine, 39, 40

Afferent neurons, 26, 38, 206

Age differences

 basilar membrane, 190

 DPOAEs, 100, 101, 183, 190, 191–192, 273

 SOAEs, 49–50

 TEOAEs, 71–74, 75, 76, 165, 277–281, 283

 traveling wave delay, 190

Air pressure, effects on OAEs, 136–140

Amplitudes, DPOAEs

 age differences, 100, 101, 183, 190, 191–192, 273

 and DPOAE phase, 92

 and ear-canal pressure, 137, 138

 ear-side differences, 96, 98

 and frequencies, 95–96, 97, 166–167, 196, 197, 312, 334, 335–337

 gender differences, 96, 99, 100

 and hearing thresholds, 102–103, 183

 and middle-ear pressure, 138

 and primary tones, 87–89, 94, 103–106, 312

 and pure-tone thresholds, 167, 169–171, 181, 195–197

 stimulus levels, 167, 184–188

Amplitudes, TEOAEs

 age differences, 74, 277–281, 283

 calculations, 112–113

 and ear canal, 133, 135, 136–137

 ear-side differences, 72, 74

 gender differences, 72, 74

 and middle-ear pressure, 138–139

 neonates, 70, 71, 142–143, 254, 273–274, 276

 stimuli, 65, 115, 135

Animal studies

 DPOAEs, 103, 206

 SOAEs, 55–56

 TEOAEs, 64

 TEOAE suppression, 125, 127

Architectural acoustics model, 5

Archiving (records), 345

Artifact control, 321

Audiometric thresholds. *See also* Hearing thresholds

 OAEs, 8, 17–18

 SOAEs, 47–48

 TEOAEs, 72, 73

Auditory-brainstem response (ABR)

 children, evaluating, 297, 299

 and eighth-nerve tumor diagnosis, 208

 frequency-specific stimulation, 9

 and hearing loss, 182, 218, 220–221

 neonatal screening programs, 236, 247–248, 251

 post-operative tests, 209, 210

 response-signal extraction, 9

Auditory microstructure, 182

Auditory neuropathy, 297

Auditory threshold sensitivity, 14–18

Averaging

 data point averaging, 320

Fast Fourier Transform (FFT), 320, 327, 335, 341
linear-time domain averaging, 327, 329
response recovery, 320
RMS (root-mean-square) averaging, 323, 327, 334
TEOAE response waveform, 111
time averaging, 198–201, 320
time-synchronous averaging, 9, 200–201
transient-suppressed time-synchronous averaging, 200
windowed signal averaging, 199–200

Band reproducibility, 254
Basilar membrane
age, effects of, 190
displacement, 34
and DPOAEs, 92, 183
location, 24
motion of, 35–36, 39, 84
and SOAEs, 50
and traveling wave, 29–30
Behavior Observation Audiometry, 292, 293
Boys Town National Research Hospital, 279

Calibration
DPOAEs, 106–107
ILO equipment, 106–107
preliminary, 315
probe-output intensity, 319
Celesta503, 308, 328
Children, evaluating, 271–272, 276–304. See also Neonatal screening programs
case studies, 292–302
cochlear changes, monitoring, 299
DPOAEs, 279, 281
ear-canal size, 286
and noise, 284–286
preparing for testing, 317, 321
sedation, 285
TEOAEs, 71, 72, 277–281

Chinchillas (and SOAEs), 55–56
Cleft Palate Clinic, 288, 298
Click stimuli
compared with tonal stimulation, 9
data collection, 12, 13
frequency-specific OAE recordings, 281
intensity and response, 65
TEOAE masking, 111, 113, 114–118, 121–122, 125, 127
TEOAEs, 63, 75, 76, 280–281
Cochlear amplifier, 36, 39, 46, 63, 84, 103
Cochlear anatomy, 23–28
Cochlear function during surgery, 208–211
Cochlear implant, 226–227
Cochlear microphonic potential, 32–33, 36, 64, 65
Cochlear partition, 24–25, 28–29, 39
Cochlear response and frequency specificity, 9
Cochlear Sounder, 2
Combination tones, 30
Common Procedural Terminology (CPT), 237
Compound action potential, 38, 41
Compression utility software, 345
Computers
external-isolation transformer, 335
platforms, 318
safety standards, 335
Conductive hearing loss, 132, 133, 246, 287
Congenital peripheral auditory dysfunction. See Neonatal screening programs
Crossed olivo-cochlear bundle (COCB), 17, 120
CUBeDIS, 200, 308, 329

Database management, 250–251, 344–346
Data point averaging, 320
Deafness. See also Hearing loss
central deafness, 165
theories of, 7

Decibel levels, 14–18
Deconvolution, 322–324
Differential nonlinear response, 322, 323
Discriminant analysis, 191
Distortion product OAEs. *See* DPOAEs
DP-audiogram, 18, 89, 167
DP-grams, 89, 95, 167, 312, 314, 334, 336, 337, 339
DP-gram templates, 342
DPOAE clinical applications, 166–175. *See also* DPOAEs
  bitonal stimulation, 166–167
  children, 279, 281
  dips, monotonic, 194, 197
  eighth cranial-nerve lesion, 228
  eighth cranial-nerve tumor diagnosis, 207
  hearing aids, 224
  hearing loss, 166, 172, 173, 201
  hearing thresholds, 100, 102–103, 167, 171, 173, 181, 183, 186
  neonatal screening programs, 234, 236, 255–256, 261, 273–274, 276, 281
  noise floor, effect of, 187–189
  noise immunity, 182
  nulls, 194
  pure-tone thresholds, 167, 169–172, 181, 182, 185, 190–197
  reporting results, 175, 176, 177
  standard scores, 175
  test protocols, 167, 168
  zone of uncertainty, 169
DPOAEs, 83–107. *See also* Amplitudes, DPOAEs; DPOAE clinical applications; EOAEs; Frequencies, DPOAEs; Measurement methods
  and afferent neurons, 206
  age differences, 100, 101, 183, 190, 191–192, 273
  animal studies, 103, 206
  and cochlear response observation, 13–14
  detection threshold, 89
  and ear-canal pressure, 137
  ear side, 96, 98
  equipment for measuring, 84–87, 106–107, 308
  false positives, 188
  first recordings, 2, 5
  gender differences, 96, 99, 100
  growth function, 133, 171–172, 184–185, 190, 194
  input/output function, 89–91, 133, 134, 190, 312–313, 315
  measurement, 10–11, 19, 84–91
  and middle-ear fluid, 140
  multiple, 13
  onset latency, 88, 91–92
  and outer hair cells, 182
  phase, 91, 92, 189, 196
  prevalence, 95
  response forms, 87–94
  and SOAEs, 58, 176, 195
  stimulus calibration, 106–107
  suppression, 92–94
  and TEOAEs, 15, 173–175
  TEOAE technology, compared with, 12–14
  tuning curves, 92, 94
  two-tone stimulation, 9, 10–11
Drivers (transducers), 318
DSP processor, 84, 86, 334, 335

Ear canal
  and backward transmission, 133–134
  and calibration problems, 319
  closing to maximize OAE level, 7–8
  developmental changes, 141, 142
  examining prior to testing, 315
  recording SOAEs, 46
  size in children, 286
  spectral average of noise in, 47
Ear-canal air pressure, effect on OAEs, 136–137, 144–146
Ear-canal probes. *See* Probe assemblies
Eardrum
  developmental changes, 142
  and OAEs, 7, 133
  perforations, 140–141
Ear-side differences
  DPOAEs, 96, 98

SOAEs, 49
TEOAEs, 72, 74, 75, 76
Eighth cranial-nerve lesion, 228
Eighth cranial-nerve neurons, 26–27, 40, 41, 42
Eighth cranial-nerve tumors, 206–211
Endocochlear potential, 4, 28, 32
Endolymph, 23, 25, 28, 32, 34
Energy loss and auditory functioning, 3–4
EOAEs, 205–230. *See also* DPOAEs; TEOAEs
    assessing normal cochlear functioning, 229
    children, evaluating, 271–272, 276–304
    and cochlear function during surgery, 208–211
    and cochlear lesions, 212
    preneural origins, 206
    and sudden hearing loss, 211–214
Evoked otoacoustic emissions. *See* EOAEs

Fast Fourier Transform (FFT)
    averaging, 320, 327, 335, 341
    ILO 88 display, 253–254, 281
    and noise floor, 187, 200, 201
    and sampling rate, 340–341
    SOAEs, 309
    TEOAEs, 310
FFT. *See* Fast Fourier Transform (FFT)
Filtering (signal processing), 9, 198
Fourier transform (FT), 198–199
Frequencies, DPOAEs
    and age, 190
    and amplitudes, 95–96, 97, 166–167, 196, 197, 312, 334, 335–337
    and hearing loss, 172
    and hearing thresholds, 181
    and noise, 187
    primary tones, 183–184, 312
    and traveling waves, 189
Frequencies and cochlear partition, 28–29
Frequency selectivity
    early observations, 6

hair cells, 41
near SOAEs, 57
TEOAEs, 64
Frequency specificity, 3, 9, 181, 281

Ganglion. *See* Spiral ganglion
Gaussian distribution, 96
Gender differences
    DPOAEs, 96, 99, 100
    hearing sensitivity, 153
    SOAEs, 49, 53, 153
    TEOAEs, 72, 74, 75–76
Glycerol, 165, 172
Gold, Thomas, 3, 4, 46
Growth function
    DPOAEs, 133, 171–172, 184–185, 190, 194
    TEOAEs, 133, 159
GSI60, 308, 327

Hair cells, 24–26. *See also* Inner hair cells; Outer hair cells
    frequency selectivity, 41
    innervation patterns, 26
    interactions of inner and outer, 39–40
    motility, 5, 6
    nonlinearities, 38–39, 84
    and potassium, 32, 34–35
    potentials, 32–34, 35, 36, 40
    stimulus to, 30
    synapses, 40
    and TEOAEs, 65
    transduction, 30–31, 34–35, 40–41
    transmitters, 31, 35, 40
Hamming window, 199
Healthy People 2000, 234, 246
Hearing
    place theory of, 3
    telephone theory of, 3
Hearing aids, 224, 297, 298–299
Hearing Health Institute, Fort Worth, 237–238
Hearing loss. *See also* Deafness; Sensorineural hearing loss
    conductive, 132, 133, 246, 287
    and DPOAEs, 166, 172, 173, 201
    infant, 218, 220–221

noise-induced, 173
prevalence data, neonates, 240
and SOAEs, 48
sudden hearing loss, 164, 211–220
and TEOAEs, 156–166
and viral neuritis, 227–228
Hearing thresholds, 14–18. *See also*
Audiometric thresholds
DPOAEs, 100, 102–103, 167, 171, 173,
181, 183, 186
EOAEs, 287, 303
OAEs, 8
SOAEs, 153–154
TEOAEs, 65, 156, 158, 159, 161, 165–
166, 173
High-frequency sensorineural hearing
loss, 159, 160
HISCREEN (software), 251
HITRACK (software), 251
Hypoxia, 48

IBM computers, 86, 318
Idiopathic sudden hearing loss. *See*
Sudden hearing loss
ILO equipment, 308, 330
display, 66–69, 252–255
frequency components analysis, 281,
282
ipsilateral suppression of TEOAEs,
121
low-cut filter option, 286
neonatal screening programs, 242–
243
Quickscreen option, 254, 256, 261,
286
stimulus calibration, 106–107
TEOAEs, 75, 80, 236
Implants, cochlear, 226–227
Inner hair cells
afferent fibers, 34, 36
potentials, 42
pure tone stimulation, 35
stimulated by fluid, 30
Input impedance, 132, 141
Input/output function
DPOAEs, 89–91, 133, 134, 190, 312–
313, 315

TEOAEs, 114–115, 132–133, 280
Instrumentation. *See* Measurement
methods
Intermodulation distortion. *See*
DPOAEs
Ipsilateral fatiguing stimuli, 53
Ipsilateral suppression of TEOAEs,
110–128. *See also* TEOAEs
animal studies, 125, 127
contralateral masking, 122, 123–124
efferent-mediated effects, 127
forward masking, 121–123, 124, 125
simultaneous masking, 111–112, 116,
118

Joint Committee on Infant Hearing,
237, 241, 245

Kemp, David, 2, 46, 63–64, 151
Koop, C. E., 234

Linear time-domain averaging, 327, 329
Logan Regional Hospital, 245, 247–
252, 255, 256, 257, 262, 265–266
Loop diuretics, 20, 64

Macintosh computers, 86, 318
Magnitude reflectance data, 182, 197
Maximum length sequences, 324–325
Mayo Clinic, 207, 237
Measurement methods, 307–331. *See
also* ILO equipment
DPOAEs, 312–313, 320, 325, 327,
333–342
equipment available, 308
SFOAEs, 313–314
SOAEs, 309, 310
TEOAEs, 309–312, 324
Medial olivocochlear system (MOCS),
120–121, 125, 127
Ménière's disease, 161, 162, 163, 165, 172
Menstrual cycles and SOAEs, 50
Mesenchyme, 141–142
Microphones, 7, 8, 307
and calibration, 319
DPOAEs, 84, 312, 333
frequency-response curve, 333

and noise floor, 187, 201
and sampling rate, 338
SOAEs, 46, 309
TEOAEs, 111
transducers, 317–318
Microstructure, DPOAE, 195–196
Microstruture audiogram, 56–57
Middle ear
    backward transmission, 133–134
    developmental changes, 141–142
    forward transmission, 132–133
    input impedance, 132
    models of function, 131–132
    muscle contraction, 53
    and OAE detection, 7
    pressure and SOAEs, 52
    reflex threshold in TEOAE masking,
        125, 126
    resonance, neonates, 71
Middle-ear disease, 130–149
    case studies, 143–149
    children, evaluating, 287
    and DPOAEs, 182
Multiple sclerosis and sudden hearing
    loss, 212, 214, 216, 217, 218

National Consortium on Newborn
    Hearing Screening, 256
National Institutes of Health
    Consensus Statement, 241, 245
Neonatal screening programs, 233–
    268. *See also* Neonates
    age of identification of hearing
        impairment, 233–234
    data interpretation, 255–257, 283
    data management, 250–251
    DPOAEs, 234, 236, 255–256, 261,
        273–274, 276, 281
    equipment needed, 243–245
    financing, 237–239
    flowchart, 247
    high-risk approach, 233
    noise and testing, 188–189, 254, 255–
        256, 262–264, 274
    outpatient, 291
    pass-refer criteria, 255–256, 281, 283,
        291

preparation for, 239–246
preterm infants, 240, 276
rescreening, 250, 265
skills test, 249
TEOAEs, 69–71, 80, 234–236, 247–
    250, 255–256, 276–277
test validity, 255, 258–260, 287, 291
training personnel, 246–249, 264–
    265
Neonates. *See also* Neonatal screening
    programs
    EOAE amplitudes, 70, 71, 142–143,
        254, 273, 276
    and frequency energy, 274–275
    OAEs compared with adults, 50,
        234, 272–273
    SOAEs, 50, 71
Nerve fibers, 25–27
    afferent, 34
    efferent, 27–28
    and frequency information, 41–42
    on inner hair cells, 36
    responses, 40–43
    and transmitter, 35, 40
Neural networks, 191, 193–194
Newborns. *See* Neonatal screening
    programs; Neonates
Noise
    artifact reject, 321
    and averaging time, 200, 286, 320–
        321, 341
    and children, testing, 284
    and DPOAE detection, 187–189
    neonatal screening programs, 188–
        189, 254, 255–256, 262–264, 274
    and OAE response, 11–12
    rejection, 201, 286, 341
    and SOAEs, 46
    and waveform reproducibility, 321
Noise, ambient, 257, 262, 284
Noise estimation, 200–202
Noise-induced hearing loss, 173
Nonlinearity
    hair cells, 38–39, 84
    OAE generation, 19
    OAE measurement, 10
    traveling waves, 4, 10, 11

OAE-audiometric threshold gap, 18
OAEs. *See also* DPOAEs; EOAEs;
    SOAEs; TEOAEs
    air pressure, effects of, 136–140
    and audiometric outcomes,
        comparing, 151–152
    and audiometric thresholds, 8, 17–18
    and cochlear functioning, 14, 17, 18
    and developmental changes in ear,
        141–143
    history of technology, 1–7
    latency, 10, 11, 19
    and middle-ear pathologies, 140–141
    nature of, 7–8
    otitis media, effects of, 140
    recording, 8–12
    reporting test outcomes, 175, 176
Objective tinnitus. *See* Tinnitus
Organ of Corti
    effect of outer-hair-cell motility, 39
    motility in, 4
    and OAE generation, 7
    and SOAEs, 48
    supporting cells, 24
    and tectorial membrane, 30, 31
    and traveling waves, 3
    viewed from cochlear duct, 26
O-T gap, 18
Otitis media, effects on OAEs, 134,
    136, 140
Otoacoustic emissions. *See* OAEs
Otosclerosis, 132, 141
Ototoxic drugs, 48, 159, 173
Outer hair cells
    afferent innervation, 43
    and afferent neurons, 26, 38
    displacement of stereocilia, 30
    and DPOAEs, 182
    efferent innervation, 39, 43, 52–53
    electrical stimulation of, 37, 38
    electromotility, 38–39
    and OAE generation, 19, 205
    potentials, 32, 36, 40
    and SOAEs, 46–47
    and TEOAE generation, 164
    and TEOAE tuning curves, 120
Oval window, 24

Perilymph, 23, 24, 28
P-e tubes, 287
Place theory of hearing, 3
Pneumatization (temporal bone), 142
Potassium (endolymph), 23, 32, 34–35
Primary tones, 83–84. *See also* Pure
    tones
    and DPOAE amplitudes, 87–89,
        103–106, 183–186, 312
    and DPOAE tuning curve, 94
    and frequencies, 87–89, 183–186, 312
    and input/output function, 91
    multiple pair presentations, 337
    and multiple SOAEs, 54
Probe assemblies, 8
    cleaning, 244
    design, 317
    examining, 316
    insertion, 261–262, 263, 319
    and noise, 334
    speakers, 333
Probe tips
    cleaning, 244–245, 316
    fitting, 257, 317
    and noise, minimizing, 257, 284
Psychoacoustic auditory phenomena
    map, 5
Psychophysical tuning curves, 57–58
Pure-tone average, 209
Pure tones. *See also* Primary tones
    and compound action potential, 38
    and inner hair cells, 35
    and SFOAEs, 313
    and SOAEs, 51–52
    stimulus, 9, 14, 27
    two-tone stimulus, 8, 9, 10–11
Pure-tone threshold microstructure,
    195–196
Pure-tone thresholds
    and DPOAEs, 167, 169–172, 181, 182,
        185, 190–197
    and TEOAEs, 74, 76, 157

Racial differences (SOAEs), 49, 153
Radio technology, 3
Ranger OAE, 308
Record archiving, 345

Reflectance data, 182, 197
Reproducibility scores, 71, 136, 158, 159, 161, 162, 176, 283
Response extraction design, 9–10
Response waveform, 111, 253–254, 255
Resting potential, 28, 32
Rhode Island Hearing Assessment Program, 237, 240, 241, 248, 257, 291
Rippling phenomenon, 182, 197
RMS (root-mean-square) averaging, 325, 327, 334
Round window, 24

Sampling rate (DPOAEs), 337–341
Scala tympani, 23–24
Scala vestibuli, 23–24
Scout OAE system, 308, 326
Sensorineural hearing loss
    case studies, 223–227
    children, 280
    and DPOAEs, 105, 172, 201
    neonates, 246
    and SOAEs, 153
    and TEOAEs, 156, 159, 164, 206–207, 298
SFOAEs
    measurement methods, 313–314
    neonatal screening programs, 234
Side links, 24, 30
Signal processing methods, 197–201
Signal-to-noise ratio
    DPOAEs, 95, 186, 320, 335, 341, 342
    OAE recording, 11–12, 320–321, 327
SOAE clinical applications. *See also* SOAEs
    hearing loss, 48, 153
    hearing thresholds, 153–154
    high-level SOAEs, 153–154
    low-level SOAEs, 153
    neonatal screening programs, 234
    pathological states and SOAEs, 154
    prevalence and normal hearing, 153
    tinnitus, 54–55
SOAEs, 46–59. *See also* SOAE clinical applications
    age differences, 49–50
    amplitude, 51, 52, 136
    animal studies, 55–56
    and audiometric thresholds, 47–48
    contralateral stimulation, 52–53
    cycles, 50–51
    and DPOAEs, 58, 176, 195
    and ear-canal pressure, 136
    ear side, 49
    equipment for measuring, 308
    first recordings, 5
    frequencies, 50–51, 52, 153–154
    frequency selectivity, 57
    gender differences, 49, 53, 153
    multiple, 53–54
    neonates, 50, 71
    and overactivity, 4
    prevalence figures, 48–50
    and pure tones, 51–52
    racial differences, 49, 153
    recording, 46, 343
    spectral peaks, 46, 310
    and TEOAEs, 58, 80, 114–115, 120, 176
    tuning curves, 51–52, 57–58
    vulnerability to cochlear insults, 48
Speech Awareness Thresholds, 288–290
Speech development, delayed, 221–223
Speech Reception Thresholds, 209
Speech Recognition Thresholds, 288–290
Spiral ganglion, 26
Spontaneous OAEs. *See* SOAE clinical applications; SOAEs
Standing waves, 4, 5, 319
Stapes footplate, 24, 28
Stereocilia, 24, 25, 30, 36
Stereociliary bundle, deflection of, 34
Stimulus frequency otoacoustic emissions. *See* SFOAEs
Stimulus level
    DPOAEs, 167, 184–188, 281
    ILO equipment, 254, 255
Stimulus protocol selection, 335–337, 338
Stimulus selection, 8–9

Stimulus waveform, 252
Stria vascularis, 28
Subjective tinnitus. *See* Tinnitus
Sudden hearing loss
    case studies, 212–220
    and TEOAEs, 164
Summating potential, 32–33, 36
Suppression technique (SFOAEs), 314

Tectorial membrane
    location, 24, 25
    and organ of Corti, 30, 31
    and outer-hair-cell motility, 39
Telephone theory of hearing, 3
Temporary threshold shift, 53
TEOAE clinical applications, 154–166.
        See also TEOAEs
    children, 71, 72, 277–281
    eighth cranial-nerve disorders,
        diagnosis of, 206–207
    hearing loss diagnosis, 156–166,
        206–207
    hearing thresholds, 65, 156, 158, 159,
        161, 165–166, 173
    neonates, 69–71, 80, 234–236, 247–
        250, 255–256, 276–277
    parameters and audiometric
        outcomes, 154–156, 158–159
    post-operative measures, 209–210
    reporting results, 175, 176
    reproducibility scores, 71, 136, 158,
        159, 161, 162, 176, 283
    skills test, 249
    tone bursts, 162–164
    zone of uncertainty, 158
TEOAEs, 63–80. *See also* Amplitudes,
        TEOAEs; EOAEs; Ipsilateral
        suppression of TEOAEs;
        Measurement methods; TEOAE
        clinical applications
    age differences, 71–74, 75, 76, 165,
        277–281, 283
    animal studies, 64
    and audiometric thresholds, 72, 73
    click stimuli, 63, 75, 76, 280–281
    and cochlear response observation,
        12–13

contralateral stimulation, 77, 79
differential nonlinear response, 322
    and DPOAEs, 15, 173–175
    DPOAE technology, compared with,
        12–14
    and ear-canal pressure, 136
    ear side, 72, 74, 75, 76
    equipment for measuring, 111, 236,
        308
    first instrument demonstrated, 2
    first recordings, 6
    frequencies, 117–120, 159–164
    frequency-specific stimulation, 119–
        120
    gender differences, 72, 74, 75–76
    growth function, 133, 159
    input/output function, 114–115, 132–
        133, 280
    latency, 10, 115, 322
    and middle-ear fluid, 140
    and pure-tone thresholds, 74, 76,
        157
    and SOAEs, 58, 80, 114–115, 120, 176
    spectral peaks, 119, 162, 311
    tone bursts, 76–77, 80, 162–164
    tuning curves, 120
Threshold minima (and SOAEs), 56–
    57
Time averaging (signal processing),
    198–201, 320
Time-bandwidth product, 199
Time gating, 10, 13
Time-synchronous averaging, 9, 200–
    201
Tinnitus, 4, 5, 54–55, 212, 216
Tip links, 24, 34, 36
Tonal stimulation
    compared with click stimuli, 9
    DPOAE recording, 13
Tone bursts
    suppression of responses, 64
    in TEOAE masking, 111, 114–118
    TEOAEs, 76–77, 80, 162–164
Training, neonatal screening, 246–249,
    264–265
Transdcuction, 30–31, 34–35, 40–41
Transducers, 8, 317–318, 319

Transient evoked OAEs. *See* TEOAEs
Transient stimulus, 8, 9, 10
Transient-suppressed time-
    synchronous averaging, 200
Traveling wave, 28–30
    discovery, 3
    and DPOAE latency, 92
    and hearing threshold, 14
    and nonlinearity, 4, 10, 11
    and pure tones, 27
    reverse, 4–5, 48
    and stimulus frequencies and levels,
        10–11
Traveling wave delay, 10, 189–190, 196
Tuning curves
    DPOAEs, 92, 94
    iso-suppression, 93, 112, 116–119
    nerve fibers, 42
    psychophysical, 57–58
    SOAEs, 51–52, 57–58
    suppression phenomenon, 64
    TEOAEs, 120
Two-tone stimulus, 8, 9, 10–11
Tympanic membrane, 319
Tympanometry, 18, 132

University of Kansas Medical Center,
    284
Utah's High-Risk Hearing Screening
    Program, 233–234
Utah State University, 245, 248–252

Validity, neonatal testing, 255, 258–
    260, 287, 291
Viral neuritis and hearing loss, 227–
    228
Virtual (Model 300), 86, 308, 331
Visual Reinforcement Audiometry,
    221, 222, 292, 293, 300–302
Von Bekesy, G., 3, 4, 35–36

Wave reproducibility, 254, 321
Windowed signal averaging, 199–200
Women and Infants' Hospital of
    Rhode Island, 238, 240–241, 262,
    265, 283
Word recognition scores, 209

Zone of uncertainty (threshold levels),
    157, 158, 169